# Phytomedicine in Cardiovascular Health

# Phytomedicine in Cardiovascular Health

## Integrating Tradition with Modern Drug Delivery

*Edited by*

**K. Ravi Shankar**

**Dhanabal Palanisamy**

**S. Kavimani**

**Divya Narla**

**Sistla Ramakrishna**

**H.V.V.S.S. Lakshman K.**

**Venkata C. Nainala**

WILEY

Published by John Wiley & Sons, Inc., Hoboken, New Jersey.



*Library of Congress Cataloging-in-Publication Data applied for:*

Paperback ISBN: 9781394402526

Cover Design: Wiley
Cover Images: bit24/stock.adobe.com, abhijith3747/stock.adobe.com

Set in 9.5/12pt STIXTwoText by Straive, Pondicherry, India

# Contents

# List of Contributors

***Suneetha Achanti***
KVSR Siddhartha College of Pharmaceutical Sciences
Vijayawada
Andhra Pradesh
India

***Shakil Akthar***
Department of Pharmacy
Central University of South Bihar
Gaya
Bihar
India

***Ramesh Alluri***
Vishnu Institute of Pharmaceutical Education and Research
Narsapur
Andhra Pradesh
India

***Sadhe Amala***
Aditya College of Pharmacy
Jawaharlal Nehru Technological University
Surampalem
Andhra Pradesh
India

***Lakshmana Rao Atmakuri***
V. V. Institute of Pharmaceutical Sciences
Gudlavalleru
Andhra Pradesh
India

***Anupama Baratam***
KVSR Siddhartha College of Pharmaceutical Sciences
Vijayawada
Andhra Pradesh
India

***Rudolf Bauer***
Institute of Pharmaceutical Sciences
University of Graz
Austria

***Veera R. Bitra***
Department of Pharmacology
School of Pharmacy
Faculty of Health Sciences
University of Botswana
Gaborone
Botswana
South Africa

***Mohan Gandhi Bonthu***
Department of Pharmaceutical Analysis
JSS College of Pharmacy
JSS Academy of Higher Education and Research
Ooty, The Nilgiris
Tamil Nadu
India

***M. V. N. L. Chaitanya***
School of Pharmaceutical Sciences
Lovely Professional University
Phagwara
Punjab
India

***Pavan Kumar Chintamaneni***
Department of Pharmaceutics, GITAM School of Pharmacy
GITAM (Deemed to be) University
Hyderabad
Telangana
India

***Nakkala Danamurthy***
QIS College of Pharmacy
Prakasam District
Ongole
Andhra Pradesh
India

***Kamal Dua***
Graduate School of Health, Faculty of Health
University of Technology Sydney
Sydney, New South Wales
Australia

***Alluri Pavani Gayatri***
Department of Pharmacology
JSS College of Pharmacy
JSS Academy of Higher Education and Research
Ooty, The Nilgiris
Tamil Nadu
India

***Sree Geetha A***
Aditya College of Pharmacy
Surampalem
Andhra Pradesh
India

*Gowri Gollu*
Department of Pharmaceutical Analysis
Raghu College of Pharmacy
Andhra University
Visakhapatnam
Andhra Pradesh
India

*Saurabh Gupta*
Chameli Devi Institute of Pharmacy
Rajiv Gandhi Proudyogiki Vishwavidyalaya University
Indore
Madhya Pradesh
India

*N. Harikrishnan*
Faculty of Pharmacy
Dr. M.G.R. Educational and Research Institute
(Deemed to be University)
Chennai
Tamil Nadu
India

*Anu Pravallika Janipalli*
Department of Pharmaceutical Technology
Aditya College of Pharmacy
Surampalem
Andhra Pradesh
India

*S. M. Khamanga*
Faculty of Pharmacy
Rhodes University
Makhanda
Eastern Cape
South Africa

*Asapu Hema KIranmayi*
Aditya College of Pharmacy
Jawaharlal Nehru Technological University
Surampalem
Andhra Pradesh
India

*Garlanka Venkata Naga Kiranmayi*
Department of Pharmacology, Faculty of Pharmacy
Dr. M.G.R. Educational and Research Institute
Chennai
Tamil Nadu
India

*Gnaneswari Kodi*
Aditya College of Pharmacy
Surampalem
Andhra Pradesh
India

*Surya Prakasarao Kovvasu*
College of Pharmacy
Western University of Health Sciences
Pomona
CA
USA

*Dasari Santhi Krupa*
Department of Pharmacology
Krishna University College of Pharmaceutical Sciences and Research
Machilipatnam
Andhra Pradesh
India

*Kumar CSP*
Department of Pharmaceutics, School of Pharmacy
Aditya University
Surampalem
Andhra Pradesh
India

*Arya Lakshmi Marisetti*
School of Pharmaceutical Sciences
Delhi Pharmaceutical Sciences and Research University
New Delhi
India

*Madhavi Latha Samala*
Department of Pharmaceutical Technology
Aditya College of Pharmacy
Surampalem
Andhra Pradesh
India

*Nalini Mathala*
Department of Pharmacology
Raghu College of Pharmacy
Andhra University
Visakhapatnam
Andhra Pradesh
India

*Dhanalekshmi Unnikrishnan Meenakshi*
Department of Pharmacology and Biological Sciences
College of Pharmacy
National University of Science and Technology
Muscat
Sultanate of Oman

*Long Chiau Ming*
School of Medical and Life Sciences
Sunway University
Sunway City
Malaysia

***Naga Venkata Lakshmi Sirisha Mulukuri***
Department of Pharmacognosy,
Nitte College of Pharmaceutical Sciences
Nitte University (Deemed to be University)
Bengaluru
Karnataka
India

***Sathyamoorthy Nandhakumar***
Department of Pharmaceutics, Faculty of Pharmacy
Dr. M.G.R. Educational and Research Institute
Chennai
Tamil Nadu
India

***Raghuveer Pathuri***
Department of Pharmaceutics, GITAM School of Pharmacy
GITAM (Deemed to be) University
Hyderabad
Telangana
India

***Gummadi Veda Priya***
Aditya College of Pharmacy
Jawaharlal Nehru Technological University, Kakinada
Surampalem
Andhra Pradesh
India

***Karri Swathi Priya***
Srinivasarao College of Pharmacy
Andhra University
Visakhapatnam
Andhra Pradesh
India

***Sarikonda Tripura Venkata Raghavamma***
Chalapathi Institute of Pharmaceutical Sciences
Acharya Nagarjuna University
Guntur
Andhra Pradesh
India

***Pathuri Raghuveer***
School of Pharmaceutical Sciences
GITAM University
Hyderabad
Telangana
India

***Talluri Sesha Rajeswari***
Ernest Mario School of Pharmacy
Rutgers University
Piscataway
New Jersey
USA

***Bodapati Raju***
Department of Pharmaceutical Chemistry
Aditya College of Pharmacy
Surampalem
Andhra Pradesh
India

***Gummadi RamaKrishna***
Department of Pharmaceutics, School of Pharmacy
Aditya University
Surampalem
Andhra Pradesh
India

***Ponakampalli Rambabu***
Department of Pharmacognosy
Krishna University College of Pharmaceutical Sciences and Research
Machilipatnam
Andhra Pradesh
India

***K. Ravi Shankar***
Aditya College of Pharmacy
Aditya University
East-Godavari District
Andhra Pradesh
India

***Thirumala Devi Siriki***
Aditya College of Pharmacy
Surampalem
Andhra Pradesh
India

***Akshintala Sree Gayatri***
Department of Pharmaceutical Chemistry
Aditya College of Pharmacy
Surampalem
Andhra Pradesh
India

***Karumanchi Srikanth***
Institute of Pharmaceutical Sciences and Research for Girls
Dattakala Shikshan Sanstha's Institute of Pharmaceutical Science & Research
Dr. Babasaheb Ambedkar Technical University
Pune
Maharashtra
India

***Grandhi Srikar***
Department of Pharmaceutical Sciences
Vignan's Foundation for Science
Technology and Research
Guntur
Andhra Pradesh
India

***Evelyn Sharon Sukumaran***
Department of Pharmacology
Faculty of Pharmacy
Dr. M.G.R. Educational and Research Institute
Chennai
Tamil Nadu
India

***Balakrishna Talamanchi***
Department of Pharmaceutics
VV Institute of Pharmaceutical Sciences
Gudlavalleru
Andhra Pradesh
India

***Thummala Udaya Kumar***
Department of Pharmaceutics, School of Pharmacy
Aditya University
Surampalem
Andhra Pradesh
India

***Bondada N.B. Vaidehi***
Department of Pharmaceutical Chemistry
Aditya College of Pharmacy
Surampalem
Andhra Pradesh
India

***Thangavel Mahalingam Vijayakumar***
Department of Pharmacy Practice
SRM College of Pharmacy
SRM Institute of Science and Technology
Kattankulathur
Tamil Nadu
India

***Haya Khader Ahmed Yasin***
Department of Pharmaceutical Sciences
College of Pharmacy and Health Sciences
Ajman University
Ajman
United Arab Emirates

# Preface

Cardiovascular diseases are leading cause for morbidity and mortality posing persistent challenge to public health system and clinical management. The modern medicine has made remarkable progress in diagnostics, therapeutic preventive strategy, they quest for safer, accessible and holistic treatment options remains ongoing. The phytomedicine rooted in centuries of traditional practices has emerged as promising complement to cardiovascular care.

This unique book "*Phytomedicine in Cardiovascular Health: Integrating Tradition with Modern Drug Delivery*" explores the rich potential of plant based therapies along with innovations of modern pharmaceutical technologies. By bridging traditional wisdom with advanced drug delivery system highlight herbal bioactives that can be transformed into scientifically validated, effective and therapeutic agents for cardiovascular wellbeing.

The various chapters provide comprehensive understanding of cardiovascular pathology, important phytoconstituents with cardio-protective effects and cutting edge delivery platforms like nanoparticles, liposomes, phytosomes and control release systems.

This specialized book is designed for Researchers, Academicians, Clinicians, Industry Professionals and Postgraduate Students who are involved in natural product research, cardiovascular drug development and pharmaceutical technology. This book encourages interdisciplinary collaboration and can address the growing burden of cardiovascular disorders paving the integrative cardiovascular therapeutics.

# Acknowledgments

We express our deepest gratitude to all those who contributed the development of this book "*Phytomedicine in Cardiovascular Health: Integrating Tradition with Modern Drug Delivery*". Their support, guidance and encouragement have been invaluable throughout the journey their expertise in Pharmacology, Phytochemistry and Drug Delivery served as strong foundation for this book. We are grateful to colleagues and fellow academicians who share their knowledge and supported the scientific discussions that enriched the contents of this book. Our heartfelt appreciation to the institution, library that offered resources and research environment for completing this work. Their unconditional support made it possible to explore the diverse dimensions of phytomedicine and cardiovascular therapeutics. Finally, we acknowledge all the authors whose contribution to the field of herbal medicines, modern medicines have paved the way for scientific advancements that this book explored the highlight.

# Introduction to Cardiovascular Diseases and Herbal Medicine

CHAPTER 1

**Gnaneswari Kodi[1], Suneetha Achanti[2], Thirumala Devi Siriki[1], and Sree Geetha A[1]**

[1] *Aditya College of Pharmacy, Surampalem, Andhra Pradesh, India*

[2] *KVSR Siddhartha College of Pharmaceutical Sciences, Vijayawada, Andhra Pradesh, India*

## 1.1 INTRODUCTION

### 1.1.1 CARDIOVASCULAR DISEASES

Cardiovascular diseases (CVDs) are a class of disorders that affect the heart and associated blood vessels and encompass a wide range of conditions that involve narrowed or blocked blood vessels, leading to a variety of conditions like peripheral vascular diseases, coronary heart disease, heart failure and heart attacks, dyslipidemias, hypertension, chest pain (Angina pectoris), or stroke, registering universal deaths of more than 17 million and accounting as a considerable burden both economically and health-wise worldwide [1]. The need for more effective preventive and treatment measures for CVDs is essential due to the increased incidence of patients suffering [2]. In the recent era, it is relatively prevalent that the incidence of these CVDs is escalating among young individuals [3, 4]. The main evolution of CVDs is due to the vascular smooth muscle cell (VSMC) impairment, inflammation, and dysfunction of the endothelium, which becomes a paramount offender with absolute cardiovascular risk, leading to atherosclerosis, thrombosis, high blood pressure, coronary vasoconstriction, and myocardial ischemia [5]. Endothelial cell dysfunction is important because this phenomenon could be reversed, and it is stated that a healthy endothelium could reveal vasodilatory and anti-inflammatory properties [5].

### 1.1.2 EPIDEMIOLOGY OF CARDIOVASCULAR DISEASES

Despite drawing attention to healthy lifestyle encouragement, studies in 2019 estimated that 17.9 million deaths were observed due to the risk of CVDs, representing all-inclusive deaths of 32% globally [6, 7]. According to WHO 2024, diseases of the cardiac system remain the prime source of death, increasing to 18.5 million collapses each year, portraying comprehensive deaths of 35%, among which 85% are owing to myocardial infarction, heart attack, or stroke. Low- and middle-income populations are mainly affected, and lifestyle changes, inadequate healthcare infrastructure, and late diagnosis are the main trends. The demographic data [8] reveals that men are more prone to early onset of CVDs, and women in the post-menopause period are also at risk. Mortality from CVDs is highest in developed countries due to an increased workload on the nervous system that leads to hypertension, as well as a sedentary lifestyle, like lack of exercise and poor diet, which ultimately leads to atherosclerotic plaque deposition in blood vessels, heart attacks, or possibility of stroke [3].

#### 1.1.2.1 Epidemiological Models and Assessment Tools

The important epidemiological models for risk assessment include:

- Framingham risk score for evaluating the probability of cardiac attacks based on blood pressure, cholesterol, diabetes, smoking, etc.
- WHO/ISH (International Society of Hypertension) risk prediction charts that guide the interventions based on regional CVD risks [9].
- QRISK (QRESEARCH Cardiovascular Risk Algorithm) and ASCVD (atherosclerotic cardiovascular diseases) are risk estimators that include socioeconomic status and family history, along with more accurate predictors.

### 1.1.3 RISK FACTORS OF CARDIOVASCULAR DISEASES

The leading determinants of CVDs are categorized into environmental, metabolic, and behavioral risk factors like systolic blood pressure, low-density lipoprotein (LDL) cholesterol, body mass index, fasting plasma glucose, kidney dysfunction, diet, smoking, consumption of alcohol, physical activity, pollution, and temperature. [10] Rare and emerging risk factors like vitamin D, homocysteine, plasma concentration of uric acid, gut microbiota, sleep duration, and apnea are also being linked to the development of cardiovascular threat [11].

**Adaptable Determinants**

- Exalted blood pressure
- Hyperlipidemia
- Tobacco consumption

- Diabetes mellitus
- Adiposity
- Quiescence
- Processed foods
- Intemperate alcohol consumption
- Psychosocial stress

**Unalterable Risk Factors**

- Age and gender [12]
- Ancestry and heredity
- Ethnicity

#### 1.1.3.1 Risk Factor Clustering

This involves a cluster of metabolic conditions like obesity, hypertension, dyslipidemia, and insulin resistance that act synergistically to raise the risk of CVDs and the social determinants of health that influence the risk distribution [12].

#### 1.1.3.2 Strategies to Prevent the Risk Factors

- Salt reduction
- Tobacco cessation
- Public campaigns for physical activity and healthy diets
- Early screening for hypertension, diabetes, and dyslipidemia
- Preventive pharmacotherapy (antihypertensive drugs, statins) [9]
- Counseling regarding lifestyle

### 1.1.4 MAJOR TYPES OF CARDIOVASCULAR DISEASES

Heart diseases are allied to the transgression of blood supply to the heart muscles, violation of ions like potassium, sodium, and calcium, infringement of the heart's nerve fibers. Owing to changes in the permeability of blood vessels, vascular diseases originate.

#### 1.1.4.1 Hypertension

Hypertension is a dominant player in the advent of heart disorders like atherosclerosis, stroke, artery diseases, and heart failure [13]. It is also referred as a silent killer due to the delayed onset of symptoms until advanced stages of the disease. Hypertension is defined as tenacious escalation of arterial blood pressure exceeding systolic pressure of 140 mmHg and a diastolic pressure of 90 mmHg [14]. An unmanaged and elevated blood pressure can influence changes like arterial remodeling, potentially making the walls narrower by thickening and causing them to lose their elasticity. This mechanism is termed arteriosclerosis, which can trigger target organ damage [15, 16], affecting brain, kidney, retina, and so on [17, 18].

**1.1.4.1.1 Pathophysiology** The two principal elements of hypertension involve cardiac output and systemic vascular resistance that elevate the blood pressure. Sodium intake, renal system function, and mineralocorticoids are the key contributors to an amplified cardiac output. The sympathetic nervous system, renin–angiotensin system, local autoregulation, and humoral factors are the main influencers of vascular resistance [19]. Activation of the sympathetic and renin–angiotensin systems cause vasoconstriction and sodium retention, along with humoral mediators like angiotensin, endothelin, and catecholamines [20], thus ultimately altering blood viscosity and flow, increasing stiffness of the vascular wall, and promoting oxidative stress in vascular smooth muscle and endothelial cell proliferation [21].

#### 1.1.4.2 Atherosclerosis

Atherosclerosis is a chronic progressive disease of the arterial wall that leads to conditions like coronary artery disease (CAD), peripheral vascular disease, and stroke. It is not only a risk factor but also a major contributor to the incidence of heart disease.

**1.1.4.2.1 Pathophysiology** It is characterized by inflammation arising from the impairment of endothelial cells, permitting accumulation of LDLs within the intima of the vessel wall, which are converted into oxidized LDL. These oxidized LDL particles initialize and expose cell adhesion molecules of the endothelium and recruit more inflammatory leukocytes into the sub-endothelial space [22]. Interleukins, cytokines, and reactive oxygen species (ROS) are secreted by these inflammatory blood cells, forming an inflamed arterial wall microenvironment. This microenvironment creates buildup of matrix, proliferation of VSMCs, and deposition of lipids, forming an atherosclerotic plaque [23–26]. In the course of time, progressive thickening occurs, persistently expanding and provoking occlusion of blood flow to other organs, and ensuing disorders like myocardial infarction, unstable angina, or stroke [27, 28].

Figure 1.1a,b illustrates the core pathological events underlying the development and progression of CVDs, with various predisposing factors such as hypertension involving alterations in cardiac output and systemic vascular resistance that initiate pathological changes primarily through endothelial injury and VSMC (Vascular Smooth Muscle Cell) dysregulation. Inflammatory stimuli initiate endothelial injury, leading to the accumulation of LDLs (low density lipids) within the vascular intima and their subsequent oxidation to oxidized LDL. The presence of oxidized LDL triggers endothelial cell activation, promoting the expression of cell adhesion molecules that attract and bind leucocytes. Activated immune cells release interleukins, cytokines, and ROS (reactive oxygen species), creating pro-inflammatory microenvironment within the arterial wall. This cascade stimulates VSMC proliferation and lipid deposition, resulting in intimal thickening and plaque development. Progressive plaque growth narrows the vessel lumen, reducing blood flow and leading to severe cardiovascular complications such as myocardial infarction, angina, stroke, and sudden cardiac death.

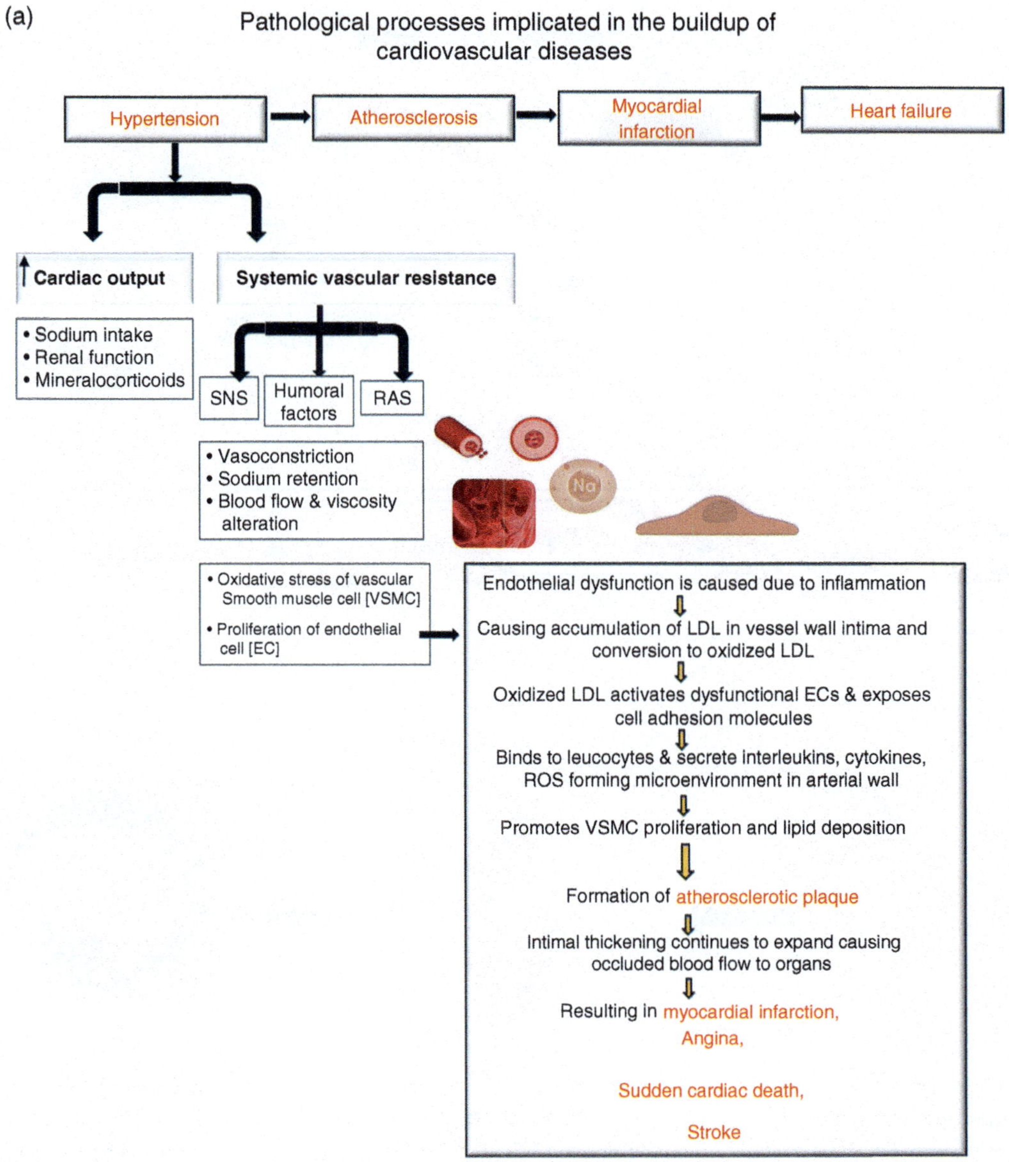


**FIGURE 1.1** (a) Core pathological events during cardiovascular diseases (CVDs); (b) pathological processes implicated in the buildup of cardiovascular diseases.

### 1.1.4.3 Coronary Artery Disease/Ischemic Heart Disease (IHD)

In this state of disease, plaque builds up in the coronary arteries, which supply the heart with sufficient blood, thereby leading to diminished blood flow.

#### 1.1.4.3.1 Pathophysiology

- Atherosclerosis and arteriosclerosis (plaque accumulation)
- Constriction of arteries resulting in diminished oxygen and blood supply
- Ischemia, angina pectoris, and myocardial infarction [29]

**Symptoms:**

- Chest discomfort (angina)
- Shortness of breath (dyspnea)
- Fatigue, with pain radiating from the shoulder to the palm
- Heart attack (blockage of an artery) [30]

**Causes: [31]**

- High lipid profiles
- Smoking
- Hypertension
- Diabetes
- Lack of exercise

**Diagnosis:**

- ECG
- Treadmill test

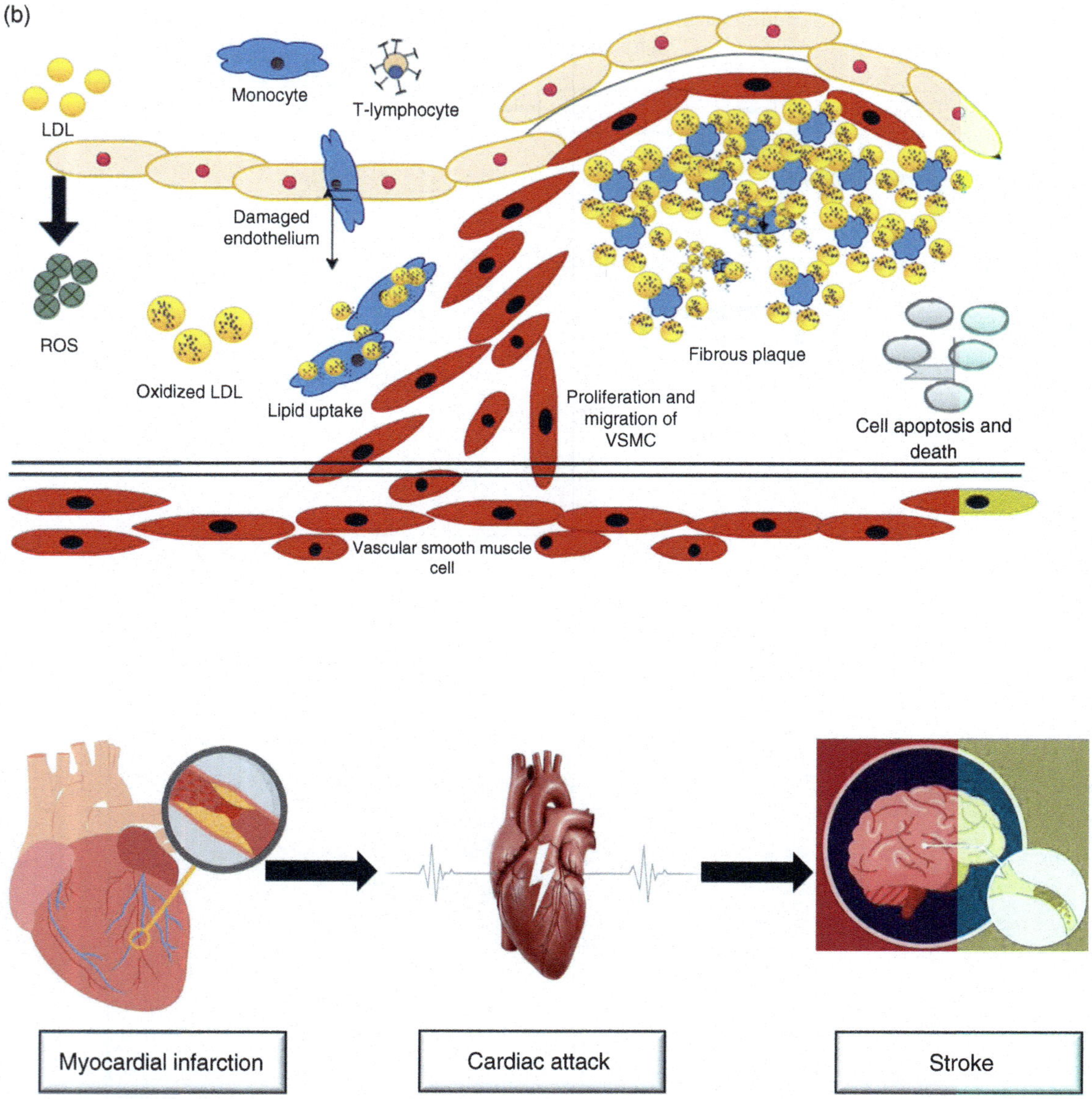


FIGURE 1.1 (Continued)

- Coronary angiography
- Cardiac biomarkers (troponin)

### 1.1.4.4 Cerebrovascular Diseases

Stroke or transient ischemic attacks are provoked owing to influence of the blood flow and circulation to the brain, leading to temporary or permanent neurological dysfunction [32]. There are few types like

- Ischemic stroke (blockage in cerebral blood vessels)
- Hemorrhagic stroke (bleeding in and around the brain)
- Transient ischemic attack (temporary blockage and warning for stroke)

**Symptoms:**

- Numbness or weakness
- Confusion and difficulty in speaking
- Blurred vision
- Loss of balance or coordination

**Risk factors:**

- Hypertension (abnormal levels of blood pressure)
- Atrial fibrillation
- Diabetes
- Smoking
- Elevated lipid profiles

**Diagnosis:**

- Computed tomography (CT) (or) magnetic resonance imaging (MRI) of the brain
- Carotid ultrasound
- Cerebral angiography

#### 1.1.4.5 Heart Failure (HF)

This is an important clinical diagnosis in which the heart cannot meet the requirements of the body, attributable to the blood-pumping efficiency of the heart.

**Types:**

- Left-sided heart failure (very common – pulmonary symptoms)
- Right-sided heart failure (peripheral edema)
- Systolic heart failure (reduced ejection fraction)
- Diastolic heart failure (preserved ejection fraction but impaired filling)

**Symptoms:**

- Dyspnea
- Somnolence
- Swelling of the legs and abdomen
- Orthopnea

**Causes:**

- CADs
- Hypertension
- Cardiomyopathy
- Valve disease
- Arrhythmias

**Diagnosis:**

- Echocardiogram
- Chest X-ray
- ECG
- BNP levels (B-type natriuretic peptide)

#### 1.1.4.6 Peripheral Arterial Disease (PAD)

This is a distinguished circulatory condition in which the blood flow specifically to the legs is diminished due to narrowed arteries [33].

**Symptoms:**

- Claudication (leg pain followed by cramping during walking)
- Numbness
- Weakness
- Coldness in the foot

**Causes:**

- Atherosclerosis and arteriosclerotic diseases
- Smoking
- Diabetes
- High blood pressure and lipid profiles

**Diagnosis:**

- Doppler ultrasound
- Angiography (computed tomography (CT)/MRI)
- Ankle-brachial index

#### 1.1.4.7 Rheumatic Heart Disease (RHD)

This is a chronic condition that causes damage to the heart valves as a result of rheumatic fever and streptococcal throat infection [34, 35].

**Pathophysiology:**

- Autoimmune reaction targeting the heart, joints, and brain
- Most commonly affecting the mitral and aortic valves

**Symptoms:**

- Severe breathlessness
- Chest pain
- Swelling of limbs
- Heart murmur

**Diagnosis:**

- Echocardiography [36]
- Jones criteria for rheumatic fever
- ASO titer (anti-streptolysin O)

#### 1.1.4.8 Congenital Heart Disease (CHD)

This results in structural abnormalities of the heart or great vessels present at the time of birth [37].

**Types:**

- Atrial septal defect
- Ventricular septal defect
- Tetralogy of Fallot
- Patent ductus arteriosus (PDA)
- Coarctation of the aorta

**Symptoms:**

- These symptoms vary based on type and severity
- Cyanosis (bluish skin)
- Poor feeding or growth
- Shortness of breath
- Heart murmur

**Diagnosis:**

- Prenatal ultrasound (fetal echo)
- Echocardiography
- Cardiac catheterization

#### 1.1.4.9 Deep Vein Thrombosis and Pulmonary Embolism

The condition of deep vein thrombosis is associated with a blood clot [38] in deep veins (typically in the legs), showing symptoms like swelling, pain, redness, and warmth, and possible risks are immobility, surgery, and inherited clotting disorders.

In pulmonary embolism, a clot from deep vein thrombosis travels to the lungs, causing severe blockage [39], and the symptoms observed are sudden chest pain, shortness of breath, and a rapid heart rate, which can be life-threatening.

**Diagnosis:**

- D-dimer test
- Venus Doppler ultrasound
- CT pulmonary angiography

## 1.2 CONVENTIONAL MANAGEMENT OF CARDIOVASCULAR DISEASES

Conventional management of heart diseases refers to the standard medical practices and important therapies implemented to prevent, treat, and manage different CVDs [9]. All these approaches were established and endorsed by international guidelines, in particular those from the American Heart Association, the European Society of Cardiology, and the World Health Organization. Contemporary healthcare regulations focus on preventing and minimizing the likelihood of heart disease [40], minimizing adverse outcomes, and addressing the major risk factors of cardiovascular disorders. For instance, in the condition of atherosclerosis, therapeutic approaches focus on modulating hemostasis, controlling hyperlipidemia, or modulating thrombotic complications [41]; hence, they rely on reducing LDLs using statins [40, 42, 43] or combinational drugs depending on patients' response. Modern and multiple antihypertensive drugs are employed to control elevated blood pressure in hypertensive patients [44]. Due to the availability of numerous antihypertensive agents, physicians are able to prescribe highly effective drug combinations for reducing blood pressure and protecting target organs [45].

### 1.2.1 GOALS OF MANAGEMENT [46]

- Reduce morbidity and mortality
- Prevent disease progression
- Relieve symptoms (angina, dyspnea)
- Improve quality life
- Prevent complications (heart failure, stroke)

### 1.2.2 MAJOR ASPECT OF TRADITIONAL CARDIOVASCULAR DISEASE MANAGEMENT

#### 1.2.2.1 Lifestyle Modification

This is implemented along with pharmacological therapy for the prevention of CVD. In this, dietary management is much needed to improve an individual's lifestyle [47] by suggesting low-sodium, low-fat diets, reducing saturated fats, increasing fiber intake, and encouraging the individuals to opt for nourishing foods like fruits, veggies, and whole grains, thereby curbing convenience foods and added sugars.

The individual is advised to increase physical activity through moderate exercise for three hours per week and complete cessation of smoking, thus reducing the risk of recurrent CVD [48]. Alcohol intake is very much restricted for men and women, with a limitation of one drink per day, along with increasing mindfulness, incorporating relaxation techniques, and seeking therapy for anxiety and depression, thereby reducing unwanted stress.

#### 1.2.2.2 Pharmacological Management

This is very important and particularly is prescribed based on the type and severity of CVDs.

a. **Antihypertensives**:
   These are the medicaments used to control abnormally high blood pressure, which is a key factor in CVD. Beta-blockers (e.g., Metoprolol) lower the blood pressure and heart rate [49], inhibitors like calcium channel blockers (like amlodipine) dilate blood vessels, angiotensin-converting enzyme inhibitors (such as losartan) reduce afterload and mortality, and diuretics (e.g., hydrochlorothiazide) help by reducing fluid overload [50].
b. **Antiplatelet and anticoagulant therapies:**
   This class of drugs is used to prevent clot formation and recurrent events. Aspirin is considered the cornerstone for secondary platelet prevention [51]. Clopidogrel–ticagrelor dual therapy is used after stenting or acute coronary syndrome, and Warfarin [52] is used for deep vein thrombosis, atrial fibrillation, and pulmonary embolism.
c. **Lipid lowering drugs:**
   These class of drugs are used to manage hyperlipidemia, statins (atorvastatin, rosuvastatin) lower LDL cholesterol and stabilize plaques [53]. Ezetemibe and PCSK9 (proprotein convertase subtilisin/kexin type 9) inhibitors are mainly employed in statin-intolerant patients showing significant reduction of bad LDLs.
d. **Antianginal and antiarrhythmic drugs:**
   These are mainly used against all types of angina pectoris [54] and CADs and are also used to treat arrhythmias. Nitrates [55–57], including nitroglycerine, act as a vasodilator, and quinidine and amiodarone are used to control arrhythmias [58–60].

Figure 1.2 presents an overview of major pharmacological classes used in managing cardiovascular disorders, including

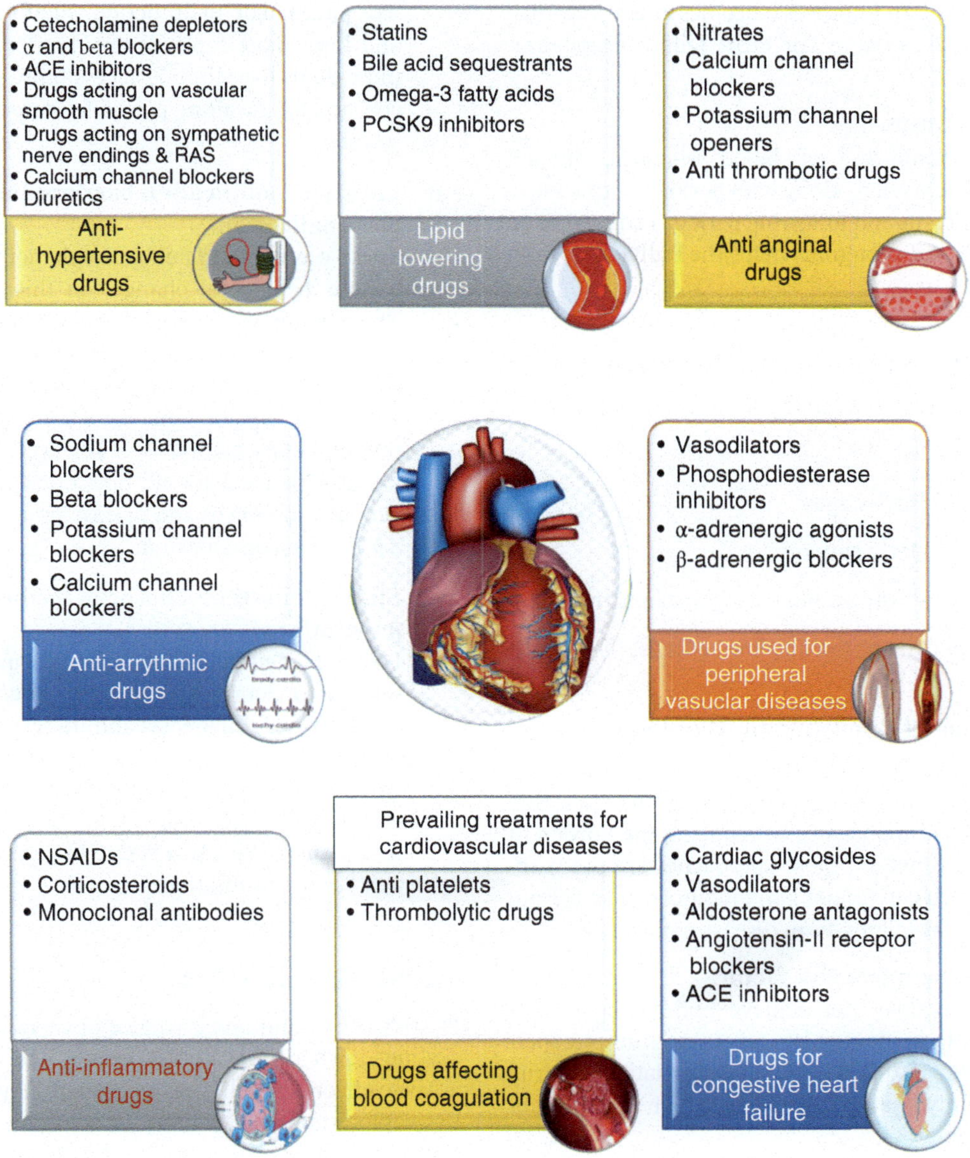


**FIGURE 1.2** Pharmacological treatment strategies for cardiovascular diseases.

antihypertensives, antianginal agents, anticoagulants, and lipid-lowering drugs.

#### 1.2.2.3 Surgical and Interventional Management

a. **Percutaneous coronary intervention (PCI):**
This includes angioplasty and stenting, used in acute coronary syndrome as well coronary artery stenosis [61, 62].

b. **Coronary artery bypass grafting (CABG):**
This surgical technique is for open-heart surgery to bypass blocked arteries and is also performed in multi-vessel disease or in diabetic patients [63, 64].

c. **Valve repair or replacement:**
This is specific to surgical or transcatheter aortic valve replacement [65] and also for valvular stenosis or regurgitation.

d. **Implantable devices:**
These include pacemakers for AV block or bradycardia, and implantable cardioverter defibrillators [66], which are opted for perilous arrhythmic patients.

e. **Cardiac resynchronization:**
This therapy is advantageous for patients with heart failure associated with dyssynchrony [67, 68].

f. **Thrombolytic therapy:**
This is used for the emergency treatment of ischemic stroke and myocardial infraction [68]. Drugs like streptokinase and alteplase are advised.

g. **Cardiac rehabilitation:**
This is a designed program, wherein training exercises and counseling are specified for patients to reduce unwanted stress and strain and to support individuals in making behavioral changes, resulting in improved outcomes in

patients with CVD. It improves outcomes after myocardial infarction, bypass grafting, or heart failure hospitalization [69–71].

h. **Long-term monitoring**:
Continuous monitoring of blood pressure, glucose levels, and lipid profiles, along with periodical checkups, with the physicians and following patient's education on warning signs and symptoms helps the individuals from CVDs [72].

#### 1.2.2.4 Challenges in Conventional Management

There are few challenges that are highly focused on [73, 74]:

- Poor medication
- Underdiagnosis in early stages
- Polypharmacy in elderly patients
- Gender disparities with reference to diagnosis and treatment
- Limited access in rural or low-income settings

#### 1.2.2.5 Limitations of Conventional Therapies

Lifestyle modifications, pharmacological treatment, and different surgical procedures are the conventional therapies that have acquired clinical importance in reducing the burden of various CVDs [74]. However, these approaches are not without limitations, which can hinder patient outcomes in certain populations, as well as in long-term disease control.

a. **Control of incomplete risk factor:**
Several patients may not achieve optimal control of hypertension, hyperlipidemia, and diabetes despite their treatment. This is due to individual variation in drug response, mainly pharmacogenetics, which leads to suboptimal outcomes.

b. **Medication-related limitations:**

- Therapeutic drugs may have few side effects, and tolerability varies among individuals. Patients receiving statins experience myopathy and elevated liver enzymes. Similarly, patients treated with beta-blockers and ACE blockers may experience fatigue, depression, erectile dysfunction, cough, angioedema.
- Polypharmacy is very common in elderly or comorbid patients and may lead to drug–drug interactions, noncompliance, and possible increased risk of adverse effects.
- Lifelong medication regimens result in poor adherence in about 50% of population. Other reasons include cost, side effects, complex dosing schedules, and lack of symptoms.

c. **Surgical or interventional therapy limitations:**
CABG and PCI are invasive with high risks of bleeding, infection, and other complications. In angioplasty, restenosis can occur even with stenting, and device failures, like pacemaker malfunction, require close monitoring and immediate replacement. Low- and middle-income individuals have limited accessibility because of the high cost and long waiting period for surgery in public health systems.

d. **Lifestyle modification barriers and lack of personalization:**
These are very difficult to implement and sustain with various behavioral changes in this real-world setting. The individuals dietary habits are shaped by factors such as socioeconomic status, education, mental health and cultural food preferences. Limited access to nutritious foods can further challenge their ability to maintain proper dietary compliance. The acceptable conventional therapy "one-size fits all" does not account for individual genetic differences and disease progression, resulting in a lack of personalization.

e. **Limitations of psychosocial factors and certain populations:**
Lack of mental health support and poor outcomes related to depression, anxiety, and stress integration result in underdiagnosis and undertreatment in cardiac management [75]. Often certain populations like women, elderly, and frail patients cannot tolerate standard doses or aggressive therapies. Ethnic disparities in treatment cause barriers due to genetics, access-related, and cultural limitations.

## 1.3 HERBAL MEDICINE

Despite the ubiquitous existence of therapeutic regimens for scaling down cardiovascular events, their probably critical adverse effects are still areas of concern. Thus, this has evoked the exploration of alternative and complementary therapies for the enhanced oversight of CVDs [2]. There is an expanding awareness of the role of herbs in anticipating their use [76]. Herbal medicine, also termed as phytotherapy or botanical medicine, specifically refers to the use of plants or plant-derived substances to prevent or cure various diseases and maintain proper health. This is one of the ancient forms of medicine and remains a key element of traditional and complementary medicinal systems in the world. This herbal medicine includes whole-plant (leaves, seeds, fruit, bark, and roots) extracts, tinctures [77], and herbal formulations (teas, ointments, etc.).

### 1.3.1 HISTORICAL BACKGROUND

Historically herbs are interpreted as any form of plants or plant products [78]. Plants with healing properties were first medicaments used, and extracts from plants served as the foundation of the foremost drugs [79]. Herbal medicine is one of the most ancient medicinal systems, which can be tracked thousands of years ago [80], and has been practiced for many years across different civilizations.

Indisputably, nature is a paramount source in discovering new drugs that lead the way for the treatment of various diseases [81]. The chronicles of natural drug inception were established in Mesopotamia (nearly 2600 BC) and demonstrated the utilization of around 100 plant-acquired compounds. The Egyptian Ebers Papyrus (from 1500 BC) provides one of the best records of the use of more than 700 natural medicines. Fifty-two natural medicinal preparations from the Chinese *Materia Medica* (1100 BC) (for example, ginseng and liquorice root) and 800 natural extracts (Ashwagandha, turmeric) were recorded in the Indian Ayurvedic record [81, 82]. Greek medicine and indigenous medicine systems were also accomplished across Africa, America, and Australia. In 1985, the WHO estimated that about 65% of the world's inhabitants would depend on herb-derived traditional medicaments and identified 122 compounds, with different host countries using 94 plant species for ethnomedicinal treatment [83]. Despite favorable outcomes of bringing natural products into practice, the focus of drug discovery shifted due to the proceedings in combinatorial chemistry [81]. Nonetheless, naturally derived compounds are the major sources of new drugs due to the elucidation of contemporary published scientific data, technological breakthroughs, and research trends [82, 84].

### 1.3.2 PRINCIPLES OF HERBAL MEDICINE

- Herbal medicine operates based on several principles like holistic approach, which considers lifestyle, environment, and emotional aspects of whole person, and mainly aims to restore balance and support the individual's healing capacity.
- Herbal medicine provides synergistic action [2], with different active constituents present in the whole plant potentiating its therapeutic effect and reducing toxicity compared with a single-compound drug.
- Herbal medicine treatment is often tailored to individual needs as per the symptoms and constitution and is often prevention-oriented, supporting immunity, promoting general wellness, and improving resistance to stress.
- Herbal and plant remedies not only contain thousands of bioactive compounds with therapeutic significance but are also considered economical [85].

### 1.3.3 FORMS OF HERBAL PREPARATIONS

- Chamomile is available in the forms of teas and infusions
- Ginger root is available in decoction form
- Echinacea is available in the form of tincture
- *Ginkgo biloba* is available in the form of tablets and capsules
- Arnica is best used in the form of ointments and cream for skin or joints

### 1.3.4 ROLE AND SAFETY OF HERBAL MEDICINE IN MODERN WORLD

The role of herbal medicine in the modern era is increasing tremendously over synthetic drugs due to prospective natural remedies with no side effects. The WHO supports amalgamation of traditional and herbal medicines into national healthcare systems. Some important pharmaceuticals which are derived from plants include aspirin from willow bark, digoxin from foxglove, and artemisinin from *Artemisia annua*. It is a very well-known fact that not all herbs and medicinal plants are safe [1], few may be toxic or interact with conventional drugs like ephedra. Further, the quality-control aspects, along with the standardization process, remain a big challenge in the manufacturing of herbal drugs. Important regulatory bodies, like the United States Food and Drug Administration (USFDA), the European Medicines Agency (EMA), and many countries' pharmacopeias, have classified these herbs as dietary supplements and listed them as herbal formulations.

### 1.3.5 ADVANTAGES, CHALLENGES, AND LIMITATIONS OF HERBAL MEDICINE

Notable advantages of herbal medicine are

- Natural and generally well-tolerated
- Rich source of bioactive compounds
- Can mark chronic or functional disorders (stress and digestion)
- Affordable and accessible, especially in rural or developing areas

However, these are a few challenges and limitations ahead for these herbal medicines, which include:

- Lack of clinical trials for many herbal formulations
- Risk regarding misidentification, contamination, or adulteration
- Herb–drug interactions [1]
- Dosage and potency

### 1.3.6 HERBAL MEDICINE IN CARDIOVASCULAR HEALTH

CVDs like hypertension, atherosclerosis, arteriosclerosis, myocardial infarction, cardiac arrhythmias, cardiac failure, and stroke are the leading causative factors for death worldwide. Conventional therapies, though effective, have limitations, with side effects, cost, and drug resistance [86]. The role of herbal medicine is gaining popularity as an integrative and revolutionary approach to effective CVD therapy due to its natural origin, multi-target effects, and fewer side effects when used meticulously.

#### 1.3.6.1 Mechanism of Action of Cardiovascular Herbs

The herbal medicines used in CVDs exhibit different mechanisms by targeting pathophysiological processes and exerting synergistic effects. The primary mechanism of these cardiovascular herbs are as follows:

i. **Antioxidant activity:** Oxidative stress plays crucial role in the pathogenesis of atherosclerosis and myocardial infraction. Herbs like turmeric, green tea, and grapes seed extract, which are very rich in polyphenols, flavonoids, and curcuminoids, neutralize free radicals reducing LDL cholesterol, and protecting endothelial cells from damage, thereby improving nitric oxide availability for vasodilation [87].

ii. **Anti-inflammatory effect:** Chronic inflammation is a key factor in CVDs, including atherosclerosis and hypertension. Herbs like turmeric, boswellia, and ginger [87] inhibit enzymes such as tumor necrosis factor-alpha (TNF-α), interleukin 6 (IL-6), and ERP, pro-inflammatory cytokines, and cyclooxygenase 2 (COX-2), as well as nuclear factor-kappa B (NF-κB) pathways.

iii. **Hypolipidemic effect:** Several herbs [1] reduce plasma cholesterol and triglyceride levels, supporting dyslipidemia management. Garlic and guggul lower total and LDL cholesterol, increase high-density lipoprotein (HDL) levels, inhibit HMG Co-A (3-hydroxy-3-methylgl utaryl-coenzyme A reductase) reductase, and enhance bile acid excretion.

iv. **Antihypertensive effect:** Many herbs exhibit vasodilatory and diuretic activities to help control high blood pressure [88]. *Hibiscus sabdariffa*, garlic, and olive leaf [89] exhibit angiotensin-converting enzyme inhibition, calcium channel-blocking property, enhanced nitric oxide synthesis, and promotion of renal sodium excretion (natriuresis).

v. **Antiplatelet and anticoagulant activity:** Thrombosis and platelet aggregation [90] are the two factors that contribute to myocardial infraction and stroke. Few herbs act as natural blood thinners; for example, garlic, ginger, and *G. biloba* inhibit platelet aggregation, suppress thromboxane $A_2$ synthesis, and enhance fibrinolytic activity [91] with potential interactions with all connectional anticoagulants.

vi. **Vasodilatory and endothelial effects:** Herbs like ginseng, hawthorn improve vascular tone and endothelial function by enhancing blood flow and reducing vascular resistance [92]. These herbs increase endothelial nitric oxide production, inhibit endothelin-1, and protect VSMCs from any possible vascular stress.

vii. **Cardiotonic effect:** *Terminalia arjuna* increases myocardial contractility, supporting the management of mild to moderate heart failure. This herb strengthens heart muscle contraction and improves cardiac output [93], providing digitalis-like effects with improved safety.

viii. **Antiarrhythmic effect:** Herbs like motherwort (*Leonurus cardiaca*) and arjuna (*T. arjuna*) stabilize cardiac rhythm by acting on ion channels or by reducing myocardium excitability [94, 95]. These two medicinal herbs modulate calcium and potassium channels and exhibit mild sedative effects, thereby reducing stress-induced arrhythmias.

ix. **Diuretic effect:** Dandelion and celery seed are herbs with natural diuretic properties [96] helping in the management of hypertension and fluid retention. These two medicinal herbs promote excretion of sodium and water, reducing blood volume and pressure.

x. **Anti-atherosclerotic activity:** Turmeric, garlic, and guggul are medicinal herbs that inhibit plaque formation, enhance lipid clearance [97], and reduce vascular inflammation. These herbs enhance cholesterol efflux [98] from macrophages and inhibit foam cell formation.

Figure 1.3 presents selection of medicinal plants that are traditionally and scientifically recognized for their beneficial effects on the cardiovascular system. The illustration emphasizes the integrated role of plant-derived compounds in preserving endothelial function, enhancing myocardial performance, and preventing vascular damage associated with oxidative stress and inflammation. The illustration underscores the significance of traditional medicinal knowledge as a foundation for developing natural, plant-based cardioprotective therapies.

#### 1.3.6.2 Clinical Evidence and Research

Various medicinal herbs have shown different clinical evidence that supports future research.

- **Garlic (*Allium sativum*):** Meta-analysis shows significant reductions in blood pressure and LDL cholesterol, and it also exhibits a mild antiplatelet effect.
- **Hawthorn (*Crataegus* spp.):** Clinical trials suggest this drug is beneficial in mild heart failure with improvements in exercise capacity and symptom relief.
- **Turmeric (*Curcuma longa*):** This herb is shown to reduce inflammatory markers (C-reactive protein (CRP), TNF-α) and improve endothelial function in some small clinical studies.
- **Green tea (*Camellia sinensis*):** Due to its antioxidant and lipid-lowering properties, long-term consumption of green tea reduces cardiovascular mortality [99].
- **Arjuna (*T. arjuna*):** In heart failure patients, this herbal medicine demonstrated significant improvement in left ventricular ejection fraction in a few Indian clinical trials.

The findings outlined in Table 1.1 represent the different plant species used in the management of various CVDs.

Table 1.1 summarizes various medicinal plants employed in the prevention and treatment of cardiovascular disorders. It lists the herbs and their therapeutic roles, collectively

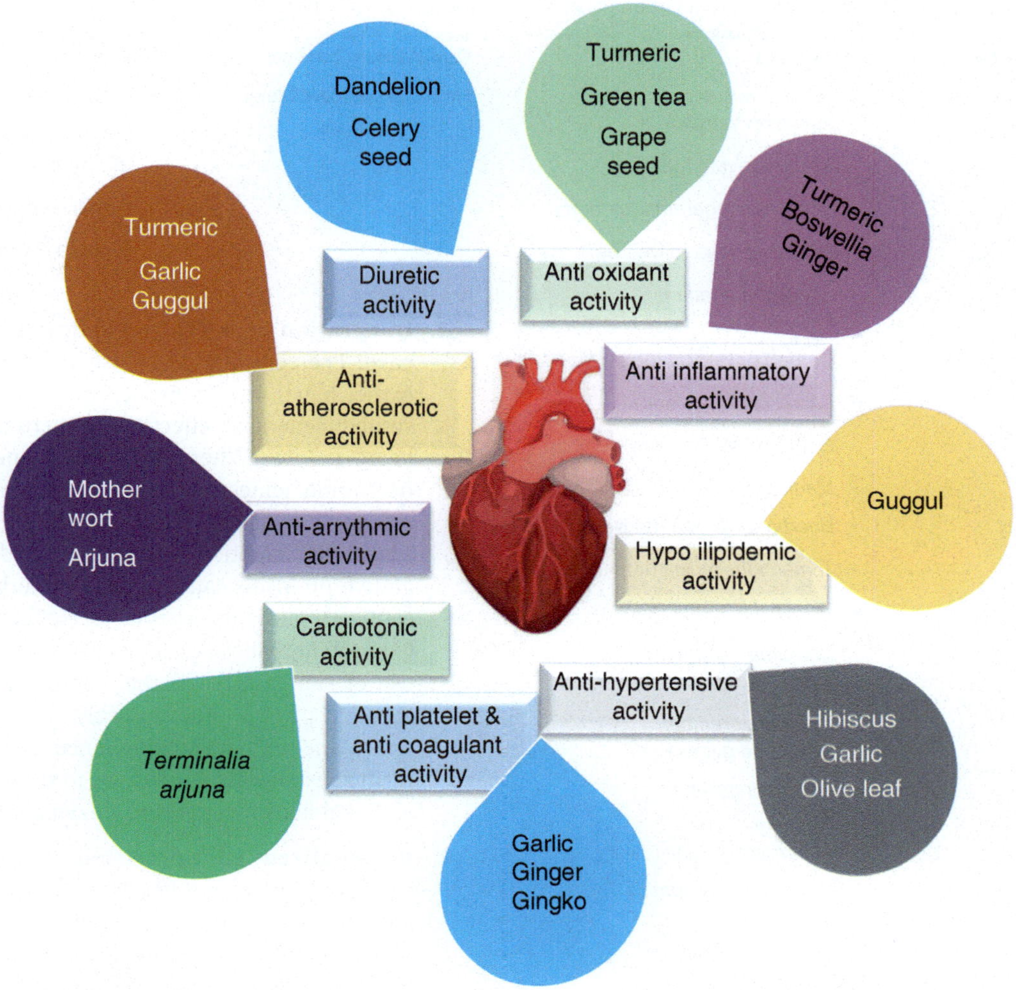


**FIGURE 1.3** Significance of traditional medicinal knowledge for their therapeutic effects on the cardiovascular system.

demonstrating the potential of phytotherapy as a complementary approach to conventional cardiovascular treatment.

### 1.3.6.3 Advantages of Herbal Medicine in Cardiovascular Diseases

Several herbal medicines offer many advantages, including multi-target actions [100], better affordability and accessibility, exhibiting mild side effects, and cultural acceptability in traditional medicinal systems like Ayurveda and traditional Chinese medicine [101].

### 1.3.6.4 Safety Concerns and Limitations

- Proper attention needs to be focused on the safe use of herbal medicines in terms of herb–drug interactions. The examples are:
  - Garlic + anticoagulants – increased bleeding risk
  - *G. biloba* + aspirin – risk of intracranial hemorrhage
- There is a great concern related to herbal medicine standardization issues with variations in active compound content, dosage, and formulation between the products.
- The wide usage of herbal medicines is limited due to a lack of large-scale trials and the possibility of misuse and overdose, particularly in self-medication.

### 1.3.6.5 Assimilation with Conventional Therapy

This herbal medicine is best used as a complementary therapy for critical interventions. The use of phytopharmaceuticals [102] and standardized extracts is being developed to bridge the gap between herbal medicine and conventional drugs.

Collaboration between herbalists, pharmacists, and physicians is essential to ensure safe and effective use.

### 1.3.6.6 Conjunctional and Anticipation in Cardiovascular Health

i. **The need for integrative approaches:** Despite significant advancements in modern medicine, CVD remains the leading cause of mortality and morbidity worldwide. This has led to growing interest in integrative healthcare models that unify conventional medicine, herbal medicine, lifestyle interventions, technological innovations like digital health and artificial intelligence, and finally precision and personalized medicine [102].

**Table 1.1** Plant species used in the treatment of various CVDs.

| Cardiovascular condition | Plant species |
|---|---|
| Reduction of blood pressure | • *Achillea millefolium* (common yarrow)<br>• *Allium sativum* (garlic)<br>• *Berberis integerrima* (barberry)<br>• *Olea europaea* (olive tree)<br>• *Silybum marianum* (milk thistle) |
| Management of angina | • *Camellia sinensis* (green tea)<br>• *Panax spp.* (ginseng)<br>• *Ginkgo biloba* (ginkgo)<br>• *Medicago sativa* (alfalfa) |
| Antioxidant activity | • *Boerhavia diffusa* (hogweed)<br>• *Tamarindus indica* (tamarind)<br>• *Terminalia arjuna* (arjuna)<br>• *Curcuma zedoaria* (white turmeric)<br>• *Zingiber zerumbet* (shampoo ginger) |
| Treatment of blocked arteries | • *Anthemis gayana* |
| Cardiomyopathies | • *Apium graveolens* (celery) |
| Congenital heart disease | • *Strychnos nux-vomica* (poison nut) |
| Heart attack prevention | • *Carthamus tinctorius* (safflower)<br>• *Inula helenium* (elecampane) |
| Reduction of blood lipid levels | • *Coriandrum sativum* (coriander)<br>• *Lactuca sativa* (lettuce)<br>• *Mentha spicata* (spearmint)<br>• *Senna alexandriana* (Alexandrian senna),<br>• *Sesamum indicum* (sesame)<br>• *Trigonella foenum-graecum* (fenugreek) |
| Cardiac arrhythmias | • *Ulmus glabra* Hudson |
| Improvement of venous blood flow | • *Melilotus indicus* |
| Anti-inflammatory (cardioprotective support) | • *Curcuma longa* (turmeric)<br>• *Withania somnifera* (Ashwagandha)<br>• *Ocimum sanctum* (holy basil)<br>• *B. diffusa* (punarnava)<br>• *Tinospora cordifolia* (guduchi) |
| Heart failure (cardiotonic) | • *Nerium indicum* (oleander)<br>• *Crataegus oxyacantha* (hawthorn)<br>• *A. sativum* (garlic)<br>• *Emblica officinalis* (amla) |

ii. **Integration of herbal medicine in cardiovascular care:** The complimentary use of important herbs like garlic, hawthorn, turmeric, and arjuna have demonstrated beneficial effects in hypertension, IHD, and heart failure. When integrated appropriately, these herbal medicines can enhance conventional therapies, reduce side effects, and improve quality of life [103]. The implementation of structured, evidence-based integrative protocols safely combines herbal and pharmaceutical treatments. A key factor is effective collaboration between herbalists, cardiologists, and pharmacists. The use of standardized herbal extracts and the development of phytopharmaceuticals ensure dose accuracy, safety, and regulatory compliance. Standardized herbal medicines may act as adjuncts to statins, beta-blockers, and angiotensin-converting enzyme inhibitors [104].

iii. **Personalized and precision medicine:** Genomic studies are revealing genetic predispositions to CVD, and future directions include pharmacogenomics, which identifies patients who may benefit from specific medicinal herbs. Biomarker-guided herbal formulations are helpful in targeting of information, oxidative stress, and lipid metabolism [105].

iv. **Technological integration:**

   a. **Digital health and monitoring:** Digital devices can track heart rate, blood pressure, ECG, and physical activity, helping herbal and lifestyle interventions [106]. Mobile apps and telemedicine can guide the use of herbal supplements and diet.

   b. **Artificial intelligence:** Artificial intelligence models can analyze the patients' data to recommend personalized integrative treatment plans [106]. Further, machine learning can identify synergistic herb–drug combinations and predict adverse interactions.

v. **Emerging research and innovations:** The recent trends and innovations include:

- Nanotechnology [107], which is being explored to enhance the bioavailability and targeted delivery of herbal compounds.
- Medicinal herb-based nutraceuticals, which are being designed to serve as both food and medicine.

Examples include cardioprotective teas and fortified oils.

- Active research, which is focused on herb combinations with synergistic effects (polyherbal formulations).

vi. **Regulatory and education framework:** WHO guidelines are very crucial, particularly for the global harmonization of herbal medicine standards.

- Pharmacovigilance systems [108] should be enhanced to monitor herb–drug interactions and different adverse events.
- Intensive training for medical practitioners should be provided to facilitate safe and more effective use in integrative cardiology practice.

vii. **Challenges and rationale**
According to the data presented in Table 1.2, the major challenges associated with the use of herbal medicines in cardiovascular care, along with the rationale supporting their continued exploration, are being demonstrated [86]. The table emphasizes the need for standardized formulations and improved quality control measures to enhance the credibility and therapeutic reliability of herbal products in CVD management.

**Table 1.2** Major challenges associated with the use of herbal medicines in cardiovascular care.

| Principal drawbacks | Scientific rationale |
|---|---|
| Insufficient safety and efficacy evidence | Herbal products are introduced into the market without rigorous preclinical or clinical validation to establish safety and therapeutic efficacy in contrast to conventional pharmaceutical agents. |
| Use in vulnerable populations | Clinical evaluation of herbal formulations in pediatric and pregnant populations is largely absent. Consequently, their administration is discouraged in children, pregnant or lactating women, and those planning conception due to potential risk of adverse outcomes. |
| Contamination and unintentional substitution | Instances of product mislabeling, where listed botanicals are replaced with alternative or incorrect plants, have been documented. Furthermore, contamination with synthetic drugs or other adulterants poses additional safety concerns. |
| Inconsistent active constituents | The pharmacologically active components of many herbal preparations remain unidentified, and in cases where they are known, their concentration may exhibit significant variability among different formulations. |
| Absence of specific antidotes | Improper use of herbal medicines such as excessive dosing or prolonged administration can result in serious toxic effects or organ damage. Currently, no specific antidote therapies are available to mitigate such toxicities. |

viii. **Future vision:**
Proper focus and attention are needed on the following aspects [109]:

- Holistic cardiovascular care model including
  - Conventional pharmacotherapy
  - Standardized herbal treatments
  - Lifestyle medicine (diet, exercise, stress management)
  - Digital tools (apps, artificial intelligence algorithms)
- Continuous focus on preventive cardiology using herbal medicines and dietary phytochemicals.
- Cross-disciplinary research involving botany, pharmacology, genomics, and artificial intelligence will define CVD management.

## 1.4 CONCLUSION

Millions of people worldwide are affected by a broad spectrum of cardiovascular disorders with distinct pathophysiological mechanisms, risk factors, and clinical presentations. However, risk factors such as hypertension, smoking, obesity, and physical inactivity are commonly shared. Understanding, addressing, and analyzing both adaptable and unalterable risk factors are very crucial in preventing and controlling CVDs. Different public health policies through integrated health systems and educating the individuals might reduce the risk components of these diseases. The conventional management of CVDs is based on a well-established combination of lifestyle interventions, pharmacological therapy, surgical procedures, and continuous clinical monitoring. The emergence of futuristic therapies like gene therapy and artificial intelligence-based models and the traditional methods remain core strategies in reducing cardiovascular morbidity and mortality. Though conventional therapies are the backbone of CVD management, they still have a few limitations in terms of effectiveness, accessibility, and long-term adherence. These gaps highlight the need for innovative, integrative, and personalized approaches like smart drug delivery systems, digital health monitoring, and genomics. All these strategies are effectively being explored in futuristic CVD management.

Herbal medicine is a highly valuable healthcare source with potential therapeutic use. This interest in integrity and complementary medicine, ensuring scientific validation, quality assurance, and safe practice, is essential for the effective implementation into the mainstream medicine. Herbal medicine acts as a promising adjuvant in CVD management, particularly in prevention and early intervention. There are several herbs that show clinical relevant benefits and the need for high-quality research, standardization of products, and confirmation of safety and efficacy. Professional collaboration is essential for these medicines. As might be expected, the entire future lies in modern approaches that combine the strengths of herbal and modern medicine.

The therapeutic application of herbal medicines in the management of CVDs remains insufficiently supported by robust scientific evidence. Although certain herbal agents exhibit activity on biological pathways associated with cardiovascular function, existing clinical investigations are generally limited by small sample size and lack statistically significant effects on major clinical outcomes. Consequently, the current body of evidence is inadequate to endorse the clinical use of herbal medications for cardiovascular conditions. Furthermore, potential adverse effects, including drug–herb interactions, contamination and substitution with other compounds, present additional safety concerns. It is therefore imperative that physicians enhance their understanding of herbal pharmacology to critically evaluate their clinical implications, effectively counsel patients regarding their potential risks and benefits, and emphasize that natural origin does not inherently equate to safety. Further well-structured clinical studies with larger participant samples are essential to clarify the therapeutic potential and mechanistic pathways of various medicinal plants in CVDs.

Amalgamating herbal medicine into mainstream cardiovascular care holds transformational potential, with advancements in innovative technology, pharmacology, and data science. The future of cardiovascular health lies in holistic scaffolding that values both tradition and innovation.

## REFERENCES


1. Shaito, A., Thuan, D.T., Phu, H.T. et al. (2020). Herbal medicine for cardiovascular diseases: efficacy, mechanisms, and safety. *Front. Pharmacol.* 11: 422.
2. Liu, C. and Huang, Y. (2016). Chinese herbal medicine on cardiovascular diseases and the mechanisms of action. *Front. Pharmacol.* 7: 469.
3. Sakhanda, I. and Kosyachenko, K. (2018). Assortment of herbal medicines of the treatment of cardiovascular diseases. *Wiadomosci Lekarskie (Warsaw, Poland : 1960)* 71 (5): 1104–1108.
4. Gaziano, T., Reddy, K.S., Paccaud, F. et al. (2006). Cardiovascular disease. In: *Disease Control Priorities in Developing Countries*, 2ee (ed. D.T. Jamison, J.G. Breman, A.R. Measham, et al.). Washington (DC): The International Bank for Reconstruction and Development / The World Bank New York: Oxford University Press.
5. Celermajer, D.S. (1997). Endothelial dysfunction: does it matter? Is it reversible? *J. Am. Coll. Cardiol.* 30 (2): 325–333.
6. Cimmino, G., Natale, F., Alfieri, R. et al. (2023). Non-conventional risk factors: "fact" or "fake" in cardiovascular disease prevention? *Biomedicine* 11 (9): 2353.
7. Joseph, P., Lanas, F., Roth, G. et al. (2025). Cardiovascular disease in the Americas: the epidemiology of cardiovascular disease and its risk factors. *Lancet Reg. Health Am.* 42: 100960.
8. Townsend, N., Kazakiewicz, D., Lucy, W.F. et al. (2022). Epidemiology of cardiovascular disease in Europe. *Nat. Rev. Cardiol.* 19 (2): 133–143.
9. Sulashvili, N. and Nimangre, R.R. (2025). Manifestation of some aspects of cardiovascular diseases, implications, pharmacotherapeutic strategies, effects, impacts and potential hazards in general. *Junior Res.* 3 (1): 1–27.
10. Lindstrom, M., DeCleene, N., Dorsey, H. et al. (2022). Global burden of cardiovascular diseases and risks collaboration, 1990–2021. *J. Am. Coll. Cardiol.* 80 (25): 2372–2425.
11. Lacey, B., Herrington, W.G., Preiss, D. et al. (2017). The role of emerging risk factors in cardiovascular outcomes. *Curr. Atheroscler. Rep.* 19 (6): 28.
12. Ungvari, A., Gulej, R., Patai, R. et al. (2025). Sex-specific mechanisms in vascular aging: exploring cellular and molecular pathways in the pathogenesis of age-related cardiovascular and cerebrovascular diseases. *Geroscience* 47 (1): 301–337.
13. Sawicka, K., Szczyrek, M., Jastrzebska, I. et al. (2011). Hypertension–the silent killer. *J. Pre-Clin. Clin. Res.* 5 (2): 43–46.
14. Muntner, P., Carey, R.M., Gidding, S. et al. (2018). Potential US population impact of the 2017 ACC/AHA high blood pressure guideline. *J. Am. Coll. Cardiol.* 71 (2): 109–118.
15. Triantafyllidi, H., Tzortzis, S., Lekakis, J. et al. (2010). Association of target organ damage with three arterial stiffness indexes according to blood pressure dipping status in untreated hypertensive patients. *Am. J. Hypertens.* 23 (12): 1265–1272.
16. Fan, X., Zhu, M., Chi, C. et al. (2017). Association of arteriosclerosis and/or atherosclerosis with hypertensive target organ damage in the community-dwelling elderly Chinese: the Northern Shanghai Study. *Clin. Interv. Aging* 12: 929–936.
17. Mensah, G.A. (2016). Hypertension and target organ damage: don't believe everything you think! *Ethn. Dis.* 26 (3): 275.
18. Abegaz, T.M., Tefera, Y.G., and Befekadu, A.T. (2017). Target organ damage and the long term effect of nonadherence to clinical practice guidelines in patients with hypertension: a retrospective cohort study. *Int. J. Hypertens.* 2017 (1): 2637051.
19. Dibona, G.F. (2013). Sympathetic nervous system and hypertension. *Hypertension* 61 (3): 556–560.
20. Oparil, S., Zaman, M.A., and Calhoun, D.A. (2003). Pathogenesis of hypertension. *Ann. Intern. Med.* 139 (9): 761–776.
21. Rodrigo, R., González, J., and Paoletto, F. (2011). The role of oxidative stress in the pathophysiology of hypertension. *Hypertens. Res.* 34 (4): 431–440.
22. Davies, M.J., Gordon, J.L., Gearing, A.J. et al. (1993). The expression of the adhesion molecules ICAM-1, VCAM-1, PECAM, and E-selectin in human atherosclerosis. *J. Pathol.* 171 (3): 223–229.
23. Tabas, I., Williams, K.J., and Borén, J. (2007). Subendothelial lipoprotein retention as the initiating process in atherosclerosis: update and therapeutic implications. *Circulation* 116 (16): 1832–1844.
24. Moore, K.J. and Tabas, I. (2011). Macrophages in the pathogenesis of atherosclerosis. *Cell* 145 (3): 341–355.
25. Al-Shehabi, T.S., Iratni, R., and Eid, A.H. (2016). Anti-atherosclerotic plants which modulate the phenotype of vascular smooth muscle cells. *Phytomedicine* 23 (11): 1068–1081.
26. Martinet, W., Coornaert, I., Puylaert, P., and De Meyer, G.R. (2019). Macrophage death as a pharmacological target in atherosclerosis. *Front. Pharmacol.* 10: 306.
27. Douglas, G. and Channon, K.M. (2014). The pathogenesis of atherosclerosis. *Medicine* 42 (9): 480–484.
28. Virmani, R., Burke, A.P., Kolodgie, F.D., and Farb, A. (2002). Vulnerable plaque: the pathology of unstable coronary lesions. *J. Interv. Cardiol.* 15 (6): 439–446.
29. Givertz, M.M. and Haghighat, A. *Clinical Manifestations, Diagnosis, and Management of High-Output Heart Failure.* UpToDate 2025.

30. Sheraliev, A. (2025). Pathophysiology of heart failure, hemodynamic changes and their consequences. *Mod. Sci. Res.* 4 (5).
31. Shams, P., Malik, A., and Chhabra, L. (2025). *Heart Failure (Congestive Heart Failure)*. Treasure Island, FL: Stat Pearls.
32. Mcginigle, K.L. (2024). Peripheral vascular disease. *Prim. Care* 51 (1): 83–93.
33. Mandaglio-Collados, D., Marin, F., and Rivera-Caravaca, J.M. (2023). Peripheral artery disease: update on etiology, pathophysiology, diagnosis and treatment. *Medicina* 161 (8): 344–350.
34. Simpson, M.T., Kachel, M., Neely, R.C. et al. (2023). Rheumatic heart disease in the developing world. *Struct. Heart* 7 (6): 100219.
35. Dass, C. and Kanmanthareddy, A. (2023). *Rheumatic Heart Disease*. Treasure Island, FL: Stat Pearls Publishing.
36. Dougherty, S., Okello, E., Mwangi, J., and Kumar, R.K. (2023). Rheumatic heart disease: JACC focus seminar 2/4. *J. Am. Coll. Cardiol.* 81 (1): 81–94.
37. Meng, X., Song, M., Zhang, K. et al. (2024). Congenital heart disease: types, pathophysiology, diagnosis, and treatment options. *MedComm* 5 (7): e631.
38. Navarrete, S., Solar, C., Tapia, R. et al. (2023). Pathophysiology of deep vein thrombosis. *Clin. Exp. Med.* 23 (3): 645–654.
39. Glazier, C.R. and Baciewicz, F.A. Jr. (2024). Epidemiology, etiology, and pathophysiology of pulmonary embolism. *Int. J. Angiol.* 33 (02): 076–081.
40. Reiner, Ž., Laufs, U., Cosentino, F., and Landmesser, U. (2019). The year in cardiology 2018: prevention. *Eur. Heart J.* 40 (4): 336–344.
41. Weber, C. and Noels, H. (2011). Atherosclerosis: current pathogenesis and therapeutic options. *Nat. Med.* 17 (11): 1410–1422.
42. Ridker, P.M., Everett, B.M., Thuren, T. et al. (2017). Antiinflammatory therapy with canakinumab for atherosclerotic disease. *N. Engl. J. Med.* 377 (12): 1119–1131.
43. Aday, A.W. and Ridker, P.M. (2018). Anti-inflammatory therapy in clinical care: the CANTOS trial and beyond. *Front. Cardiovasc. Med.* 5: 62.
44. Guerrero-García, C. and Rubio-Guerra, A.F. (2018). Combination therapy in the treatment of hypertension. *Drugs Context* 7: 212531.
45. Stewart, M.H., Lavie, C.J., and Ventura, H.O. (2019). Emerging therapy in hypertension. *Curr. Hypertens. Rep.* 21 (3): 23.
46. Elmakki, E. (2025). The role of lifestyle modifications in preventing and managing systemic hypertension: current guidelines and future directions. *Ann. Afr. Med.* 24 (1): 1–8.
47. Alyafei, A. and Daley, S.F. (2025). *The Role of Dietary Lifestyle Modification in Chronic Disease Prevention and Management*. Stat Pearls Publishing.
48. Wang, Y. and Magliano, D.J. (2025). New trends in diabetes, hypertension, and cardiovascular diseases—2nd edition. *Int. J. Mol. Sci.* 26 (2): 449.
49. Sayer, M., Webb, D.J., and Dhaun, N. (2025). Novel pharmacological approaches to lowering blood pressure and managing hypertension. *Nat. Rev. Cardiol.* 1–5.
50. Wang, N., Salam, A., Pant, R. et al. (2025). Blood pressure-lowering efficacy of antihypertensive drugs and their combinations: a systematic review and meta-analysis of randomised, double-blind, placebo-controlled trials. *Lancet* 406 (10506): 915–925.
51. Ozyuncu, N. (2025). Antiplatelet therapy in heart disease. *Rev. Cardiovasc. Med.* 26 (6): 36522.
52. Jabbar, K., Advani, R.S., Kirmani, S.A. et al. (2025). Advances in antithrombotic therapy: a review of new antiplatelet and anticoagulant medications in cardiovascular disease. *Indus J. Biosci. Res.* 3 (4): 69–78.
53. Cheng, Q., Sun, J., Zhong, H. et al. (2024). Research trends in lipid-lowering therapies for coronary heart disease combined with hyperlipidemia: a bibliometric study and visual analysis. *Front. Pharmacol.* 15: 1393333.
54. Kayani, T., Ahmad, B., Chang, R.S. et al. (2024). Beyond statins: novel lipid-lowering agents for reducing risk of atherosclerotic cardiovascular disease. *Pharmacoepidemiology* 3 (1): 117–168.
55. Prabhakar, A.P., Vedamurthy, D., and Kalra, D.K. (2025). Impact of lipid lowering therapies on the primary prevention of atherosclerotic cardiovascular disease. *Curr. Cardiovasc. Risk Rep.* 19 (1): 12.
56. Montelaro, B.M., Ibrahim, R., Thames, M., and Mehta, P.K. (2024). Optimal medical therapy for stable ischemic heart disease: focus on anti-anginal therapy. *Med. Clin.* 108 (3): 455–468.
57. Karan, V. and Madhumitha, S. (2025). Novel drugs approach in treatment of angina. *Int. J. Sci. Res. Technol.* 2 (3): 477–482.
58. Deoker, A., Lehker, A., and Mukherjee, D. (2020). Updates in antianginal and anti-ischemic therapies for acute coronary syndromes. *Curr. Cardiol. Rep.* 22 (10): 126.
59. Larson, J., Rich, L., Deshmukh, A. et al. (2022). Pharmacologic management for ventricular arrhythmias: overview of anti-arrhythmic drugs. *J. Clin. Med.* 11 (11): 3233.
60. Martínez-Rubio, A., Romiti, G.F., and Dan, G.A. (2025). Clinical significance and management of arrhythmias. In: *Antiarrhythmic Drugs*, 343–377. Cham: Springer Nature.
61. Hoole, S.P. and Bambrough, P. (2020). Recent advances in percutaneous coronary intervention. *Heart* 106 (18): 1380–1386.
62. Dehdar Karsidani, S., Farhadian, M., Mahjub, H., and Mozayanimonfared, A. (2022). Intelligent prediction of major adverse cardiovascular events (MACCE) following percutaneous coronary intervention using ANFIS-PSO model. *BMC Cardiovasc. Disord.* 22 (1): 389.
63. Raja, S.G. (2025). Postoperative management of coronary artery bypass grafting. *Heart Surg. Forum* 28 (6): E462–E475.
64. Thuan, P.Q., Chuong, P.T., Nam, N.H., and Dinh, N.H. (2025). Coronary artery bypass surgery: evidence-based practice. *Cardiol. Rev.* 33 (4): 344–351.
65. Baddour, L.M., Esquer Garrigos, Z., Rizwan Sohail, M. et al. (2024). Update on cardiovascular implantable electronic device infections and their prevention, diagnosis, and management: a scientific statement from the American Heart Association. *Circulation* 149 (2): e201–e216.
66. Jalandhra, G.K., Srethbhakdi, L., Davies, J. et al. (2025). Materials advances in devices for heart disease interventions. *Adv. Mater.* 37: 2420114.
67. Aristizábal, J.M. (2025). Cardiac resynchronization therapy: an opportunity for the right moment. *Revista Colombiana de Cardiología (English Edition)* 32 (2): https://doi.org/10.24875/RCCARE.M25000151. Universidad CES.
68. Wiedmann, F., Ince, H., Stellbrink, C. et al. (2023). Single beta-blocker or combined amiodarone therapy in implantable cardioverter-defibrillator and cardiac resynchronization therapy—defibrillator patients: insights from the German DEVICE registry. *Heart Rhythm* 20 (4): 501–509.
69. Thomas, R.J. (2024). Cardiac rehabilitation—challenges, advances, and the road ahead. *N. Engl. J. Med.* 390 (9): 830–841.
70. Zaree, A., Dev, S., Yaseen Khan, I. et al. (2023). Cardiac rehabilitation in the modern era: optimizing recovery and reducing recurrence. *Cureus* 15 (9): e46006.
71. Tessler, J., Ahmed, I., and Bordoni, B. (2025). *Cardiac Rehabilitation*. Treasure Island, FL: Stat Pearls Publishing.
72. Shiwani, M.A., Chico, T.J., Ciravegna, F., and Mihaylova, L. (2023). Continuous monitoring of health and mobility indicators in patients with cardiovascular disease: a review of recent technologies. *Sensors* 23 (12): 5752.

73. Samanidis, G. (2024). Current challenges in diagnosis and treatment of cardiovascular disease. *J. Pers. Med.* 14 (8): 786.
74. Du, Z. and Qin, Y. (2023). Dyslipidemia and cardiovascular disease: current knowledge, existing challenges, and new opportunities for management strategies. *J. Clin. Med.* 12 (1): 363.
75. Thomas, R.J., Sapir, O., Gomes, P.F. et al. (2023). Advances, challenges, and progress in cardiac rehabilitation in chronic CVD management. *Curr. Atheroscler. Rep.* 25 (6): 247–256.
76. Li, L., Zhou, X., Li, N. et al. (2015). Herbal drugs against cardiovascular disease: traditional medicine and modern development. *Drug Discov. Today* 20 (9): 1074–1086.
77. Villaescusa, L., Zaragozá, C., Zaragozá, F., and Tamargo, J. (2023). Herbal medicines for the treatment of cardiovascular diseases: Benefits and risks–a narrative review. *Int. J. Cardiol.* 385: 44–52.
78. Tachjian, A., Maria, V., and Jahangir, A. (2010). Use of herbal products and potential interactions in patients with cardiovascular diseases. *J. Am. Coll. Cardiol.* 55 (6): 515–525.
79. Nichols, M., Townsend, N., Scarborough, P., and Rayner, M. (2014). Cardiovascular disease in Europe 2014: epidemiological update. *Eur. Heart J.* 35 (42): 2950–2959.
80. Harvey, A. (2000). Strategies for discovering drugs from previously unexplored natural products. *Drug Discov. Today* 5 (7): 294–300.
81. Cragg, G.M. and Newman, D.J. (2013). Natural products: a continuing source of novel drug leads. *Biochim. Biophys. Acta Gen. Subj.* 1830 (6): 3670–3695.
82. Otvos, R.A., Still, K.B., Somsen, G.W. et al. (2019). Drug discovery on natural products: from ion channels to nAChRs, from nature to libraries, from analytics to assays. *SLAS Discov.* 24 (3): 362–385.
83. Farnsworth, N.R., Akerele, O., Bingel, A.S. et al. (1985). Medicinal plants in therapy. *Bull. World Health Organ.* 63 (6): 965.
84. Davison, E.K. and Brimble, M.A. (2019). Natural product derived privileged scaffolds in drug discovery. *Curr. Opin. Chem. Biol.* 52: 1–8.
85. Pan, S.Y., Zhou, S.F., Gao, S.H. et al. (2013). New perspectives on how to discover drugs from herbal medicines: CAM'S outstanding contribution to modern therapeutics. *Evid. Based Complement. Alternat. Med.* 2013 (1): 627375.
86. Liperoti, R., Vetrano, D.L., Bernabei, R., and Onder, G. (2017). Herbal medications in cardiovascular medicine. *J. Am. Coll. Cardiol.* 69 (9): 1188–1199.
87. Adegbola, P., Aderibigbe, I., Hammed, W., and Omotayo, T. (2017). Antioxidant and anti-inflammatory medicinal plants have potential role in the treatment of cardiovascular disease: a review. *Am. J. Cardiovas. Dis.* 7 (2): 19.
88. Meher, S.K., Das, B., Panda, P. et al. (2016). Uses of *Withaniasomnifera (Linn) Dunal (Ashwagandha)* in Ayurveda and its pharmacological evidences. *Res. J. Pharmacol. Pharmacodyn.* 8 (1): 23.
89. Suprabha, D., Avilash, R., Paul, A. et al. (2023). Food and medicinal properties of hibiscus (*Hibiscus sabdariffa* & *Hibiscus rosa-sinensis*). *Sustain. Agri Food Environ. Res.* 12 (1).
90. Damdhar, P., Pawara, K., and Valvi, A. A comprehensive review of currently researched medicinal herbs with anticoagulant potential. *Int. Res. J. Pharm. Med. Sci. ISSN (Online)* 2581–3277.
91. Liao, L., Li, X., Xu, H. et al. (2025). Systematic analysis of the interaction mechanism between platelets and coronary heart disease: from molecular pathways to new strategies for plant based antiplatelet therapy. *Front. Pharmacol.* 16: 1586265.
92. Vijayakumar, A., Park, J.H., and Kim, J.H. (2025). The role of ginseng and *ginsenosides in ROS* and cardiovascular disease. *J. Ginseng Res.*.
93. Janbaz, K.H., Hamid, I., Mahmood, M.H., and Gilani, A.H. (2011). Bronchodilator, cardiotonic and spasmolytic activities of the stem barks of *Terminalia arjuna*. *Can. J. Appl. Sci.* 3: 104–120.
94. Yarnell, E. and Abascal, K. (2003). Botanicals for regulating heart rhythms. *Altern. Complement. Ther.* 9 (3): 125–129.
95. Wojtyniak, K., Szymański, M., Matławska, I., and Leonuruscardiaca, L. (2013). (Motherwort): a review of its phytochemistry and pharmacology. *Phytother. Res.* 27 (8): 1115–1120.
96. El-Tantawy, W., Temraz, A., and Mohamed, S.A. (2024). Herbal extracts acting as diuretics: a comprehensive review. *Egypt. J. Chem.* 67 (3): 387–399.
97. Eqbal, K., Alam, M.A., Asjad, M. et al. (2022). Hypolipidemic activity of medicinal plants: an overview. *Hippocrat. J. Unani Med.* 17 (1): 6–11.
98. Selvi, P.T. (2023). A review on anti-hyperlipidemic properties of some important medicinal plants. *Indian J. Natl. Sci.* 14 (81): International Bimonthly (Print) – Open Access ISSN: 0976 – 0997.
99. Singh, A. (2024). Herbal-based nutraceuticals in management of lifestyle diseases: experience from Indian population. *Future Integr. Med.* 3 (2): 106–115.
100. Kshirsagara, A., Gnanadeebam, D.S., Deshmukh, M.V. et al. (2023). Role of herbal medicine in cardiovascular activities. *J. Adv. Zool.* 44: 278–283.
101. Saggar, S., Mir, P.A., Kumar, N. et al. (2022). Traditional and herbal medicines: opportunities and challenges. *Pharmacogn. Res.* 14 (2): 107–114.
102. Wang, Y., Li, G., Yang, L. et al. (2022). Development of innovative biomaterials and devices for the treatment of cardiovascular diseases. *Adv. Mater.* 34 (46): 2201971.
103. Ullah, A., Kumar, M., Sayyar, M. et al. (2023). Revolutionizing cardiac care: a comprehensive narrative review of cardiac rehabilitation and the evolution of cardiovascular medicine. *Cureus* 15 (10): e46469.
104. Al-Worafi, Y.M. (2025). Evidence-based complementary, alternative, and integrated medicine and efficacy and safety: angina and myocardial infarction. In: *Handbook of Complementary, Alternative, and Integrative Medicine* (ed. Y.M. Al-Worafi), 55–76. CRC Press.
105. Sethi, Y., Patel, N., Kaka, N. et al. (2023). Precision medicine and the future of cardiovascular diseases: a clinically oriented comprehensive review. *J. Clin. Med.* 12 (5): 1799.
106. Avoke, D., Elshafeey, A., Weinstein, R. et al. (2024). Digital health in diabetes and cardiovascular disease. *Endocr. Res.* 49 (3): 124–136.
107. Smith, B.R. and Edelman, E.R. (2023). Nanomedicines for cardiovascular disease. *Nat. Cardiovasc. Res.* 2 (4): 351–367.
108. Patel, N.M., Stottlemyer, B.A., Gray, M.P. et al. (2022). A pharmacovigilance study of adverse drug reactions reported for cardiovascular disease medications approved between 2012 and 2017 in the United States Food and Drug Administration Adverse Event Reporting System (FAERS) database. *Cardiovasc. Drugs Ther.* 36 (2): 309–322.
109. Chintya, Y. (2024). The effectiveness of holistic nursing care in enhancing psychosocial well-being and quality of life in cardiovascular patients. *J. Acad. Sci.* 1 (8): 964–978.

# Phytochemical-Based Interventions for Cardiovascular Complications: Mechanistic Insights and Therapeutic Promise

CHAPTER 2

**Lakshmana Rao Atmakuri[1], Kamal Dua[2], Ramesh Alluri[3], and Anupama Baratam[4]**

[1] *V. V. Institute of Pharmaceutical Sciences, Gudlavalleru, Andhra Pradesh, India*

[2] *Graduate School of Health, Faculty of Health, University of Technology Sydney, Sydney, New South Wales, Australia*

[3] *Vishnu Institute of Pharmaceutical Education and Research, Narsapur, Andhra Pradesh, India*

[4] *KVSR Siddhartha College of Pharmaceutical Sciences, Vijayawada, Andhra Pradesh, India*

## 2.1 INTRODUCTION

Cardiovascular diseases (CVDs) still remain a global threat and make a significant percentage of morbidity and mortality in all socioeconomic regions. Causing deaths of almost every three individuals in the world, diseases such as ischemic heart disease, cerebrovascular accidents, and heart failure are causing enormous pressure on national economies and healthcare systems [1]. The increased rates of sedentary lifestyles, poor diet, obesity, and the epidemic of chronic stress are further contributing to the escalation in the epidemic of CVD, and it is not only a health but also a major societal issue (Figure 2.1).

Although the up-to-date pharmacological and procedural interventions have managed to increase the survival rates and quality of life, they are not devoid of limitations. Most first-line treatments, which include statins, betablockers, calcium channel blockers, and angiotensin-converting enzyme (ACE) inhibitors, among others, have adverse effects that could prevent patient compliance [2–8]. These include fatigue and electrolyte imbalances. Besides, cardiovascular patients tend to be obese (a comorbidity) and need treatment of such conditions as diabetes, dyslipidemia, and renal disease, which will result in polypharmacy. This increases the danger of drug–drug interactions, reduces adherence, and complicates long-term treatment of the disease. Despite the efficacy of the available and most practitionable care, a considerable number of patients remain highly susceptible to further cardiovascular events.

Indeed, the use of phytochemicals – bioactive chemicals in plants – as cardioprotective agents is one such arena that has been drawing the attention of more and more cardioprotective health practitioners. In contrast with most synthetic drugs that have individual targets, many phytochemicals tend to affect various cellular and molecular mechanisms that play a role in cardiovascular health. These are antioxidant defense mechanisms, anti-inflammatory signaling, regulation of endothelial phenomena, lipid and glucose metabolism.

Furthermore, the agents have been linked with a good safety aspect, particularly when they are taken as one of the numerous elements of a balanced diet. They have special appeal as alternative or complementary therapeutic options because they are so accessible and inexpensive [2, 9–20]. An illustration comparing conventional cardiovascular drugs and phytochemical-based therapies, with their respective advantages, disadvantages, and mechanisms, is shown in Table 2.1.

Genetic engineering of phytochemicals through artificial intelligence (AI), such as to perform virtual screening, molecular docking, and personalized design nutraceuticals, only increases the pace of discovery and translation within cardiovascular medicine.

## 2.2 CLASSIFICATION, DIETARY SOURCES, AND THERAPEUTIC POTENTIAL

Phytochemicals, representing a wide variety of bioactive plant-derived compounds, are more energetically understood to be of therapeutic importance in cardiovascular medicine. These phytochemicals, found in abundance in fruits, vegetables, herbs, and whole grains, have vast biological effects that touch on several essential mechanisms associated with the complications and onset of CVDs.

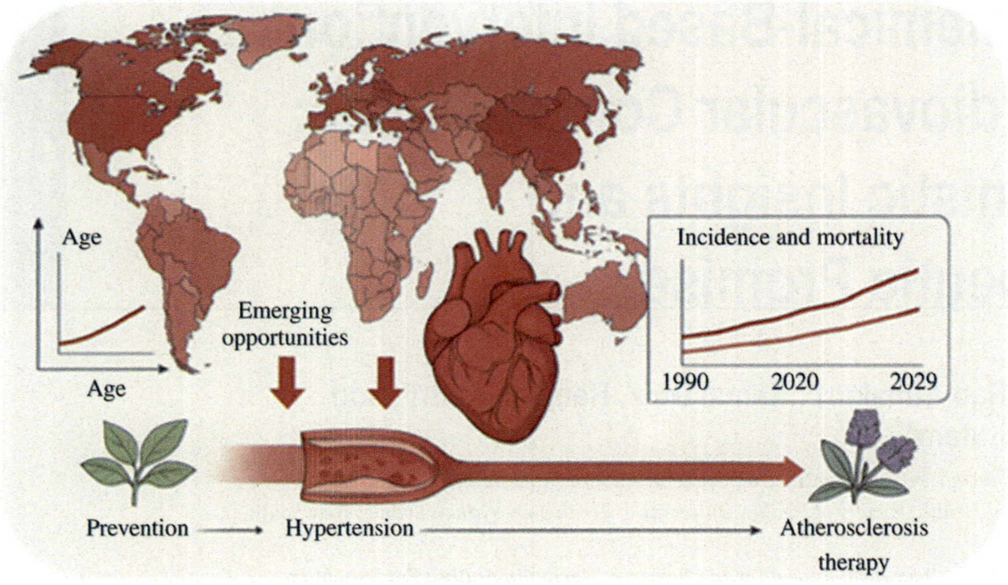


**FIGURE 2.1** Global burden of cardiovascular disease and unmet therapeutic needs.

**Table 2.1** Comparative overview: conventional cardiovascular drugs vs. phytochemicals.

| Aspect | Conventional therapies | Phytochemical-based approaches |
|---|---|---|
| Source | Synthetic, chemically engineered compounds | Natural, plant-derived bioactives |
| Mechanistic focus | Target-specific (e.g., cholesterol reduction, BP control) | Multi-pathway modulation (antioxidant, anti-inflammatory, etc.) |
| Adverse effects | Common (e.g., myalgia, hypotension, gastrointestinal issues) | Generally minimal, better tolerability profile |
| Polypharmacy risk | High in comorbid cases | Lower potential for drug–drug interactions |
| Affordability and access | High cost, insurance-dependent | More accessible, often culturally accepted |
| Scope of action | Primarily symptom control and risk factor modification | Prevention-focused; addresses underlying pathophysiology |
| Clinical evidence base | Extensive, with large RCTs | Emerging clinical data; strong preclinical foundation |
| Personalized therapy potential | Limited customization | High potential with AI and nutrigenomic integration |
| Regulatory status | Well-defined approval pathways | Variable; regulatory harmonization needed |

Compounds of different classes are structurally different, with particular molecular targets and pharmacological effects. The group of flavonoids has been extensively studied, and it is usually disseminated in citrus fruits, berries, onions, and tea. The compounds normalize the endothelial nitric oxidase synthase (eNOS) activity, suppress reactive oxygen species (ROS), and hamper the tumor necrosis factor-alpha TNF-α and nuclear factor kappa-light-chain-enhancer of activated B cells (NF-κB), inflammatory mediators. Examples of alkaloids include berberine and reserpine, and are known to affect the lipid metabolism, sympathetic activity, and vascular tone [21–26].

Among polyphenols are resveratrol and lignans, which are abundant in grapes, olive oil, flaxseed, and cocoa, and are associated with an anti-atherogenic/anti-inflammatory effects. Terpenoids occurring in turmeric (curcumin), ginger, and ginseng have an antioxidant, vasodilatory activity, antithrombotic properties. Finally, saponins obtained through legume, soy, and such plants as *Panax ginseng*, have a role in cholesterol binding, immune adjustment, and vascular protection.

Mediterranean diet, which is enriched in extra-virgin olive oil, nuts, legumes, vegetables, and red wine, and DASH diet, that is more specific focusing on fruits, whole grains, and low-fat dairy, are high in phytochemicals [27]. These diets have been repeatedly linked to better blood pressure, lipid profile, endothelial function, as well as markers of inflammation, which is mainly due to their phytochemical composition. Table 2.2 summarizes the main phytochemical classes, most frequent plant sources they are found in, and some of their cardiovascular effects [28–30].

**Table 2.2** Phytochemical classes, common sources, and associated cardioprotective roles.

| Phytochemical class | Common sources | Cardioprotective effects |
|---|---|---|
| Flavonoids | Citrus fruits, berries, onions, green tea, red wine | Antioxidant activity, vasodilation via eNOS, anti-inflammatory, platelet inhibition |
| Alkaloids | *Berberis*, *Rauwolfia*, capsicum, *Catharanthus* | Lipid regulation, blood pressure reduction, autonomic modulation |
| Polyphenols | Grapes, olives, cocoa, flaxseed, whole grains | Anti-inflammatory, anti-atherogenic, improves lipid profiles, inhibits platelet aggregation |
| Terpenoids | Turmeric, ginseng, ginger, rosemary | Antioxidant, antithrombotic, plaque stabilization, endothelial protection |
| Saponins | Legumes, soybeans, *Panax ginseng*, *Tribulus terrestris* | Cholesterol-lowering, immune modulation, anti-inflammatory |

## 2.3 MOLECULAR TARGETS IN CARDIOVASCULAR PATHOLOGY

The connections among targets need to be elucidated on a mechanistic level, as more broad-acting therapeutic approaches can be developed that employ phytochemicals [31–34], which have the ability to induce multi-targeted effects on a lower adverse effect basis.

***Nitric oxide imbalance and oxidative stress:*** The changed redox equilibrium caused by an overload of ROS, known as oxidative stress, is central to the development and advancement of cardiovascular pathology. The main sources of generation of ROS include mitochondrial dysfunction, Nicotinamide Adenine Dinucleotide Phosphate (NADPH) oxidase and imbalances of the enzymes in the vascular wall. Such reactive species kill endothelial cells, oxidize lipids, and also disrupt vasodilation. At the same time, ROS decrease the supply of a nitric oxide (NO) adaptor (eNOS), a vasoprotective agent formed by endothelial nitric oxide synthase (eNOS).

***Chronic inflammation and immune stimulation:*** Other than oxidative stress, chronic low-grade inflammation is key in the process of atherogenesis and other CVDs. Due to endothelial injury, TNF-α, interleukin6 (IL-6), and monocyte chemoattractant protein-1 (MCP-1) are upregulated as a way of inflammatory mediators. These cytokines induce signaling and expression of NF-κB [35], and they induce expression of adhesion molecules, which allow residence of leukocytes within the vascular intima. This immune process, over a period, results in the formation of foam cells, extracellular matrix breakdown, and the vulnerability of plaques.

***Atherogenesis and endothelial dysfunction:*** Endothelial homeostasis requires healthy endothelial function. Oxidation and inflammatory injuries to the endothelium, however, impair endothelial integrity, thereby deranging NO biosynthesis and augmenting vasoconstriction through production of endothelin1. The dysfunctional endothelium will also be more permeable and sticky to the circulating immune cells, which will make it quicker for lipids to infiltrate and form plaques.

***Disorder of metabolism:*** Insulin resistance, central obesity, dyslipidemia, and hypertension, constituting metabolic syndrome, make the latter a very high cardiovascular risk. High amounts of triglycerides and low-density lipoprotein cholesterol (LDL-C) [36–38], as well as low high-density lipoprotein cholesterol (HDL-C), cause a propensity for lipid buildup in the walls of the arteries and consequent formation of plaques. Transcriptional control of lipid metabolism at the molecular level occurs through transcriptional regulators of lipid disruption, which include peroxisome proliferator-activated receptors (PPARs) and AMP-activated protein kinase (AMPK). These are pathways of specific interest in phytotherapy, where a few plant-derived compounds have been found promising in regulating their activities and bringing the metabolism back into balance.

***Pathological cardiac remodeling fibrosis:*** A heart undergoes structural remodeling, which involves cardiomyocyte hypertrophy, activation of fibroblasts, and overdevelopment of extracellular cells, after ischemic injury or when extensive hemodynamic load has strained it. Such alterations undermine myocardial elasticity and contractility, which lead to heart failure [39]. TGF-β, connective tissue growth factor (CTGF), and renin–angiotensin system are the central mediators of fibrotic responses.

## 2.4 PHYTOCHEMICAL CARDIOPROTECTION MECHANISMS

Phytochemicals are cardioprotective since they work via complex pathways of molecular actions that respond to multifactorial aspects of CVDs.

***Antioxidant response in Nrf2:*** Activation of the nuclear factor erythroid 2-related factor 2 (Nrf2) signaling axis is one of the key ways phytochemicals battle oxidative stress. Nrf2 is retained in the cytoplasm under basal conditions through Keap1. Nrf2 then translocates to the nucleus in response to oxidative stimuli or binding by phytochemicals, binds the AREs, and promotes the expression of protective genes against oxidative stress, such as heme oxygenase-1 (HO-1), glutathione S-transferase (GST), and NAD(P)H: quinone oxidoreductase 1 (NQO1).

***NF-κB and inflammatory cytokine pathways inhibition:*** The major role in regulating the expression of inflammatory genes involved in CVD, such as TNF-α, interleukin-1 beta (IL-1β), interleukin 6 (IL-6), and C-reactive protein (CRP), during inflammation is performed by transcription factor NF-kappa B. NF-κB exists in the form of a complex with an inhibitor of kappa B (IκB) in the cytoplasm. Upon stimulation, IκB is degraded, allowing NF-κB to translocate into the nucleus and promote the expression of pro-inflammatory genes [40–46].

***Activation of eNOS and nitric oxide bioavailability:*** eNOS plays a vital role in the production of vasodilator and antithrombotic NO molecule, which is required to regulate vascular homeostasis. In CVD, characteristics of impaired nitric oxide signaling include abnormal eNOS performance and reduced nitric oxide levels. Various phytochemicals, especially resveratrol, have been demonstrated to increase the expression or activity of eNOS in several ways, such as through SIRT1 activation, by binding to calcium–calmodulin, and by phosphorylation via the phosphoinositide 3-kinase/protein kinase B (PI3K/Akt) pathway.

***PPARs and AMPK regulation in metabolism modulation:*** PPAR-alpha and PPAR-gamma are nuclear receptors that control lipid metabolism, glucose consumption, and infection. AMPK is an energy sensor activated in response to cellular stress conditions, and therefore it is complementary to PPAR activity because it increases fatty acid oxidation and enhances insulin sensitivity [47].

***PI3K/Akt and mitogen-activated protein kinase (MAPK)pathways in cellular survival and repair:*** PI3K/Akt promotes endothelial cell survival, angiogenesis, and cardiomyocyte protection. Upon activation, Akt acts on downstream proteins that facilitate proliferation of cells, antiapoptosis, and protein translation. The familial responses of MAPK are actualized by stress stimuli and particularize inflammation, fibrosis, and hypertrophy [48].

## 2.5 PROMINENT PHYTOCHEMICALS AND THEIR THERAPEUTIC PROFILES

These bioactives work by a variety of molecular mechanisms and have been the subject of preclinical and emerging clinical research.

***Modulator (resveratrol) of endothelial function and longevity pathways:*** Resveratrol is a polyphenolic stilbene present in grapes, red wine, and berries that has cardioprotective effects through Sirtuin 1 (SIRT1) activation. SIRT1 is a nicotinamide adenine dinucleotide $(NAD)^+$-dependent deacetylase involved in stress and metabolic processes. This stimulation increases the activity of the eNOS, which induces vasodilation and endothelial well-being [49].

***Dual Regulation of oxidative and inflammatory pathways:*** Curcumin, the major *Curcuma longa* curcuminoid, shows a specific modulation of oxidative and inflammatory processes. It also induces the Nrf2–ARE pathway, stimulates transcription of antioxidants such as HO-1 and NQO1, and at the same time prevents NF-κB signaling to attenuate production of pro-inflammatory cytokines [50–55].

***Antihypertensive and vasoprotective bioflavonoid:*** Quercetin is a flavonol that is very widely found in onion, apple, berries, and tea. Its cardiovascular effects and advantages are strong antihypertensive effects due to enhanced endothelial function and increased eNOS expression, with consequent augmented bioavailability of nitric oxide. Quercetin also suppresses ACE, which leads to relaxation of vessels.

***Metabolic modulator with cardiovascular promise:*** Berberine is a metabolic regulator and an isoquinoline alkaloid obtained from *Berberis* species. This medicament has become one of the most effective metabolic regulators associated with cardiovascular protection. It stimulates AMPK, thus improving glucose uptake, improving insulin sensitivity, and lowering hepatic lipid accumulation. Berberine also increases the expression of LDL receptors, which results in better lipid profiles and reduced LDL-cholesterol levels [56–58].

***Inflammation control and antithrombotic action:*** Broad-spectrum cardiovascular effects are seen in epigallocatechin-3-gallate (EGCG), the more abundant catechin in green tea, and citrus-derived flavonoids like naringenin and hesperidin. EGCG has been found to inhibit the signaling pathway of NF-κB, decrease the levels of CRP, and suppress the proliferation of vascular smooth muscle.

## 2.6 STRATEGIES TO ENHANCE PHYTOCHEMICAL DELIVERY

Plants produce a huge number of chemicals, and a small proportion of phytochemicals have attracted substantial interest over their powerful cardioprotective effects. These bioactives work through a variety of molecular mechanisms and have been the subject of preclinical and emerging clinical research [59–65].

***Bioavailability Challenges of phytochemicals:*** Phytochemicals like curcumin, resveratrol, and quercetin have immense *in vitro* activity but low system availability after oral consumption. Organic conversion: An example is curcumin, which is highly glucuronidated and sulfated in the body and will have little or no plasma concentration, unless appropriately formulated with delivery and enhancement.

***Revolutionizing phytochemical delivery:*** Nanostructured matrixes protect them against enzymatic degradation. The nanoformulations that can be used are polymeric nanoparticles (e.g., based on poly(lactic-co-glycolic acid) [PLGA]) that provide controlled delivery of drugs and enhance cellular intake of flavonoids and alkaloids. Liposomes made out of biocompatible lipid bilayers can be used to enclose both water-soluble and fat-soluble phytochemicals and at the same time help improve absorption. The complexation of phytochemicals with phospholipids significantly increases membrane permeability and systemic bioavailability, particularly for compounds such as silybin and quercetin, in the form of phytosomes.

***Use of bioenhancers and synergistic combinations:*** Co-administration of bioenhancers can also be used as an approach to increase phytochemical bioavailability via enhanced absorption and minimized metabolism. An example is piperine, a black pepper alkaloid, which increases curcumin bioavailability by more than 2000-fold by inhibiting glucuronidation.

## 2.7 PRECLINICAL AND CLINICAL EVIDENCE

Cardiovascular research on the benefits of phytochemicals has also been assisted by a growing amount of preclinical evidence based on an increasing number of experimental models.

**Table 2.3** Selected clinical trials on phytochemicals in cardiovascular therapy.

| Phytochemical/plant source | Study design/phase | Target condition | Key findings | Reference/trial ID |
|---|---|---|---|---|
| Resveratrol (grapes, red wine) | RCT, double-blind, placebo-controlled (phase II) | Endothelial dysfunction in hypertension | Improved flow-mediated dilation; reduced systolic BP | Timmers et al., 2011 (ClinTrials.gov: NCT01173654) |
| Curcumin (turmeric) | Randomized, placebo-controlled, crossover trial | Metabolic syndrome, inflammation | Reduced CRP, IL-6, and triglyceride levels | Panahi et al., 2016 |
| Berberine (*Berberis* spp.) | Multicenter, double-blind randomized controlled trial (RCT) (phase III) | Hyperlipidemia and type 2 diabetes | Lowered LDL-C and glycated hemoglobin (HbA1c); improved lipid profiles | Zhang et al., 2008 |
| Omega-3 fatty acids (fish oil) | Systematic review and meta-analysis | Atherosclerotic cardiovascular disease | Lowered risk of cardiac death and recurrent myocardial infarction (MI) | Mozaffarian & Rimm, 2006 |
| Quercetin (onions, apples) | Randomized, placebo-controlled, parallel-group trial | Stage 1 hypertension | Decreased systolic and diastolic blood pressure | Edwards et al., 2007 |
| Green tea catechins (EGCG) | Randomized, placebo-controlled trial | Obesity-related cardiovascular risk | Improved LDL oxidation and vascular reactivity | Basu et al., 2010 |
| Coenzyme Q10 (Ubiquinone) | Meta-analysis of RCTs | Heart failure | Improved ejection fraction and exercise capacity | Fotino et al., 2013 |

In models that simulate pathological conditions of issues like atherosclerosis, myocardial infarction, hypertension, and metabolic syndrome, animal-based studies have established that a plethora of plant-based substances possess multitargeting potential that can curb the progress of the disease [66, 67].

Phytochemicals have demonstrated promise in maintaining endothelial integrity, mitigating deposition of lipids, inhibiting oxidative and inflammatory processes that contribute to atherosclerotic plaque formation in the setting of atherosclerosis models. The antioxidative stress-reducing and endothelial-improving effects of compounds like resveratrol, as well as the modulation of inflammatory signaling pathways and the promotion of endogenous antioxidant levels by curcumin, have been witnessed.

Investigations conducted in models of hypertension and metabolic disorders depict that certain phytochemicals reduce vascular tone and improve metabolic conditions. These components also increase the release of AMPK, a key regulator of glucose and lipid homeostasis, such as berberine [68–73], and enhance the availability of endothelial nitric oxide while lowering blood pressure. These conclusions show the systemic effects of phytochemical activity and their potential role in healthcare of cardiovascular disorders.

Although the evidence of cardiovascular efficacy of phytochemicals in the human population is still developing, clinical research has provided sufficient evidence in favor of this hypothesis. Resveratrol interventions have found positive changes in endothelium-dependent vasodilation and a slight lessening of systolic blood pressure. The use of curcumin supplements, especially in combination with substances that increase its bioavailability (e.g., piperine), has been demonstrated to exhibit beneficial results in terms of the inflammatory marker profile and lipid metabolism. Berberine has come into the limelight for its twofold lipid- and glucose-lowering effects, as its effects are similar to those of pharmacotherapies. Quercetin and EGCG have had variable results in clinical trials, and this may well be due to individual variations in metabolism, existing health conditions, and dose.

Although these findings are promising, there are still significant constraints when it comes to the clinical use of phytochemicals. There are also problems such as differences in trial design, small sample sizes, short intervention duration, and lack of standardized formulations [74]. Also, a significant number of phytochemicals are have poor oral availability because of limited solubility, susceptibility to enzymatic degradation, and rapid systemic clearance, which can make them ineffective in clinical trials or in practice, even though they show good results in preclinical settings.

Standardization of extraction procedures, formulation, and administration should be enhanced in order to translate phytochemical studies into more standard approaches to therapy. There must also be sufficient and extensive studies to prove long-term safety and efficacy in large, randomized, and controlled trials. Nevertheless, existing literature indicates that phytochemicals may have great potential as adjunctive agents in cardiovascular treatment. Their action on several molecular targets can go hand in hand with the multifactorial etiology of CVDs, which justifies their inclusion in more comprehensive preventive and therapeutic approaches [75–81]. Clinical trials involving resveratrol, curcumin, berberine, quercetin, and EGCG have yielded promising results across diverse cardiovascular endpoints, as summarized in Table 2.3.

## 2.8 ARTIFICIAL INTELLIGENCE IN PHYTOCHEMICAL RESEARCH

Although traditional methods of phytochemical research are fundamental, they are often costly, time-consuming, and limited by complexity of natural product mixtures [82].

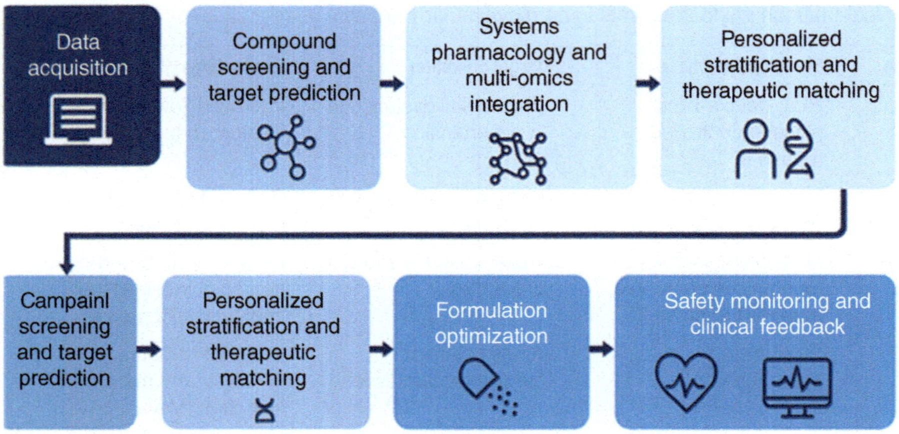


**FIGURE 2.2** AI-assisted pipeline for phytochemical discovery and personalized application.

In contrast, AI-powered software is characterized by its increased speed, accuracy, and scalability in processing large databases, identifying new bioactivities, and customizing therapeutic responses to specific patient settings.

Machine learning and deep learning models are becoming mainstream in the prediction of pharmacodynamic and pharmacokinetic properties of phytochemicals. This software can be used to screen through large natural product libraries to identify lead compounds in a short time by virtualizing their interactions with cardiovascular targets like PPARs, eNOS, or NF-κB signaling pathways.

The merger of the multi-omics data (including genomics, transcriptomics, proteomics, and metabolomics) with the systems pharmacology frameworks is also an important development made possible by AI. The AI-supported systems pharmacology assists in understanding the synergistic effects of phytochemicals and identifying pivotal points in disease pathways.

Alongside this, AI is introducing a more precise method of patient stratification. CVDs are highly heterogeneous due to the interaction effects of genetic polymorphisms, microbiome structure, metabolome, and environmental factors, which necessitate personalized therapy. Machine learning methods have the potential to interpret vast clinical and molecular data to stratify patients into subgroups with responsive conditions. This capacity forms the foundation of the advent of ultra-precise phytotherapy, which is a new horizon in medicine that is hinged on the integration of personalized medicine with evidence-based plant therapeutics.

Optimization of delivery systems is being carried out through the use of neural networks/predictive modeling tools, with consideration of variables/parameters like particle size, solubility, stability, and drug behavior, like release kinetics. With the help of these models, one can develop nanoformulations or approaches to encapsulation, and synergistic adjuvants that can greatly increase the bioavailability and efficacy of a treatment.

AI will bridge the gap between computational and botanical sciences, rationalizing the creation of next-generational phytomedicines that can be made to address the complexity of human biology. Despite some obstacles related to data quality, model validation, and regulatory acceptance, the trend at present indicates that AI will be one of the cornerstones of further promotion of phytochemical-based approach to cardiovascular health. The integration of computational tools, such as machine learning, molecular docking, and multi-omics analysis, has accelerated the discovery of phytochemicals with cardiovascular activity. A schematic overview of this AI-assisted discovery pipeline is illustrated in Figure 2.2.

## 2.9 REGULATORY FRAMEWORK AND STANDARDIZATION

The regulatory environment associated with phytochemicals to be used in cardiovascular interventions is extremely fragmented and remains in a transitional stage across the world. There are varying schemes of classification used in different jurisdictions [83]. A phytochemical can be controlled and regulated as a drug, a dietary supplement, a nutraceutical, functional food, or a traditional medicine depending on the country and designation. This variation presents significant challenges with international harmonization and market access, particularly where the drug stuff has divergent safety and efficacy standards, taking into consideration that the same compound is involved.

Phytochemicals added to dietary supplements in the United States are examples, and they are regulated by the Dietary Supplement Health and Education Act (DSHEA),which does not require premarket approval. Conversely, the European Union frequently regulates these compounds as medicinal products in the event of health claims, subjecting them to much more rigorous requirements with regard to both safety and efficacy as medicines. In Asian nations, such as India, China, and Japan, phytochemicals can be part of a traditional system such as Ayurveda, which have their own systems of regulation and documentation requirements.

As opposed to synthetic drugs of definite single active composition, phytochemicals are normally operating as mixtures, rendering routine randomized controlled tests even more demanding. Moreover, other aspects, like bioavailability, pharmacokinetics, and herb interactions with drug interactions should also be properly assessed on preclinical and clinical models that should be validated [84].

Control of quality and uniformity is still a key condition for regulatory approval. To ensure reliability and consistency with batch-to-batch variations, phytochemical profiles are authenticated using analytical techniques, like high-performance liquid chromatography (HPLC), liquid chromatography–tandem mass spectrometry (LC–MS/MS), gas chromatography (GC), and nuclear magnetic resonance (NMR) spectroscopy, to a great extent. Chemometric methods offer benefits to QC by facilitating fingerprinting and multivariate analysis of phytochemical compositions, assessing their consistency, variation, and distinguishing features.

Being internationally compliant with the manufacturing standards is an added advantage besides analytical validation. Such guidelines in the area of assuring phytochemical products' quality, safety, and traceability –such as Good Agricultural and Collection Practices (GACP) and Good Manufacturing Practices (GMP) – are becoming mandatory. Such practices consist of all supply chain processes, including cultivation and harvesting, processing, and packaging, and are crucial for upholding the integrity of plant-based therapeutics. In addition, regulatory submissions are further supported by toxicological profiling comprising of acute, sub-chronic, and chronic toxicity, genotoxicity data, and reproductive toxicity data, among others, that present convincing evidence of safety for use in humans.

Even though efforts are being made, tough regulatory issues remain. Lack of worldwide harmonization, insufficient standardized phytochemical specifications, inadequate testing capacity, and poor regulatory guideline enforcement are some of the key issues.

## 2.10 INNOVATIONS IN PHYTOCHEMICAL THERAPEUTICS

Novel achievements in biomedical science have launched phytochemicals into a new realm of therapeutic potential, with a renewed scope in the world of pharmacotherapy driven by molecular novelty and translational pharmacology [85]. Phytochemicals have been recognized as epigenetic modulators. A wide number of plant-based compounds have been shown to have the capacity to affect gene expression by modifying DNA methylation, histone acetylation, and the activity of non-coding RNA. The given epigenetic interactions prove to be crucial, especially in connection with CVDs, where chronic inflammation, oxidative stress, and metabolic imbalances are frequently related to imbalanced gene expression. As an example, compounds like curcumin, sulforaphane, and resveratrol have been shown to affect epigenetic markers that regulate endothelial function, fat metabolism, and cardiac remodeling and have the potential to provide long-term alteration of the disease.

Creating hybrid therapeutics through the combination of phytochemicals and biologics is an emerging strategy in which the bioactivity of the natural products is merged with the specificity and potency of biologic therapeutics. The goal of these conjugates is to take advantage of the target delivery capacity of monoclonal antibodies, peptides, or nucleic acids and still possess the multimodal activities of phytochemicals [86]. It is proposed that such combinations may reduce off-target effects, be more selective, and achieve greater tissue penetration, especially in cardiovascular applications. As an example, conjugates between polyphenols and peptides have demonstrated efficiency in increasing myocardial uptake and stability in models of ischemia–reperfusion injury.

At the same time, there is active pursuit of novel drug delivery systems to avoid shortcomings such as poor bioavailability, rapid degradation, and clearance, which have thus far limited clinical translation of phytochemicals. New delivery systems are under development, including oral dissolvable strips, transdermal patches, and nanoparticle formulations (nanoemulsion), which offer controlled, sustained, and patient-friendly drug delivery modes. It is possible to engineer these patches to release into the systemic circulation such cardioprotective agents as berberine or EGCG and reduce their degradation in the gastrointestinal system.

These measures are further boosted by the use of nanoemulsions and other nanoparticle-based carriers that encapsulate phytochemicals in liposomal or polymeric carriers and provide increased solubility, stability, and tissue permeation. Together with the stimuli-responsive or ligand-selective modifications, nanocarriers enable a step change in precision phytotherapy.

Collectively, these innovations represent a paradigm shift in how phytochemicals are conceptualized, formulated, and administered, with respect to cardiovascular applications. These resynthesized natural products are gradually being transformed into first-line therapeutic options, which can overcome the multifactorial complications of CVD using state-of-art biomedical tools.

## 2.11 CHALLENGES AND FUTURE PERSPECTIVES

Although scientific and clinical attention to cardioprotective properties of phytochemicals is growing, and investments in research are rising, a range of critical challenges still hold back their more comprehensive clinical incorporation. Biological variability in plant species, geographical source, and conditions of harvest and extraction methods can lead to unpredictable phytochemical compositions, which may have a dramatic effect on therapeutic effectiveness and safety [87].

Moving toward convergence of regulations with common standards of efficacy, GMP, toxicological evaluation of medications, and consumer safety will not only be scientifically acceptable but also important for ensuring consumer safety.

There exist several phytochemicals that have a long history of application in systems like Ayurveda, Traditional Chinese Medicine, and Unani but have not been subjected to rigorous pharmacology research and clinical trials [88, 89]. To bridge this gap, a participatory research is needed with due respect to traditional knowledge and the application of new analytical and clinical validation instruments. This can be achieved by harmonizing dietary phytochemical intake with the individual biological profile so that optimal cardiovascular interventions can be provided.

## 2.12 CONCLUSION

The increasing evidence on the cardioprotective effect of phytochemicals indicates that they could offer a new definition to therapeutic approach to CVDs. Key targets of phytochemical activity include central signaling axes like Nrf2, NF-κB, eNOS, AMPK, and PPARs, highlighting the multimodal nature of these interventions in cardiovascular pathology.

Resveratrol, curcumin, quercetin, berberine, and EGCG are prominent examples of individual phytochemicals that have the potential to initiate homeostatic, vascular integrity, and immune modulations within cells. The formulation technology that accompanies these agents further increases their therapeutic potential through advances in nanotechnology, formulation delivery systems, and synergistic bioenhancers. Also, the application of AI and systems biology appears as one of the approaches that would help accelerate compound screening, clarify complicated processes, and tailor phytochemicals-based treatment using genetic and metabolic signatures.

The realization of phytochemicals into future clinical care models will necessitate harmonization framework that unites the traditional systems and products with modern science validation. Prerequisites to the translational success of phytochemical therapeutics are standardization of extracts, good clinical trial data, clarity in the regulatory environment, and multidisciplinary cooperation.

The focus of further research must be on large-scale, placebo-controlled clinical trials, investigation into combinatory regimens in relation to existing pharmacologies, and also into diagnostic tools that can aid in the extraction of specific phytochemicals based on patient-specific biomarkers.

## REFERENCES


1. Shaito, A., Thuan, D.T.B., Phu, H.T. et al. (2020). Herbal medicine for cardiovascular diseases: efficacy, mechanisms, and safety. *Front. Pharmacol.* 11: 422.
2. Haines, D.D., Cowan, F.M., and Tosaki, A. (2024). Evolving strategies for use of phytochemicals in prevention and long-term management of cardiovascular diseases (CVD). *Int. J. Mol. Sci.* 25 (11): 6176.
3. Bachheti, R.K., Worku, L.A., Gonfa, Y.H. et al. (2022). Prevention and treatment of cardiovascular diseases with plant phytochemicals: a review. *Evid. Based Complement. Alternat. Med.* 2022: 5741198.
4. Hossain, M.S., Wazed, M.A., Asha, S. et al. (2025). Dietary phytochemicals in health and disease: Mechanisms, clinical evidence, and applications—a comprehensive review. *Food Sci. Nutr.* 13 (3): e70101.
5. Shang, W., Li, X.H., Zeng, L.H. et al. (2025). Mechanistic insights into flavonoid subclasses as cardioprotective agents against doxorubicin-induced cardiotoxicity: a comprehensive review. *Drug Des. Dev. Ther.* 19: 5553–5596.
6. Beura, S.K., Panigrahi, A.R., Yadav, P., and Singh, S.K. (2021). Phytochemicals as potential therapeutics for SARS-CoV-2-induced cardiovascular complications: thrombosis and platelet perspective. *Front. Pharmacol.* 12: 658273.
7. Kumar, A., Nirmal, P., Kumar, M. et al. (2023). Major phytochemicals: recent advances in health benefits and extraction method. *Molecules* 28 (2): 887.
8. Situmorang, P.A., Wibowo, S., Tanjung, M. et al. (2025). Molecular mechanism of phytochemical compounds in mitigating hypertension. *Phytomed. Plus* 5 (3): 100812.
9. Młynarska, E., Hajdys, J., Czarnik, W. et al. (2024). The role of antioxidants in the therapy of cardiovascular diseases—a literature review. *Nutrients* 16 (16): 2587.
10. Arunabh, A., Dipankar, S., Jyoti, D.D. et al. (2024). Redox imbalance and cardiovascular pathogenesis: exploring the therapeutic potential of phytochemicals. *Curr. Bioact. Compd.* 20 (9): 55–78.
11. Lakshmana Rao, A. and Suneetha, D. (2010). Current trends in herbal medicines. *J. Pharm. Res.* 3 (1): 109–113.
12. Bontempo, P., Capasso, L., De Masi, L. et al. (2024). Therapeutic potential of natural compounds acting through epigenetic mechanisms in cardiovascular diseases: current findings and future directions. *Nutrients* 16 (15): 2399.
13. Majrashi, T.A., Alshehri, S.A., Alsayari, A. et al. (2023). Insight into the biological roles and mechanisms of phytochemicals in different types of cancer: targeting cancer therapeutics. *Nutrients* 15 (7): 1704.
14. Wahid, M., Saqib, F., Abbas, G. et al. (2024). Cardioprotective and hypotensive mechanistic insights of hydroethanolic extract of *Cucumis melo L.* kernels in isoprenaline-induced cardiotoxicity based on metabolomics and *in silico* electrophysiological models. *Front. Pharmacol.* 14: 1277594.
15. Kamaruddin, N.A., Abdullah, M.N.H., Tan, J.J. et al. (2022). Vascular protective effect and its possible mechanism of action on selected active phytocompounds: a review. *Evid. Based Complement. Alternat. Med.* 2022: 3311228.
16. Li, M., Wang, S., Dong, H. et al. (2022). Harnessing natural products for myocardial infarction therapy: mechanistic insights and translational opportunities. *Pharmacol. Res.* 217: 107802.
17. Park, S.H. (2024). Role of phytochemicals in treatment of aging and cancer: focus on mechanism of FOXO3 activation. *Antioxidants* 13 (9): 1099.
18. Netala, V.R., Teertam, S.K., Li, H., and Zhang, Z. (2024). A comprehensive review of cardiovascular disease management: cardiac biomarkers, imaging modalities, pharmacotherapy, surgical interventions, and herbal remedies. *Cells* 13 (17): 1471.
19. Bakrim, S., Fessikh, M.E., Elhrech, H. et al. (2025). Targeting inflammation in cancer therapy: from mechanistic insights to emerging therapeutic approaches. *J. Transl. Med.* 23: 588.
20. Prasanna, M.M., Priyanka, M., Neelothpala, N. et al. (2017). Preliminary phytochemical, pharmacognostic and physicochemical evaluation of leaf of *Gomphrenaserrata*. *Adv.Herb. Med.* 3 (2): 16–25.
21. Porfyris, O., Detopoulou, P., Adamantidi, T. et al. (2025). Phytochemicals as chemo-preventive and therapeutic agents against bladder cancer: a comprehensive review. *Diseases* 13 (4): 103.
22. Choudhari, A.S., Mandave, P.C., Deshpande, M. et al. (2020). Phytochemicals in cancer treatment: from preclinical studies to clinical practice. *Front. Pharmacol.* 10: 1614.

23. Alarabei, A.A., Aziz, N.A.L.A., Razak, N.I.A. et al. (2024). Immunomodulating phytochemicals: an insight into their potential use in cytokine storm situations. *Adv. Pharm. Bull.* 14 (1): 105–119.
24. Lekhak, N. and Bhattarai, H.K. (2024). Phytochemicals in cancer chemoprevention: preclinical and clinical studies. *Cancer Control* 31: https://doi.org/10.1177/10732748241302902.
25. Eshraghi, R., Bahrami, A., Iravanlou, F.T. et al. (2025). Cardioprotective and anti-hypertensive effects of epigallocatechin gallate: novel insights into biological evidence. *J. Clin. Hypertens.* 27 (6): e70036.
26. Francini-Pesenti, F., Spinella, P., and Calo, L.A. (2019). Potential role of phytochemicals in metabolic syndrome prevention and therapy. *Diabetes Metab.Syndr.Obes.* 12: 1987–2002.
27. Sajana, M., Gopenath, T.S., and Kanthesh, B.M. (2024). A comprehensive review of phytochemical approaches in treatment of acute myeloid leukemia: associated pathways and molecular mechanisms. *Chin. Herb. Med.* 17 (1): 41–55.
28. Kim, H.K., Seong, J.K., Gil, W.J., and Chul-Su, Y. (2025). Exploring the therapeutic potential of phytochemicals: challenges and strategies for clinical translation. *Phytomedicine* 20: 157090.
29. Abhijeet, S., Mukesh, C.S., Raman, R. et al. (2025). The evolving role of phytochemicals in cancer therapy: mechanistic insights and emerging technologies. *J. Appl. Pharm. Sci. Res.* 8 (1): 5–16.
30. Prasanth, D.S.N.B.K. and Lakshmana Rao, A. (2018). Evaluation of pharmacognostic, phytochemical and physicochemical standards of *Wedeliatrilobata*root. *J. Pharm. Res.* 2 (1): 1–6.
31. Alaa, A.A.A., Mohammad, A.O., Rasha, M.B. et al. (2025). Phytochemicals in cancer therapy: a structured review of mechanisms, challenges, and progress in personalized treatment. *Chem. Biodivers.* e202402479.
32. Khameneh, B., Eskin, N.A.M., Iranshahy, M., and Fazly Bazzaz, B.S. (2021). Phytochemicals: a promising weapon in the arsenal against antibiotic-resistant bacteria. *Antibiotics* 10 (9): 1044.
33. Tabussam, T., Smeea, F., Huma, B.U.A. et al. (2025). Role of phytonutrients in the prevention and treatment of chronic diseases: a concrete review. *ACS Omega* 10 (13): 12724–12755.
34. Ghosh, S., Basu, S., Kayal, T. et al. (2025). Computational advancements to facilitate therapeutic application of phytochemicals: where do we stand? *Discov. Appl. Sci.* 7: 491.
35. Vafadar, A., Tajbakhsh, A., Hosseinpour-Soleimani, F. et al. (2024). Phytochemical-mediated efferocytosis and autophagy in inflammation control. *Cell Death Discov.* 10: 493.
36. Shrivastav, D., Kumbhakar, S.K., Srivastava, S., and Singh, D.D. (2024). Natural product-based treatment potential for type 2 diabetes mellitus and cardiovascular disease. *World J. Diabetes* 15 (7): 1603–1614.
37. Jaberi, K.M., Alamdari-palangi, V., Amir, S. et al. (2024). Modulatory effects of phytochemicals on gut-brain axis: therapeutic implication. *Curr. Dev. Nutr.* 8 (6): 103785.
38. Peng, A., Sitong, W., Yongting, L. et al. (2022). Micronutrient supplementation to reduce cardiovascular risk. *J. Am. Coll. Cardiol.* 80 (24): 2269–2285.
39. Faisal, M.A., Sreekumar, U.A., Remya, J. et al. (2023). A potent bioactive fraction against colon cancer from *Plectranthusvettiveroides*. *Explor. Target. Antitumor Ther.* 4: 227–239.
40. Raveesha, P., Lakshmana Rao, A., Ooha Deepika, G. et al. (2020). Pharmacognosticalstudy and preliminary phytochemical investigation of *Dechaschistiacrotonifolia* Wight &Arrn. *J. Global Trends Pharm. Sci.* 11 (4): 8782–8790.
41. Przybylska, S. and Tokarczyk, G. (2022). *Lycopene in the prevention of cardiovascular diseases. Int. J. Mol. Sci.* 23 (4): 1957.
42. Omer, M., Omer, O.I., Ali, M., and Mohamed, I.O. (2025). Therapeutic potentials of phytochemicals in the treatment of ulcerative colitis: results from animal model interventional studies. *J. Am. Nutr. Assoc.* 1–13.
43. Olalekan, S.O., Okwute, P.G., Osonuga, I.O. et al. (2025). Clinical relevance of nutraceuticals in hypertension management: mechanisms, efficacy, and integration into therapeutic protocols. *Bull. Natl. Res. Cent.* 49: 35.
44. Mukherjee, S., Chopra, H., Goyal, R. et al. (2024). Therapeutic effect of targeted antioxidant natural products. *Discov. Nano* 19: 144.
45. Silva-Pinto, P.A., de Pontes, J.T.C., Aguilar-Moron, B. et al. (2025). Phytochemical insights into flavonoids in cancer: mechanisms, therapeutic potential, and the case of quercetin. *Heliyon* 11 (4): e42682.
46. Zhang, S., Xie, X., Zhao, J. et al. (2025). Andrographolide and its derivatives in cardiovascular disease: a comprehensive review. *Planta Med.* 91 (5): 259–270.
47. Pillai, M.G. and Antony, H. (2024). Harnessing the immunomodulatory potential of natural products in precision medicine—a comprehensive review. *Explor. Drug Sci.* 2: 239–260.
48. Ayoka, T.O., Ezema, B.O., Eze, C.N., and Nnadi, C.O. (2022). Antioxidants for the prevention and treatment of non-communicable diseases. *J. Explor. Res. Pharmacol.* 7 (3): 179–189.
49. Kutluay, V.M. and Diker, N.Y. (2020). Constitution of a comprehensive phytochemical profile and network pharmacology based investigation to decipher molecular mechanisms of *Teucrium polium* L. in the treatment of type 2 diabetes mellitus. *Peer J.* 8: e10111.
50. Aminabee, S.K., Lakshmana Rao, A., Suguna Rani, P. et al. (2020). Phytochemical and *in-vitro*evaluation of anti-oxidant activity of *Mansoaalliacea*leaves. *Acta Sci. Pharm. Sci.* 4 (10): 3–7.
51. Paul-Chima, U.O., Ugwu, C.N., and Alum, E.U. (2024). Integrated approaches in nutraceutical delivery systems: optimizing ADME dynamics for enhanced therapeutic potency and clinical impact. *RPS Pharm.Pharmacol. Rep.* 3 (4): rqae024.
52. Chihomvu, P., Ganesan, A., Gibbons, S. et al. (2024). Phytochemicals in drug discovery—a confluence of tradition and innovation. *Int. J. Mol. Sci.* 25 (16): 8792.
53. Muscolo, A., Mariateresa, O., Giulio, T., and Mariateresa, R. (2024). Oxidative stress: the role of antioxidant phytochemicals in the prevention and treatment of diseases. *Int. J. Mol. Sci.* 25 (6): 3264.
54. Hasan, G.M., Anwar, S., Shamsi, A. et al. (2024). The neuroprotective potential of phytochemicals in traumatic brain injury: mechanistic insights and pharmacological implications. *Front. Pharmacol.* 14: 1330098.
55. Prasanth, D.S.N.B.K., Pavani Sandhya, K., Anusha, K. et al. (2017). Preliminary phytochemical, pharmacognostic and physicochemical evaluation of *Eranthemumnigrum*leaf. *Int. J. Res. Ayush Pharm. Sci.* 1 (2): 97–105.
56. Paul, J.K., Azmal, M., Haque, A.N.M.S.N.B. et al. (2024). Phytochemical-mediated modulation of signaling pathways: a promising avenue for drug discovery. *Adv. Redox Res.* 13: 100113.
57. Mandlik, D., Adgaonkar, P., and Mandlik, S. (2025). Phytochemical modulation of mTOR signaling: emerging nanotechnology-driven therapeutics for rheumatoid arthritis management. *Inflammopharmacology* 33 (8): 4125–4165.
58. Tote, M. and Ahmed, S. (2025). *Cichoriumintybus* in translational medicine: phytochemicals, mechanisms, and therapeutic applications. *J. Drug Deliv.Ther.* 15 (5): 104–113.
59. Uti, D.E., Atangwho, I.J., Alum, E.U. et al. (2025). Natural antidiabetic agents: current evidence and development pathways from medicinal plants to clinical use. *Nat. Prod. Commun.* 20 (3).
60. Mikkili, I., Suluvoy, J.K., Thathapudi, J.J., and Krupanidhi, S. (2024). Synergistic strategies for cancer treatment: leveraging natural products, drug repurposing and molecular targets for integrated therapy. *Beni-Suef Univ. J. Basic Appl. Sci.* 13: 96.

61. Sudhakar, M., Krishnaiah, P., Lakshmana Rao, A., and Raju, D.B. (2005). Antimicrobial guided phytochemical evaluation of the pods of *Caesalpiniapulcherrima*. *Asian J. Chem.* 17 (4): 2353–2358.
62. Sadiq, S.C., Joy, M.P., Aiswarya, S.U. et al. (2024). Unlocking nature's pharmacy: an in-depth exploration of phytochemicals as potential sources of anti-cancer and anti-inflammatory molecules. *Explor. Drug Sci.* 2: 744–784.
63. Pal, D., Singh, P., Prasad, M.E., and Upadhye, V.J. (2025). Key insights on therapeutic potential of various phytochemicals against breast cancer. *Nat. Resour. Hum. Health* 5 (3): 339–353.
64. Tanny, S.Z., Shahriar, M.M., Metu, C.L.N. et al. (2025). Exploring the therapeutic promise of *Ampelocissuslatifolia*: a short review. *J. Med. Chem. Ther.* 1 (1): 1–6.
65. Gao, Y., Wang, B., Qin, G. et al. (2024). Therapeutic potentials of allicin in cardiovascular disease: advances and future directions. *Chin. Med.* 19: 93.
66. Balkrishna, A., Sharma, N., Srivastava, D. et al. (2024). Exploring the safety, efficacy, and bioactivity of herbal medicines: bridging traditional wisdom and modern science in healthcare. *Future Integr. Med.* 3 (1): 35–49.
67. Anantharaj, V., Punitha, S., Gowri, R. et al. (2024). Therapeutic potential of flavonoids: a mechanistic insight into neuroinflammation and neurodegenerative disease prevention. *Afr. J. Biomed. Res.* 27 (4s): 13552–13560.
68. Shimsa, S., Mondal, S., and Mini, S. (2024). Syringic acid: a promising phenolic phytochemical with extensive therapeutic applications. *R&D Funct. Food Products* 1 (5): 1–14.
69. Adeleye, A.E., Owolabi, M.S., and Abdulkabir, A.O. (2025). Multifunctional natural products in disease modulation: a systems perspective on cancer and cardiovascular therapies. *AROC Pharm. Biotechnol.* 5 (1): 1–8.
70. Gauttam, V.K., Munjal, K., Chopra, H. et al. (2024). A mechanistic review on therapeutic potential of medicinal plants and their pharmacologically active molecules for targeting metabolic syndrome. *Curr. Pharm. Des.* 30 (1): 10–30.
71. Vani, K., Malathi Priyanka, M., Durga Srinivas, P. et al. (2016). Phytochemical and in-vitroevaluation of antioxidant activity of *Sesamum indicum*leaves. *Indian J. Pharm. Pharmacol.* 3 (1): 7–12.
72. Priya, V.L. and Devi, M. (2025). Potential of integrating phytochemicals with standard treatments for enhanced outcomes in TBI. *Brain Inj.* 39: 904–920.
73. Khan, A., Maparu, K., and Aran, K.R. (2024). *Catharanthus roseus*: a comprehensive review of its phytochemicals, therapeutic potential, and mechanisms of action. *Nat. Cell Sci.* 2 (4): 224–237.
74. Das, A., Khan, S., Roy, S., and Das, S. (2023). Phytochemicals for mitigating the COVID-19 crisis: evidence from pre-clinical and clinical studies. *Explor. Drug Sci.* 1: 336–376.
75. Timmers, S., Konings, E., Bilet, L. et al. (2011). Calorie restriction-like effects of 30 days of resveratrol supplementation in obese humans. *Cell Metab.* 14 (5): 612–622.
76. Panahi, Y., Mahboobeh-Sadat, H., Khalili, N. et al. (2015). Antioxidant and anti-inflammatory effects of curcuminoid–piperine combination in subjects with metabolic syndrome: a randomized controlled trial and an updated meta-analysis. *Clin. Nutr.* 34 (6): 1101–1108.
77. Zhang, Y., Li, X., Zou, D. et al. (2008). Treatment of type 2 diabetes and dyslipidemia with the natural plant alkaloid berberine. *J. Clin. Endocrinol. Metab.* 93 (7): 2559–2565.
78. Mozaffarian, D. and Rimm, E.B. (2006). Fish intake, contaminants, and human health: evaluating the risks and the benefits. *JAMA* 296 (15): 1885–1899.
79. Edwards, R.L., Lyon, T., Litwin, S.E. et al. (2007). Quercetin reduces blood pressure in hypertensive subjects. *J. Nutr.* 137 (11): 2405–2411.
80. Basu, A., Sanchez, K., Leyva, M.J. et al. (2010). Green tea supplementation affects body weight, lipids, and lipid peroxidation in obese subjects with metabolic syndrome. *J. Am. Coll. Nutr.* 29 (1): 31–40.
81. Fotino, A.D., Thompson-Paul, A.M., and Bazzano, L.A. (2013). Effect of coenzyme Q10 supplementation on heart failure: a meta-analysis. *Am. J. Clin. Nutr.* 97 (2): 268–275.
82. Keshav, B., Princess, W., Ajay, T. et al. (2025). Mechanistic insights into punicalagin's cytotoxic effects on lung cancer cells: a review. *Int. J. Pharm. Sci.* 3 (4): 2670–2693.
83. Singh, D., Kharb, R., Sharma, S.K., and Kumar, V. (2024). Phytochemical and pharmacological intervention of indole and their derivatives: a comprehensive review. *Nat. Resour. Hum. Health* 4 (3): 308–317.
84. Paneni, F., Canestro, C.D., Libby, P. et al. (2017). The aging cardiovascular system: understanding it at the cellular and clinical levels. *JACC* 69 (15): 1952–1967.
85. Patel, K. and Patel, D.K. (2025). Therapeutic role of phytochemicals in gallbladder cancer: pharmacological activity and associated molecular mechanisms. *J. Enterocolitis* 4 (1): 1–8.
86. Reddy, N.S.S., Sreenu, T., and Raju, P. (2025). Phytochemical frontiers: advancing the management of metabolic syndrome. *Lett. Appl. NanoBioScience* 14 (2): 53.
87. Bharati, G. and Swati, P. (2024). Cardioprotective potential of herbal medicine: a review. *Indian J. Pharm. Sci.* 86 (4): 1218–1229.
88. Sarma, H., Sahariah, J.J., Devi, R., and Sharma, H.K. (2022). Challenges and opportunities in the management of cardiovascular diseases. *Sci. Phytochem.* 1 (1): 36–40.
89. Singh, H.V., Shahid, M.O., Ashish, J., and Akhlesh, K.S. (2024). Breast cancer: from etiology to therapeutic interventions. *Res. J. Pharmacol. Pharmacodyn.* 16 (3): 199–207.

# Traditional and Modern Strategies in Cardiovascular Therapy: Innovative Blends

CHAPTER 3

**Sathyamoorthy Nandhakumar[1], Dhanalekshmi Unnikrishnan Meenakshi[2], Thangavel Mahalingam Vijayakumar[3], and Pavan Kumar Chintamaneni[4]**

[1] *Department of Pharmaceutics, Faculty of Pharmacy, Dr. M.G.R. Educational and Research Institute, Chennai, Tamil Nadu, India*

[2] *Department of Pharmacology and Biological Sciences, College of Pharmacy, National University of Science and Technology, Muscat, Sultanate of Oman*

[3] *Department of Pharmacy Practice, SRM College of Pharmacy, SRM Institute of Science and Technology, Kattankulathur, Tamil Nadu, India*

[4] *Department of Pharmaceutics, GITAM School of Pharmacy, GITAM (Deemed to be) University, Hyderabad, Telangana, India*

## 3.1 INTRODUCTION

To concisely define cardiovascular diseases (CVD): they are a set of conditions that majorly affect the vital organs of the cardiovascular system, primarily the heart and the coronary arteries. The conditions that majorly affect the cardiovascular system and lie at the basis of CVDs are atherosclerosis, coronary artery disease, ischemic heart disease, and cardiac arrhythmias. Increase in blood pressure due to vasoconstriction and deposition of fat in the blood vessels, a condition referred to as atherosclerosis, are major reasons for the CVDs. Formation of a blood clot inside the blood vessels, a condition called thrombosis, is also one of the pathogenic conditions underlying CVDs [1]. Major mortality and morbidity are related to CVDs especially stroke and ischemic heart disease, with reported deaths of around 20 million worldwide. There are several factors contributing to the risks of having CVDs, like age, diabetic conditions, hypertension, food habits, lifestyle, obesity, working style, and stress levels. On one side, there are advancements in the available technology that can address the need for the treatment methods for preventing, curing, or treating CVDs, and on the other side urbanization, obesity, and hypertension, along with diminishing food quality and nutrition, produce many disease conditions and disorders in the human body. Consumption of alcohol, smoking, and lack of exercise contribute to the metabolic risk factors, which are also reasons for CVDs [2].

Traditionally, CVDs in South Asian regions are prevented by the use of remedies from the olden period, like ayurvedic medicines, traditional Chinese medicine (TCM), or ethnomedical practices. Such traditional medicines are even used for treating CVDs. Several other therapeutic methods like acupuncture, yoga, and meditation are employed for restoring balance in mind and body. Trust in traditional remedies is increasing because they produce fewer side effects. Traditional remedies are carried forward from generation to generation with the belief that they cure ailments and also prevent such debilitating conditions. Since traditional remedies are easy to access and indigenous to rural areas, they are widely used among many people [3]. Though modern medicines are gaining significance in claiming treatment for CVDs, traditional medicines are still maintaining their place. These medicines are used either alone or in combination with other drugs or even in combination with conventional drugs for synergetic effect. Because of the cultural values placed on traditional remedies and belief in their efficiency, they still maintain their vitality and significance [4].

For the management of CVDs, herbal plant extracts with a variety of therapeutic qualities, such as reduction of cholesterol, regulation of blood pressure, anti-inflammatory, and antioxidant effects are used. To treat conditions like hypertension, atherosclerosis, and hyperlipidemia, common herbs, such as green tea, hibiscus, garlic, hawthorn, and saffron, are used for their ability to lower low-density lipoprotein (LDL) levels, promote vasodilation, prevent angiotensin-converting enzyme (ACE) activity, and reduce oxidative stress. Recently, some clinical trials and scientific research have been conducted emphasizing the potential significance, safety, and effectiveness of herbal treatments in CVD. The safety profiles and herb–drug interactions must be evaluated for the incorporation of herbs in conventional treatment plans [5].

Currently, the treatment for CVDs aims at reducing symptoms, preventing further advancement of diseases, and controlling risk factors like diabetes, dyslipidemia, and hypertension. Yet, they fail to address the fundamental oxidative stress and mitochondrial dysfunction, which are the pathophysiological basis of cardiac injury and age-related vascular damage. These strategies are not very effective in repairing preexisting mitochondrial damage and may also have serious adverse effects that discourage cellular recovery [6]. For improving mitochondrial biogenesis, decreasing oxidative damage, and improving cardiomyocyte survival, a successful targeted treatment is the best option. Multicomponent herbal formulations and natural products offer a promising option within TCM. Antioxidants targeting mitochondria are targeted by the use of nanosystems, which also enhance bioavailability. Research shows that these methods can enhance mitochondrial function, reduce reactive oxygen species (ROS) production, and prevent injury during ischemia–reperfusion. Rather than just treating the symptoms of CVD, these methods provide hope for treatment that addresses the underlying mitochondrial pathology [7]. This chapter explores the synergistic effects of traditional and modern strategies in cardiovascular therapy and highlights the innovative approaches that bridge of ancient wisdom with contemporary science.

## 3.2 GLOBAL AND REGIONAL BURDEN OF CVD

CVD is the leading cause of the high number of premature deaths, of about 12.5 million deaths globally, as measured in DALYs (disability-adjusted life years) in 2023 compared to 1990. DALYs are a measure of disease, injury, and disability in a population. In the low- and middle-SDI (Socio-Demographic Index) regions. The burden of CVD has increased due to factors like aging, population, and modifiable risk factors, like unhealthy diets, high systolic blood pressure, air pollution, and tobacco use. On the other hand, high-income regions have seen CVD rates stabilize or slightly decrease in recent years. Despite of improvements in healthcare, diagnostics, and treatment, high-income countries continue to experience a stable or increasing burden of CVD, mainly because of ongoing exposure to risk factors and health inequalities [8]. Factors including sedentary lifestyles, high body mass index (BMI), high systolic blood pressure, and unhealthy diets, along with aging and rapid urbanization, have been the major reasons for the increasing global burden of CVD. The main causes of global burden of CVDs are elevated plasma glucose, high body mass index, and hypertension [9]. Environmental hazards such as air pollution and variations in lead exposure also influence the risk of CVDs. The worldwide trend is still one of increasing burden, even though health policies and technological advancements have recently stabilized or slightly decreased the burden in some regions, particularly in high-income countries. This is especially true in low- and middle-income countries, where changes in lifestyle, urbanization, and aging populations have outpaced advancements in healthcare interventions and prevention [10].

## 3.3 ETIOLOGY OF CARDIOVASCULAR DISEASES

The development and advancement of atherosclerosis and other cardiac pathologies are influenced by various factors by a combination of genetic, lifestyle, and environmental factors. The major risk factors of CVDs include modifiable and non-modifiable factors.

### 3.3.1 HYPERTENSION

Hypertension is defined as a chronic medical condition in which the force of blood against the arterial wall remains consistently elevated beyond the normal range. Chronic high blood pressure causes vascular changes that elevate the development of organ damage which is linked to hypertension. High blood pressure causes stiffening of blood vessels, and decreased elasticity results in the thickening of the artery wall and increased deposition of extracellular matrix components. Continuous elevation of blood pressure can directly damage the endothelium, resulting in endothelial malfunction. Vasodilators such as nitric oxide production will be reduced. The risk of cardiovascular events, including myocardial infarction (MI) and stroke, arises from the development of atherosclerosis plaques and the infiltration of inflammatory cell facilitated by endothelial damage [11]. Thickening of the heart wall due to elevated blood pressure increases cardiac workload, elevates cardiovascular risk, promotes atherosclerosis, and leads to the development of left ventricular hypertrophy (LVH).

### 3.3.2 DIABETES MELLITUS

Chronic hyperglycemia is the main symptom of diabetes mellitus linked with blood vessel and tissue damage, which results in macro vascular disorders like peripheral arterial disease, cerebrovascular disease, and coronary artery disease, as well as microvascular concerns like retinopathy, nephropathy, and neuropathy [12]. Long-term hyperglycemia increases atherosclerosis, which is the main pathophysiology underlying CVD, and promotes endothelial dysfunction, oxidative stress, and pro-inflammatory state. Moreover, diabetes coexists with obesity, hypertension, and dyslipidemia, which promote the formation and proliferation of plaque. Hyperglycemia destroys arteries and produces an environment which is conductive to thrombosis. Insulin resistance causes abnormal metabolism, which increases atherogenesis. Due to diabetic autonomic neuropathy, these processes work together to induce coronary artery disease and other macrovascular issues, often without any indicative signs, increasing the risk of myocardial infarction, stroke, and heart failure in diabetes patients [13].

### 3.3.3 OBESITY

Obesity is an independent risk factor for the development of CVD; they have a complex and multidimensional relationship. Excess adipose tissue, especially visceral fat, is the main cause of atherosclerosis, endothelial dysfunction, and cardiac

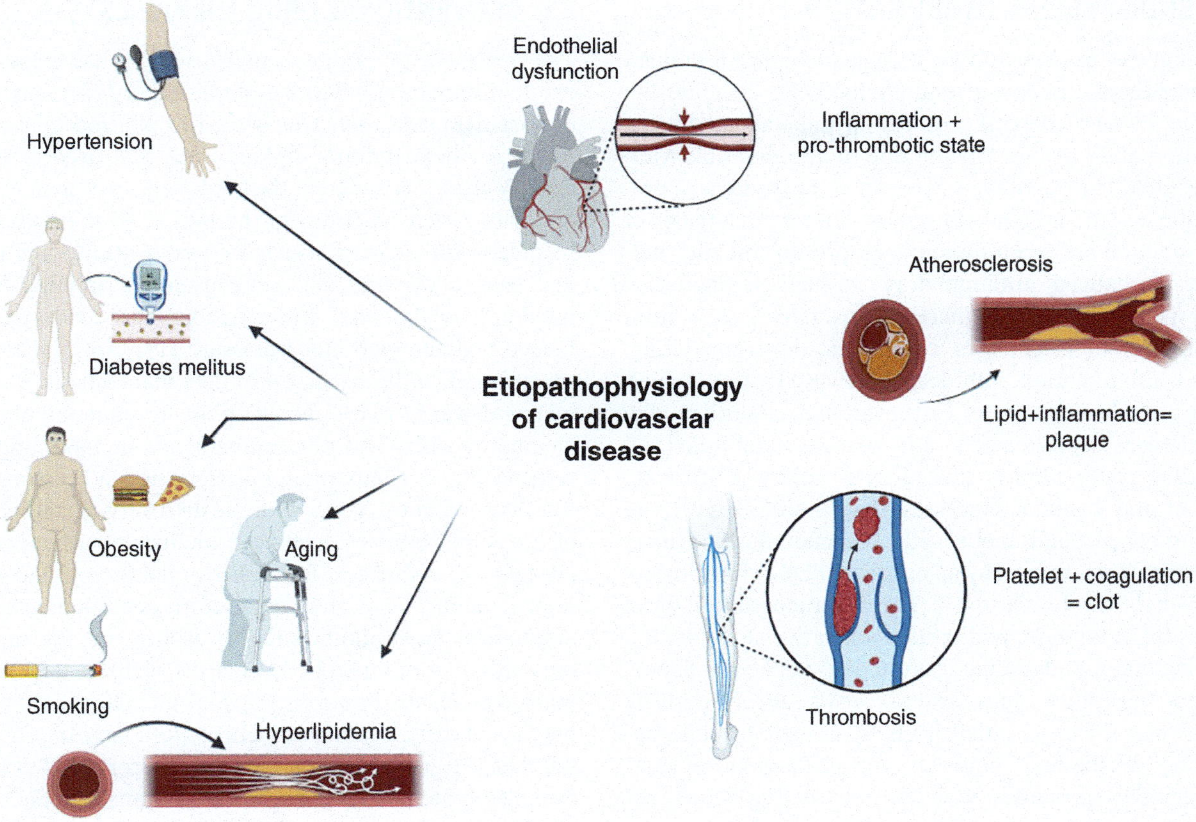


**FIGURE 3.1** Etiopathophysiology of cardiovascular disease.

remodeling, and also contributes to harmful metabolic effects such as insulin resistance, dyslipidemia, hypertension, and systemic inflammation. Worsening of vascular damage and disruption of regular heart function are associated with excess adipose tissue, which releases inflammatory mediators such as cytokines and adipokines. The risk of CVD is increased by changes in fat distribution, which affect the blood pressure and lipid profiles [14].

### 3.3.4 SMOKING

Smoking is reportedly one of the most important modifiable risk factors for CVDs. Smoking damages the endothelium lining of blood vessels and causes chronic inflammation and oxidative stress. This factor leads to the formation of atherosclerotic plaque, which causes conditions like peripheral vascular disease, coronary artery disease, and stroke. The accelerated accumulation of plaque in blood arteries due to smoking lowers high-density lipoprotein (HDL) cholesterol levels and promotes LDL oxidation [15].

## 3.4 PATHOPHYSIOLOGY OF CARDIOVASCULAR DISEASES

Endothelial dysfunction and atherosclerosis, characterized by inflammation and lipid buildup in the arterial walls, lead to plaque formation, artery narrowing, and potential rupture, which can result in heart attacks, strokes, or ischemia. These processes belong to the pathophysiology of CVD. The etiopathophysiology of CVDs is illustrated in Figure 3.1.

### 3.4.1 ATHEROSCLEROSIS

Atherosclerosis is caused by the accumulation of lipids, cholesterol, and cellular debris in the artery walls. It is a chronic inflammatory disease that can worsen blood flow and raise the risk of heart attacks and strokes by the formation of plaque. The development of plaque in arteries is caused by intricate interactions of molecular and cellular mechanisms. Atherosclerosis starts with endothelial dysfunction, which is frequently brought on by smoking, oxidative stress, dyslipidemia, and high blood pressure [12]. Inflammation in the plaque is due to release of pro-inflammatory cytokines like interleukin-1 beta (IL-1β) by the foam cells. Thrombus development is due to the inflammatory breakdown of the fibrous cap, and the high susceptibility to rupture causes plaque instability. Plaque formation starts with endothelial damage and dysfunction, which encourages monocyte adhesion and migration into the subendothelial region. This mechanism results in the formation of a complex plaque with a fibrous cap and cellular components. Inflammation weakens the cap and raises the possibility of rupture, which can cause thrombosis and blockage of an artery [13].

### 3.4.2 ENDOTHELIAL DYSFUNCTION

Endothelial dysfunction is a pathological condition defined by the impaired function of endothelial cells that line the interior of blood vessels. It requires an imbalance between vasodilation and vasoconstriction due to decreased bioavailability of nitric oxide, which is essential in the process of preserving the health and tone of arteries. The characteristics of this dysfunction are pro-inflammatory, pro-thrombotic environment, enhanced inflammatory responses, increased vascular permeability, and increased oxidative stress from excess ROS. These changes cause vascular remodeling, increased inflammation, and decreased vasodilation, which helps in the advancement of cardiovascular conditions like atherosclerosis, hypertension, and diabetes mellitus [14]. Endothelial dysfunction is caused by a variety of intricate molecular and cellular processes that interfere with the natural function of endothelial cells. The main mechanism is the oxidative stress caused by an excess of ROS, which lowers the bioavailability of nitric oxide. This obstructs vasodilation, promotes inflammation, and induces oxidative stress, which are key factors of endothelial dysfunction. Leukocyte adherence and infiltration into arterial walls are caused by inflammatory reaction, which leads to damage of endothelium. The interaction between the inflammation and oxidative stress promotes vascular remodeling, increased vascular permeability and enhances atherogenic processes. Overall, oxidative stress and inflammation synergistically impair endothelial cell function, contributing to the pathogenesis of various CVDs [16].

### 3.4.3 THROMBOSIS

Thrombosis is the formation of a blood clot inside the blood vessel, which restricts blood flow, resulting in diseases like heart attacks or strokes. Platelet activation, aggregation, pro-thrombotic molecule release, and coagulation cascade activation all interact intricately in the mechanism of action of thrombosis. Platelets adhere to exposed subendothelial matrix proteins through surface molecules such as integrin $\alpha IIb\beta 3$ and Glycoprotein VI (GPVI) when there is vascular damage. Platelet activation brought on by this adhesion results in shape change, the release of granule contents like thromboxane $A_2$ and Adenosine diphosphate (ADP), and the recruitment of more platelets. In order to create a primary platelet plug, activated platelets release surface chemicals that encourage aggregation [17]. Chemokine and lipid mediators, such as ceramides and oxidized low-density lipoproteins (ox-LDL), are released concurrently by activated platelets, which intensify inflammation and thrombotic reactions. In order to stabilize the clot, procoagulant factors also trigger the coagulation cascade, producing thrombin, which converts fibrinogen to fibrin. The development and progression of CVDs are significantly influenced by thrombosis, which contributes to arterial occlusion, plaque formation, and plaque rupture, all of which can result in myocardial infarction and stroke [18].

## 3.5 CONVENTIONAL DRUG THERAPIES

The treatment of cardiovascular disorders has changed as a result of important milestones in the history of traditional cardiovascular medication. One of the first pharmacological treatments for heart failure, digitalis, was first used in the 18th century and is derived from the foxglove plant. The introduction of antihypertensive drugs in the middle of the 20th century included beta-blockers, which lowered heart rate and myocardial oxygen demand and were useful in treating illnesses including angina and hypertension, and diuretics, which helped regulate high blood pressure [19]. An increase in the spectrum of cardiovascular disorders that could be effectively managed was observed following the introduction of calcium channel blockers and nitrate treatments in 1960s and 1970s, respectively. An important milestone in CVD management was attained in the 1980s with the discovery of statins, a class of drugs that inhibit 3-hydroxy-3-methylglutaryl-coenzyme A (HMG-coA) reductase, lower LDL cholesterol, and thereby reduce the incidence of atherosclerotic conditions. The use of antiplatelet medications, such as aspirin, for the secondary prevention of thrombotic events, as well as targeted lipid management, also began during this time. The safety and effectiveness of these treatments were continuously improved over following decades, and they eventually formed the basis of evidence-based pharmacological management, which significantly reduced cardiovascular morbidity and mortality globally [1]. These developments have created a fundamental aspect of contemporary cardiovascular medicine and paved the way for further innovation in the battle against the prevalence of cardiovascular illnesses worldwide.

### 3.5.1 LIPID-LOWERING AGENTS

These are agents which prevent atherosclerosis by lowering the triglyceride and cholesterol levels in blood. This in turn reduces the occurrence of CVD. Table 3.1 summarizes the profile of some lipid-lowering agents.

### 3.5.2 ANTIHYPERTENSIVE DRUGS

These are hypotensive agents belonging to different categories, each with a different mechanism of action. These drugs include calcium channel blockers (prevent calcium from entering vascular and cardiac muscles); diuretics (lower blood volume by promoting water and salt excretion); beta-blockers (lower heart rate and cardiac output); ACE inhibitors; and angiotensin II receptor blockers (dilate blood vessels by blocking the renin–angiotensin system). Table 3.2 summarizes the profile of some antihypertensive drugs.

### 3.5.3 ANTITHROMBOTIC THERAPY

These are agents intended to prevent or break up thrombosis, or blood clots, which can otherwise cause heart attacks, strokes, and pulmonary embolisms. The following Table 3.3 summarizes the profile of some antithrombotic drugs.

**Table 3.1** Summary of antilipidemic agents in cardiovascular disease management.

| Class | Common drugs | Mechanism of action | Use in cardiovascular disease |
|---|---|---|---|
| Bile acid sequestrants | Cholestyramine, colestipol, colesevelam, colestimide, sevelamer | In the intestine, bind negatively charged bile acids to increase bile acid excretion and hepatic conversion of cholesterol to bile acids. Additionally, this increases LDL receptors [20] | It reduces LDL-C by 10–20% and is most effective when used in conjunction with statins to treat hypercholesterolemia [21]. |
| Fibrates | Bezafibrate, ciprofibrate, clofibrate, fenofibrate, gemfibrozil, pemafibrate | Stimulate Apolipoprotein A - ApoA-I and ApoA-II production to increase HDL levels; activate Peroxisome proliferator activated receptor alpha (PPAR-$\alpha$) to elevate lipoprotein lipase activity and enhance the breakdown of particles rich in triglycerides [22]. | It is used to treat metabolic syndrome, mixed dyslipidemia, and hypertriglyceridemia. Minimizes the prospect of acquiring coronary heart disease (CHD) [23]. |
| PCSK9 inhibitors | Alirocumab, evolocumab, inclisiran | Hepatic LDL receptor degradation is avoided by blocking the Proprotein convertase subtilisin kexin type 9 (PCSK9) enzyme, which raises LDL clearance and dramatically reduces LDL-C [24]. | Used to prevent major cardiovascular events in individuals with familial hypercholesterolemia and reduce LDL-C by up to 60% [25]. |
| Statins | Atorvastatin, fluvastatin, lovastatin, pitavastatin, pravastatin, rosuvastatin, simvastatin | HMG-CoA reductase, the enzyme that regulates the rate of cholesterol formation, is competitively inhibited to lower intracellular cholesterol and activates LDL receptors to enhance LDL removal [26]. | Both primary and secondary prevention of coronary heart disease are achieved with its usage by reducing the incidence of MI and stroke and 30–50% of LDL-C [27]. |

**Table 3.2** Summary of Antihypertensive agents in cardiovascular disease management.

| Class | Common drugs | Mechanism of action | Use in cardiovascular disease |
|---|---|---|---|
| ACE inhibitors | Captopril, enalapril, lisinopril, ramipril | In order to enhance bradykinin, reduce angiotensin II, inhibit the angiotensin-converting enzyme, decrease aldosterone and vasoconstriction, and promote vasodilation [28]. | Decrease morbidity and death in heart failure, post-MI, diabetic nephropathy, and hypertension [29]. |
| Angiotensin II receptor blockers (ARBs) | Irbesartan, losartan, telmisartan, valsartan | Reverse the effects of angiotensin II, block the $AT_1$ receptor, and lower aldosterone and vasoconstriction without raising bradykinin [30]. | ACE inhibitor equivalent with similar use; good for heart failure, hypertension, and post-MI [31]. |
| Beta-blockers | Atenolol, bisoprolol, carvedilol, metoprolol, propranolol | By blocking $\beta_1/\beta_2$ receptors, beta-blockers lower myocardial oxygen consumption, heart rate, contractility, and renin release [32]. | Beneficial for post-MI, angina, heart failure, hypertension, and arrhythmias; reduces cardiovascular events [33]. |
| Calcium channel blockers | Amlodipine, diltiazem, nifedipine, verapamil | Dihydropyridines cause vasodilation and reduce cardiac contractility by blocking L-type calcium channels; non-dihydropyridines alter heart rate, whereas dihydropyridines primarily widen arteries [34]. | Reduce the risk of heart failure and stroke by treating angina, hypertension, and arrhythmias [35]. |

## 3.6 TRADITIONAL SYSTEMS OF MEDICINE AND THEIR CONCEPT OF CARDIOVASCULAR HEALTH

Although the aim of all systems of medicine is well-being and good quality of life, each system approaches disease and health from a different perspective. While modern medicine, or the allopathic system of medicine, is based on the targeted and molecular approach, the traditional system of medicine views cardiovascular health as an essential component of the body's homeostatic balance. Rather than focusing on treatment, these traditional systems focus on prevention and lifestyle practices to maintain cardiovascular health. These ancient systems use natural medicines and complex herbal formulations to deal with the basic causes of disease.

**Table 3.3** Summary of Antithrombotic agents in cardiovascular disease management.

| Class | Common drugs | Mechanism of action | Use in cardiovascular disease |
|---|---|---|---|
| Factor Xa inhibitors | Apixaban, edoxaban, rivaroxaban | By blocking factor Xa, direct oral anticoagulants (also known as factor Xa inhibitors) reduce the development of fibrin and stop prothrombin from being converted to thrombin. | Used to control atrial fibrillation, prevent and treat venous thromboembolism, and lower the risk of subsequent cardiovascular events [36]. |
| Glycoprotein IIb/IIIa receptor antagonists | Abciximab, eptifibatide, tirofiban | Platelet glycoprotein (GP) IIb/IIIa receptors are blocked by GP IIb/IIIa inhibitors, which stops fibrinogen from binding and platelets from aggregating. | Used to prevent thrombosis during percutaneous coronary interventions (PCI) and acute coronary syndromes [37]. |
| Irreversible platelet aggregation inhibitor | Aspirin | Aspirin suppresses thromboxane $A_2$ and platelet aggregation via inhibiting COX-1 in platelets. | Prevents arterial thrombosis in peripheral artery disease, coronary artery disease, and stroke [38]. |
| P2Y12 ADP receptor antagonist (prodrug) | Clopidogrel | Clopidogrel reduces platelet aggregation by permanently inhibiting the platelet P2Y12 receptor once it has been activated. | Prevents acute coronary syndrome, stroke, and post-stent implantation [39]. |

#### 3.6.1.1 Cardiology from Ayurvedic Perspective

In Ayurveda, the heart is contemplated as the center of emotion and consciousness. The health of the heart is considered to be influenced by three essential bioenergetic principles or "*doshas*." They are "*vata*" (movement), "*pitta*" (metabolism), and "*kapha*" (structure). Ayurveda affirms that any imbalance in these bioenergetic principles or *doshas* shall result in CVD or "*Hridroga*." The imbalance of *doshas* leads to accumulation of toxins in the body's channels, which leads to the loss of vital essence [40]. Ayurveda therefore recommends a holistic treatment for *Hridroga*, which encompasses a healthy diet with whole grains and leafy greens, lifestyle modifications such as practicing yoga and meditation to counter stress, and including exercises such as *suryanamaskar* (Sun salutation) to enhance circulation and energy [41].

The mainstream of treatment in ayurvedic practice for CVD is the use of herbal remedies or *rasavana*. Some traditional medicines such as *Terminalia arjuna*, are revered for their ability to strengthen the heart muscle and regulate blood pressure and lipid levels in body [42]. *Curcuma longa* (turmeric) is used on a regular basis owing its blood-purifying and anti-inflammatory properties [43]. Ayurveda also recommends the usage of polyherbal formulations such as "*Triphala*" – meaning blend of three fruits – which is used to detoxify the body and clear the plaques from the blood vessels. Some of the ayurvedic formulations are listed in Table 3.4. Understanding the potential use of ayurvedic medicines in CVD such as hypocholesterolemia, antioxidant, hypotensive, and antiplatelet activities, and the validation of their uses, is being explored by the scientific community.

**Table 3.4** Ayurvedic herbal formulations for cardiovascular disease management.

| Formulation name | Main herbal components | Mechanism of action | Therapeutic use in cardiovascular disease |
|---|---|---|---|
| Arjuna Guggulu | *Commiphora wightii, Terminalia arjuna, Withania somnifera* | Increases cardiac output, safeguards the myocardium, and attenuates oxidative stress. | Used in ischemic heart disease, hypertension, and heart failure [44]. |
| Dashmoola Kwatha/decoction | *Aegle marmelos* (Bilva), *Oroxylum indicum* (Shyonaka), *Stereospermum suaveolens* (Patala) | Decreases vascular inflammation, enhances circulation, and maintains overall cardiovascular integrity. | Implemented in chronic heart failure, hypertension, and postischemic reperfusion [45]. |
| Guggulu-based formulations (e.g., Yogaraja Guggulu, Maha Yogaraja Guggulu) | *C. wightii, Emblica officinalis, Terminalia chebula, Zingiber officinale* | Functions as a cardiotonic, anti-atherosclerotic, and antioxidant; stabilizes *kapha* and *pitta dosha*. | Used in hyperlipidemia, hypertension, and coronary artery disease [46]. |
| Lavana Bhasma with herbs | *Asparagus racemosus,* rock salt, *T. chebula, W. somnifera* | Strengthens the heart, balances *vata* and *pitta dosha*, and increases vascular elasticity. | Applicable in hypertension, palpitations, and cardiovascular weakness [47]. |
| Sarpagandha Ghana/ Rauwolfia preparation | *Rauwolfia serpentina* | Exerts natural antihypertensive action through regulation of nerve-mediated vascular tone. | Applicable in chronic hypertension and cardiovascular stress [48]. |

**Table 3.5** Formulations of traditional Chinese medicine for cardiovascular disease management.

| Formulation name | Main herbal components | Mechanism of action | Therapeutic use in cardiovascular disease |
|---|---|---|---|
| Buyang Huanwu Tang | *Angelica sinensis, Astragalus membranaceus, Carthamus tinctorius, Ligusticum chuanxiong, Paeoniae rubra, Semen persicae, Rehmannia glutinosa* | Increases tissue oxygenation, promotes angiogenesis, and stimulates microcirculation. | Used in cardiac rehabilitation, paralysis, and ischemic stroke [50]. |
| Dan Shen Yin | *Amomum villosum, Salvia miltiorrhiza, Santalum album* | Lowers vascular resistance, increases blood flow, and shields cardiac tissue from ischemia damage. | Used to treat coronary artery disease, hypertension, and angina pectoris [51]. |
| Shengmai San | *Ophiopogon japonicus, Panax ginseng, Schisandra chinensis* | Increases heart energy, avoids oxidative damage, and restores the balance of *qi* and *Yin*. | Used to treat myocardial ischemia, exhaustion, and heart failure [52]. |
| Tongxinluo capsule | *Buthus martensii, Hirudo, P. ginseng, Scolopendra subspinipes, Ziziphus jujuba* | Improves vascular integrity, prevents ischemia damage, and reduces the spread of inflammation. | Used to treat myocardial infarction and coronary artery disease [53]. |
| Xuefu Zhuyu Tang | *A. sinensis, C. tinctorius, Glycyrrhiza uralensis, Ligusticum chuanxiong, Paeonia lactiflora, Rehmannia glutinosa* | Enhances myocardial oxygenation, reduces vascular blockage, and improves hemodynamics. | Used to treat ischemic heart disease, hypertension, and chest discomfort [53]. |

#### 3.6.1.2 Cardiology from Traditional Chinese Medicine Perspective

TCM theorizes heart as the emperor of all organs, which governs the circulation of blood. It is also considered the house of *Shen,* which comprehends mind, spirit, and consciousness. TCM advocates that health shall depend on the smooth flow of blood and *qi* (vital energy) through the meridians. The pathology of cardiovascular system is considered to result from a disharmony of *qi* and *yang*. This imbalance could lead to blood stasis – which is considered similar to thrombosis. The treatment in TCM often aims to restore harmony or balance by treating deficiencies and revitalizing circulation [49].

The treatment regimen in TCM involves complex multi-herb formulas called *Fufang*. In these formulations, each of the herbs is included to play a specific role, yet they work synergistically to restore the well-being of the patient. Herbs like *Salvia miltiorrhiza* are used to invigorate blood circulation and disperse plaque. *Panax notoginseng* is used to sojourn bleeding and improve circulation. Clinically validated formulas such as Shengmai San and Oishenyiqi are usually prescribed in conjunction with allopathic treatment in Asia. Some of the TCM formulations are listed in Table 3.5.

## 3.7 THE CHALLENGES OF TRADITIONAL MEDICINE

### 3.7.1 THE REGULATORY HURDLES

The major distinction between conventional cardiology and traditional medicine lies in the concept of the mind–heart connection. In recent times, although modern medicine acknowledges the role of mental well-being and stress management in CVD, it considers stress and mental health as comorbidities or risk factors. In contrast, traditional medicine locates the mind–heart connection at the center of CVD management. These systems advocate stress and mental turmoil as causes of cardiovascular pathology rather than comorbidities.

This philosophical difference in understanding CVD also extends to the research methodologies, creating a major hindrance to evidence generation. While traditional medicine focuses on deriving an efficient output from the complex interconnectivity of medicinal components, modern medicine seeks to isolate the individual molecules with defined mechanisms. Ultimately, the gold standard of Western medicine – randomized controlled trials, which is designated to evaluate the single molecules – cannot be applied to traditional medicines owing to flawed or inconclusive results. Thus, the lack of scientific evidence for traditional medicines is not merely a data gap but a methodological conflict. Figure 3.2 brings illustrates the comparison of the various features of conventional cardiology and traditional medicine [54].

Thus, despite the rich history and potential preclinical evidence, the translation of traditional medicine usage into the mainstream clinical practice has been thwarted because of deep-rooted hurdles such as lack of scientific evidence and inability to align with regulatory requirements. On dissection of these challenges, the daunting barriers to clinical translation, standardization, and safety originate from the inherent physicochemical properties of active ingredients and the complexity of the herbal formulations themselves.

### 3.7.2 BIOAVAILABILITY – A BARRIER TO CLINICAL TRANSLATION OF HERBS

A poor pharmacokinetic profile has been the main barrier that has impeded the potential bioactive molecules derived from traditional herbs from entering the modern pharmacology horizons. The complex chemical structures of these phytochemicals,

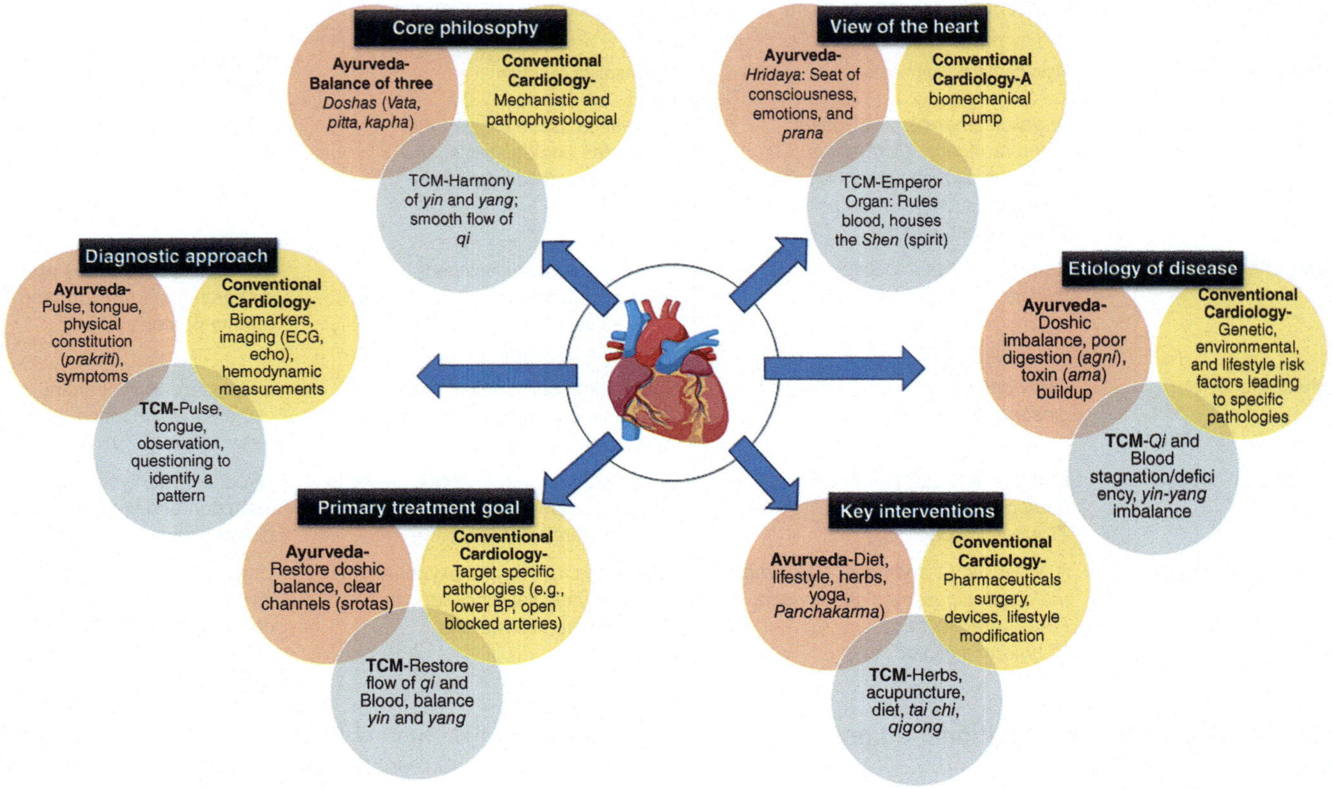


**FIGURE 3.2** Overview of Ayurveda, traditional Chinese medicine, and conventional cardiology.

which give them the power to act as antioxidants and anti-inflammatory agents, often render them unstable and poorly soluble in the gastrointestinal (GI) environment or cause them to undergo extensive first-pass metabolism. Thus, a bioactive compound which shows remarkable potential for CVD management *in vitro* experiments fails miserably under physiological conditions due to poor bioavailability and does not reach the target tissues following oral administration [55].

For instance, curcumin, the principal bioactive compound from turmeric, is a classic example of this bioavailability challenge. *In vitro* studies on curcumin have documented extensive evidence for its anti-inflammatory, antioxidant, and anti-atherosclerotic properties, making it look like an inevitable source of management of CVD. However, curcumin is highly hydrophobic, with aqueous solubility as low as 11 ng/ml at pH 5 [56]. When orally ingested, curcumin undergoes rapid degradation in the GI and rapid first pass metabolism in the liver, leaving it untraceable in plasma to elicit the pharmacological activity.

Similarly, resveratrol, a polyphenol derived from grapes, has wide-ranging cardioprotective activity. Yet, its clinical use is hampered by its poor bioavailability. Though the drug is rapidly absorbed following oral administration, it is extensively metabolized into glucuronide and sulfate conjugates in the intestine and liver. This results in bioavailability less than 1% of the compound. This is a common trend among many such potential bioactive compounds, which needs to be addressed to reap their therapeutic benefits [57].

#### 3.7.2.1 The Herb–Drug Interactions

An elusive yet significant clinical risk involved in the usage of herbal bioactive compounds is the potential interaction between herbal and prescribed cardiovascular drugs. Many compounds derived from plants have the ability to either induce or inhibit the cytochrome P4560 (CYP450) enzymes in liver, which are responsible for metabolizing most of the therapeutic molecules prescribed for patients [58]. Such interactions could have consequences of dangerous nature, where such interactions may either reduce the action of a life-saving drug or potentiate the activity of drugs to a toxic range. The list of some of the common herb–drug interactions are tabulated in Table 3.6.

#### 3.7.2.2 Nanotechnology – A Modern Approach for Overcoming Hurdles of Drug Delivery

Nano drug delivery systems are engineered carriers with particle size less than 1000 nm and surface characteristics suitable for delivering cargo to the desired site. The surface chemistry and nature of the nanoparticles can be modified to achieve both targeting ability and controlled drug release [61]. The performance of a drug in the physiological milieu is determined by its physicochemical properties which in turn affect its absorption and disposition characteristics. The discovery or synthesis of a drug with ideal pharmacokinetic properties is a rare reality. Hence, scientists opt to modify the pharmacokinetics of the payload drug by placing it in

**Table 3.6** Examples of common herb–drug interactions.

| Herbal medicine | Conventional drug/class | Nature of interaction | Proposed mechanism | Clinical recommendation |
|---|---|---|---|---|
| *Allium sativum* (garlic) | Anticoagulants (e.g., warfarin), nifedipine, Calcium channel blocker (CCB) | Synergistic | Enhanced antiplatelet activity and supplementary vasodilatory effects [12]. | Patients taking blood thinners were warned about the higher risk of bleeding, and excessive hypotension needed to be monitored. |
| *Camellia sinensis* (L.) Kuntze (green tea) | Lisinopril (ACE inhibitor), Nadolol (beta-blocker) | Antagonistic | Inhibition of organic anion transporter polypeptide (OATP) transporters results in impaired intestinal absorption [59]. | During treatment with these medications, advise patients to minimize or refrain from drinking green tea. |
| *Rauwolfia serpentina* (snakeroot) | Beta-blockers, diuretics, other Antihypertensive medication (AHM) | Synergistic | Additional pharmacodynamic effects (vasodilation, decreased sympathetic tone) [60]. | Bradycardia and severe hypotension are at high risk. Without professional supervision, co-administration is often not advised. |
| *Zingiber officinale* Roscoe (ginger) | Losartan (ARB) | Synergistic | CYP2C9-mediated metabolic inhibition, raising plasma levels of losartan [59]. | Potential for enhanced hypotensive effect. Monitor BP closely if co-administered; dose adjustment may be necessary. |

nanocarriers. When a drug is encapsulated in a nanoparticle, it increases the concentration of the drug at the tissue site, raises the cellular concentration of the drug, and improves therapeutic efficacy.

Different types of nanocarriers are developed to meet the specific requirements of the encapsulated drug and the purpose of employing them. The various nanocarriers include particulate carriers (nanoparticles, nanocarriers, dendrimers, nanocapsules, lipoproteins), nanovesicular systems (liposomes, virosomes, niosomes, immunoliposomes, pharmacosomes), and supramolecular systems (micelles). Loading a drug into the nanocarriers shall protect the drug from premature degradation, enhance the absorption, improve the intracellular penetration, and control the pharmacokinetic and distribution profile of the drug.

Many drug molecules that lack the desired pharmacokinetic profile and exhibit poor therapeutic efficacy due to absorption and disposition showed improved stability and clinical benefits when formulated as nano drug delivery systems, owing to the alteration of their pharmacokinetic properties.

## 3.8 BLENDING NANOTECHNOLOGY AND TRADITIONAL MEDICINE FOR IMPROVED CVD MANAGEMENT

Nanotechnology – a well-documented modern approach for delivering drugs to the desired site with a temporal release characteristic – could be the potential solution to overcome the challenges of traditional medicines toward their clinical translation. In order to integrate traditional medicine and modern approaches, nanotechnology could be the key factor. A well-formulated traditional medicine can overcome its pharmacokinetic hindrances such as poor solubility, first-pass metabolism, poor stability, and low bioavailability [62]. The impact of nanocarriers in overcoming the shortfalls of herbal bioactive compounds is illustrated in Figure 3.3. In the following sections, the true power of nanotechnology as an enabling platform to unlock the potential of specific traditional medicines for CVDs is illustrated.

### 3.8.1 *CAMELLIA SINENSIS*

*Camellia sinensis*, commonly identified as green tea, is a rich source of polyphenols. The major polyphonic compound of this plant that enhances cardiovascular health is epigallocatechin-3-gallate (EGCG). The active components of *C. sinensis* offer multifaceted pharmacological activities, including antiproliferative, antilipidemic, antioxidant, and anti-inflammatory actions, which together contribute to the deterrence of atherosclerosis and coronary heart disease [63]. Despite promising results in *in vitro* studies, the therapeutic potential of these bioactive compounds could not be translated to clinical use due to low bioavailability and poor stability of catechins. Catechins degrade with fluctuations in temperature and pH and hence are chemically unstable under physiological conditions. This chemical degradation contributes to the poor systemic absorption and therapeutic action [64].

Employing the nanosized carrier systems for the delivery of bioactive compounds of *C. sinensis* could be a transformative strategy to overcome its limitations. Studies have observed that polyphenols of *C. sinensis*, encapsulated in solid lipid nanoparticles (SLN) and liposomes, were able to prevent chemical degradation and improve their pharmacokinetic properties. The lipid layers of SLN and liposomes form a protective shield against the environmental and enzymatic degradation of catechins, thereby enhancing their bioavailability [65]. Green tea extract encapsulated in liposomes exhibited high encapsulation up to 97% and better stability and therefore improved the delivery of EGCG to the desired tissues [63]. The skin permeation capabilities and the stability

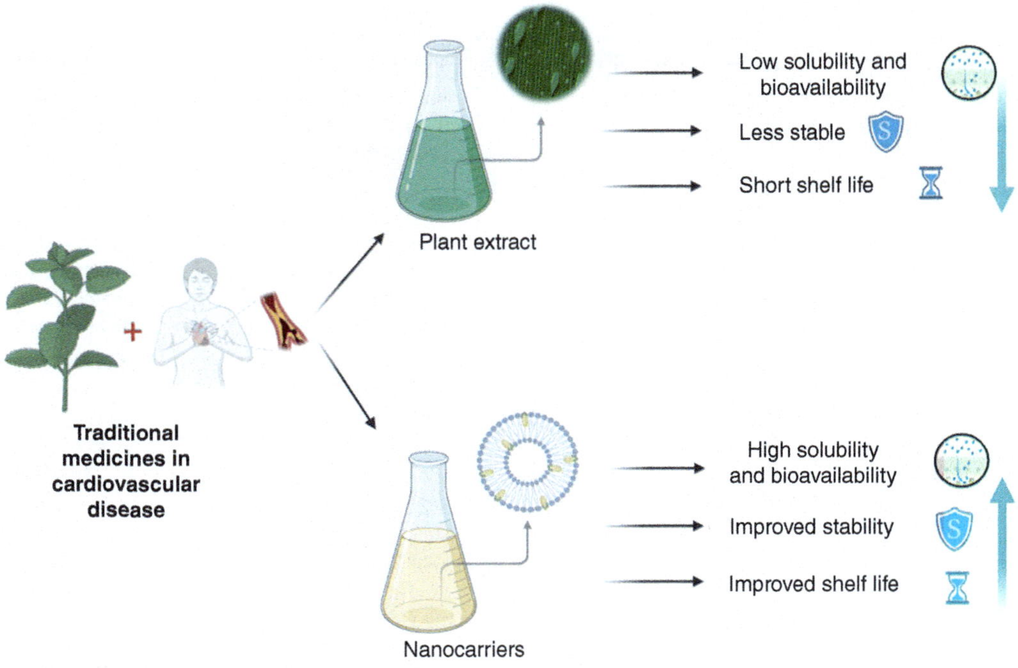


FIGURE 3.3 Illustration of the advantage of nanocarrier delivery of traditional medicine.

of the bioactive compounds of *C. sinensis* was improved when formulated as SLN-based carriers, thus supporting the topical application of these compounds for cardiovascular and transdermal use [66].

The free radical scavenging abilities of green tea polyphenols were superior when encapsulated in nanoliposomal formulations in comparison to their free form. The antioxidant activity of plant extract improved from 1.78 μg/ml for free extract to 12.49 μg/ml for the liposomally encapsulated form [65]. Another dimension of these nanocarriers that improves the absorption, release characteristics, and targeting ability of plant bioactives is their particle size – below 200 nm – and high surface area, which contribute to improved interaction with cellular membranes. Thus, the pharmacological benefits of active constituents of *C. sinensis* could be amplified by encapsulating them in nanocarriers, which holds promise to narrow down the therapeutic gap between the laboratory evidences and clinical application of catechins[67].

### 3.8.2 *CURCUMA LONGA*

The pathological foundation of atherosclerosis is chronic inflammation and oxidative stress, which cause an imbalance between the antioxidant defense and production of ROS. These factors contribute to endothelial dysfunction, accumulation of lipids in blood vessels, and plaque development [68]. The conversion of native low-density lipoproteins (LDL) to oxLDL is mediated by ROS. This sequence of events contributes to the formation of foam cell and unstable plaques, leading to stroke and myocardial infarction [69].

The potential application of *C. longa* lies in targeting the molecular pathways of atherosclerosis through its antioxidant and anti-inflammatory properties [70]. The ROS-scavenging ability of this traditional herb reduces oxidative stress and vascular inflammation. However, this remarkable benefits of *C. longa* are hindered by its lacuna in its pharmacokinetic performance, owing to instability under physiological conditions, low solubility, poor oral bioavailability, and rapid metabolism.

The applications of nanotechnology will serve to overcome challenges of curcumin, which are majorly related to drug delivery rather than the inefficiency of the compound [71]. A wide range of research was demonstrated the improvement of solubility and stability of curcumin through encapsulation in lipid vesicles, such as nanoemulsions, nanostructured lipid carriers (NLCs), and SLN [68]. The colloidal range (100–300 nm) of these nanocarriers could dodge the rapid clearance by macrophages and enhance the bioavailability and cellular interactions. The lipid nature of these carriers was favorable for encapsulating high payloads of about 70% with optimal carrier lipid material. This percentage of encapsulation could escalate to 90% with optimized formulations of NLC [69]. These nanolipid carriers, with their narrow particle size distribution and high zeta potential exhibited better physical stability over longer duration of storage.

Nanoencapsulated curcumin could contribute to cellular conditioning rather than acting solely an antioxidant supplement, by boosting native defense mechanisms of the body against oxidative stress. Curcumin in nanocarriers could upregulate the superoxide dismutase and glutathione peroxidase enzymes by activating the Nrf2 cell signaling pathway, thereby enhancing the cellular antioxidant defense of the body [68]. Modulation of the release profile of curcumin is another important contribution of nanocarriers, in addition to improving its pharmacokinetics properties. Nanoformulations release up to 90% of their curcumin payload over 48 hours, compared with the rapid clearance of free curcumin from the bloodstream. This sustained availability of the active moiety in plasma offers prolonged antioxidant shield, making it an ideal solution for chronic CVD conditions [70].

Nanoformulations, owing to their ability to improve stability, solubility, bioavailability, release and targeting ability, could enhance the clinical application of curcumin as a potent traditional therapeutic agent for the treatment of CVD.

### 3.8.3 *ALLIUM SATIVUM*

*A. sativum,* well known as garlic, has long been recognized for its medicinal value in CVD. Emerging scientific evidence also serves as a proof for its ability to manage various pathophysiological contributors to CVD, namely hyperlipidemia, thrombosis, and atherosclerosis. The organosulfur compounds of garlic that contribute to the reduction in serum lipid levels and inhibition of platelet aggregation are diallyl thiosulfinate (allicin) and its derivatives, such as diallyl disulfide (DADS) and diallyl trisulfide (DATS) [72].

The clinical applications of the bioactive compounds of garlic are hindered by their high volatility, poor solubility, chemical instability, and strong odor. These factors collectively affect bioavailability and patient compliance. Diallyl thiosulfinate is highly unstable and degrades under variable pH and high temperature. To counter the stability challenges of allicin, researchers have successfully exploited the nanodelivery systems to improve its therapeutic potential [73].

Gabriel and his colleagues utilized a top-down approach to formulate ultrasonicated nanoparticles using high-intensity probe sonication, which resulted in nanoparticles smaller than 50 nm. These nanoparticles, despite exposure to high-energy sonic waves, preserved the chemical composition of bioactive phenolic and organosulfur compounds, which was confirmed by Fourier transform infrared spectroscopy (FTIR) studies [72, 74]. They also developed nanoliposomes comprising cholesterol and lecithin to encapsulate garlic bioactives. The prepared liposomes offered both lipophilic and hydrophilic compartments, making them ideal for encapsulating the active components of *A. sativum,* which possess diverse polarity. The liposomes also had optimal size range of 100–175 nm and a zeta potential of −16 mV. The entrapment of the payload was up to 80%. These liposomes loaded with garlic bioactive compounds were able to resist GI degradation by preventing oxidation and hydrolysis in the physiological milieu and exhibited improved bioavailability [74].

SLN formulations formulated using high-pressure homogenization were found to be better carriers for lipophilic compounds like garlic oil. The size of SLNs produced was about 106 nm, with a high negative charge (−30 mV), offering good physical stability [73]. SLN formulations also offered biphasic mode of release, which is characterized by initial burst release followed by sustained release of the drug for about 72 hours, which helps in maintaining the therapeutic concentration and effective control of CVD symptoms. The *in vivo* studies on SLN formulations of garlic compounds also revealed that, owing to inverse targeting ability of these carriers, they are rapidly engulfed by the Kupffer cells of the mononuclear phagocyte system. As a result, they accumulate in the liver, the primary organ of lipid metabolism helping effective management of hyperlipidemia.

### 3.8.4 *SALVIA MILTIORRHIZA*

Tanshinone IIA (TA) and cryoptanshinone (CTS), the primary bio-constituents of *S. miltiorrhiza,* are highly regarded for their benefits in the management of coronary heart disease [75]. As with other bioactive compounds from traditional medicines, they also exhibit pharmacokinetic limitations, such as poor water solubility, short half-lives, and rapid first-pass metabolism. Various nanocarriers, especially SLN, were developed by researchers to overcome the pharmacokinetic limitations and improve their therapeutic benefits [76]. The relative bioavailability of CTS was improved by 1.86 to 2.05 times when delivered as CTS-SLN compared with CTS suspension, as evidenced in an *in vivo* pharmacokinetic study among rats. The increase in bioavailability is due to the maintenance of CTS in a supersaturable form which improves GI absorption.

NLC formulations of TA showed high entrapment efficiency up to 98% and could retain the drug during storage without drug expulsion. This property is benefited from the mixture of solid and liquid composition of NLC, which offers a less ordered inner core that provides optimal space to house the drug [75]. Nanoparticles prepared from calcium alginate and pH-responsive polymers could also increase the solubility of pure compounds of Salvia and offer controlled release [76].

Beyond improvement of solubility and stability, researchers have engineered nanocarriers to improve their cardiovascular-specific functions. TA-loaded NLCs were prepared from HDL-mimicking components, which were protein-free but mimic the native HDL in the body. These innovative nanocarriers could bind to apolipoproteins A-I (apoA-I) in HDL. As a result, the NLCs could evade the recognition by macrophages and remain in systemic circulation for extended periods. In another approach, exosome-like nanoparticles were extracted directly from *S. miltiorrhiza*. These carriers inherit the therapeutic potential of plant and promote neovascularization in the damaged heat tissues, improving cardiac function among mouse models of myocardial ischemia–reperfusion injury [77].

### 3.8.5 *WITHANIA SOMNIFERA*

*Withania somnifera* popularly, known as Ashwagandha, contains steroidal lactones called as withanolides. This primary constituent of Withania is capable of upregulating the hypothalamus–pituitary–adrenal axis and decreasing the elevated levels of cortisol levels, a positive contributor to hypertension and CVD. The low solubility and poor solubility are foreseen as the major hindrance to the clinical translation of its therapeutic potential. Nanocarriers such as liposomes, SLN, and niosomes were explored by researchers to encapsulate the Withania plant extracts to overcome their bioavailability problems [78]. Nanoliposomes (NLP) loaded with Withania extracts were reported to be exhibit more stability and improved therapeutic efficacy in *in vivo* experiments [79]. Furthermore, the sustaining ability of SLN and niosome formulations has provided a temporal release pattern for the active drug owing to the controlled release abilities of the carrier matrix [79, 80].

### 3.8.6 *GINKGO BILOBA*

The extract from *G. biloba* has been well reported for its cardioprotective properties. Such valued utilization in traditional medicine is related to its flavonoid components viz., quercetin, kaempferol, isorhamnetin, and terpene lactones, namely ginkgolides A, B, and C [81]. These flavonoid compounds protect against myocardial ischemia through vascular dilation, regulation of lipids in the blood, and inhibition of platelet aggregation. Unsurprisingly, *G. biloba* extract (GbE) is widely used in the management of peripheral arterial disease and cerebral insufficiency. Nevertheless, extensive first-pass metabolism and poor bioavailability limit their clinical efficiency. The intrinsic efficiency of this valuable traditional medicine can be utilized by overcoming these inadequacies through colloidal drug delivery.

Proliposomes composed of mannitol, sodium deoxycholate, and egg phosphatidylcholine were fabricated using spray drying technique. The incorporation of bile salts into liposomes imitates physiological lipid absorption and thereby enhances oral absorption. The oral bioavailability of flavonoids and terpenes from the plant extract was improved by 333% [81]. These proliposomes were able to passively target the active ingredients in organs relevant to CVS tissue through natural uptake by Mononuclear Phagocyte System (MPS).

Chitosan nanoparticles encapsulated with gbE were prepared by orifice ionic gelation technique. The nanoparticles formed were about 104 nm, with strong zeta potential of up to +29.3 mV, ensuring colloidal stability. These nanoparticles adhere to the mucous membrane of the GI due to their bioadhesive property and enable the epithelial absorption of GbE. SLN prepared with GbE exhibited good stability and sustained the release of the active moiety for about 72 hours, enhancing both bioavailability and mean residence time in the circulation.

### 3.8.7 *PANAX GINSENG*

*P. ginseng* is a natural cardioprotective agent recognized for its vasodilatory, antioxidant, anti-inflammatory, and anti-apoptotic activity. The pharmacological activity of ginseng is credited to the triterpene saponins called ginsenosides. Ginsenosides comprise a hydrophobic dammarane skeleton and hydrophilic side chains – an amphipathic architecture. This molecular structure of ginsenosides is responsible for their strong biological activity, yet manifests as poor absorption [82]. Ginsenosides with fewer glycosyl groups impart greater lipophilicity and better absorption [83].

Liposomes tend to be a suitable delivery system owing to their capacity to house both hydrophilic and hydrophobic payloads owing to their structural composition. Their colloidal particle size, less than 200 nm, would help to evade opsonization and phagocytosis by MPS, contributing to longer systemic circulation time and accumulation in the cardiac tissue [84]. Mixed micellar system made from phosphotidyl choline and 1,2-distearoyl-sn-glycero-3-phosphoethanolamin e polyethylene glycol 2000 utilized ginsenoside Compound K (CK) as a part of liposomal membrane by substituting the cholesterol. This structural change improved the encapsulation from 76.9% to 95.3%, along with improved membrane stability and physiological compatibility. Beyond the formulation benefits, CK also improved cardioprotective benefits by increasing nitric oxide signaling and reducing oxidative stress [84].

Targeted nanoliposomes encapsulating ginsenosides were found to reduce the oxidative stress and vascular modeling with in the atherosclerotic plaques. The sustained release of the triterpenes increases the CD31 and bFGF expressions, which are crucial for myocardial repair in post-myocardial infarction [85]. Thus, nanocarriers can transform the bioactive compounds of ginseng from a nutritional supplement into a CVS nanomedicine.

### 3.8.8 *COMMIPHORA WIGHTII*

Guggul is a resin obtained from *C. wightii*. It contains guggulsterones, a bioactive compound responsible for its anti-inflammatory and lipid-lowering effects. The plasma concentrations of the guggulsterones are hindered by their poor water solubility and low stability in physiological environment. Nanocarriers like NLC and nanovesicles were employed to overcome the bioavailability of this plant bioactive. Guggul lipid itself is employed by researches as a carrier material due to its structural similarity with cholesterol, and may offer synergistic cardioprotective activity [86]. SLN and nanovesicles formulated using Guggul lipid exhibited extended release compared to conventional formulations, PEGylation of NLC carriers encapsulated with guggulsterones could passively target the cardiac tissues owing to their enhanced circulation times in the blood [87].

## 3.9 CONCLUSION

Traditional herbs hold great potential to resolve many cardiovascular disorders. However, the clinical translation of these bioactive compounds is hindered by their pharmacokinetic properties. Nanotechnology serves as an innovative bridge between the empirical knowledge of traditional medicine and the modern approach of drug delivery. Encapsulation of herbal bioactive compounds with novel nanocarriers can overcome their physicochemical and pharmacokinetic limitations, unlocking their therapeutic potential for the management of CVDs. This integration is not about supplanting highly effective modern drugs but about augmenting them, creating a more holistic and powerful therapeutic ecosystem.

## REFERENCES


1. Singh, R., Chandi, S.K., Sran, S. et al. (2024). Emerging therapeutic strategies in cardiovascular diseases. *Cureus* 16 (7): e64388. https://doi.org/10.7759/cureus.64388.
2. Roth, G.A., Mensah, G.A., Johnson, C.O. et al. (2020). Global burden of cardiovascular diseases and risk factors, 1990–2019. *J. Am. Coll. Cardiol.* 76: 2982–3021. https://doi.org/10.1016/j.jacc.2020.11.010.
3. Susanti, R., Halimah, E., Komariah, M. et al. (2025). Traditional remedies for cardiovascular diseases in Asia: a scoping review of mind-body and herbal interventions. *J. Multidiscip. Healthcare* 18: 5249–5262. https://doi.org/10.2147/JMDH.S535719.
4. Chang, X., Zhang, T., Zhang, W. et al. (2020). Natural drugs as a treatment strategy for cardiovascular disease through the regulation of oxidative stress. *Oxid. Med. Cell. Longev.* 2020: 1–20. https://doi.org/10.1155/2020/5430407.
5. Shaito, A., Thuan, D.T.B., Phu, H.T. et al. (2020). Herbal medicine for cardiovascular diseases: efficacy, mechanisms, and safety. *Front. Pharmacol.* 11, 422. https://doi.org/10.3389/fphar.2020.00422.
6. Gao, J. and Hou, T. (2023). Cardiovascular disease treatment using traditional Chinese medicine: mitochondria as the Achilles' heel. *Biomed. Pharmacother.* 164: 114999. https://doi.org/10.1016/j.biopha.2023.114999.
7. Dai, J., Qiu, L., Lu, Y., and Li, M. (2024). Recent advances of traditional Chinese medicine against cardiovascular disease: overview and potential mechanisms. *Front. Endocrinol. (Lausanne)* 15: https://doi.org/10.3389/fendo.2024.1366285.
8. Yen, F.-S., Wei, J.C.-C., Chiu, L.-T. et al. (2022). Diabetes, hypertension, and cardiovascular disease development. *J. Transl. Med.* 20: 9. https://doi.org/10.1186/s12967-021-03217-2.
9. Fuchs, F.D. and Whelton, P.K. (2020). High blood pressure and cardiovascular disease. *Hypertension* 75: 285–292. https://doi.org/10.1161/HYPERTENSIONAHA.119.14240.
10. Gallo, G., Volpe, M., and Savoia, C. (2022). Endothelial dysfunction in hypertension: current concepts and clinical implications. *Front. Med. (Lausanne)* 8: 798958. https://doi.org/10.3389/fmed.2021.798958.
11. Renna, N.F., N, d.l.H., and Miatello, R.M. (2013). Pathophysiology of vascular remodeling in hypertension. *Int. J. Hypertens.* 2013: 1–7. https://doi.org/10.1155/2013/808353.
12. Chen, H., Zhang, Y., Aikebaier, M. et al. (2025). Decursin-loaded nanovesicles target macrophages driven by the pathological process of atherosclerosis. *Adv. Sci.* 12: 2417489. https://doi.org/10.1002/advs.202417489.
13. He, Z., Luo, J., Lv, M. et al. (2023). Characteristics and evaluation of atherosclerotic plaques: an overview of state-of-the-art techniques. *Front. Neurol.* 14: 1159288. https://doi.org/10.3389/fneur.2023.1159288.
14. Sun, H.-J., Wu, Z.-Y., Nie, X.-W., and Bian, J.-S. (2020). Role of endothelial dysfunction in cardiovascular diseases: the link between inflammation and hydrogen sulfide. *Front. Pharmacol.* 10: 1568. https://doi.org/10.3389/fphar.2019.01568.
15. Huang, Y., Song, C., He, J., and Li, M. (2022). Research progress in endothelial cell injury and repair. *Front. Pharmacol.* 13: 997272. https://doi.org/10.3389/fphar.2022.997272.
16. Higashi, Y. (2022). Roles of oxidative stress and inflammation in vascular endothelial dysfunction-related disease. *Antioxidants* 11: 1958. https://doi.org/10.3390/antiox11101958.
17. Khodadi, E. (2020). Platelet function in cardiovascular disease: activation of molecules and activation by molecules. *Cardiovasc. Toxicol.* 20: 1–10. https://doi.org/10.1007/s12012-019-09555-4.
18. Alkarithi, G., Duval, C., Shi, Y. et al. (2021). Thrombus structural composition in cardiovascular disease. *Arterioscler. Thromb. Vasc. Biol.* 41: 2370–2383. https://doi.org/10.1161/ATVBAHA.120.315754.
19. Vollset, S.E., Ababneh, H.S., Abate, Y.H. et al. (2024). Burden of disease scenarios for 204 countries and territories, 2022–2050: a forecasting analysis for the Global Burden of Disease Study 2021. *Lancet* 403: 2204–2256. https://doi.org/10.1016/S0140-6736(24)00685-8.
20. Taylor, F., Ward, K., Moore, T.H. et al. (2011). Statins for the primary prevention of cardiovascular disease. In: *Cochrane Database of Systematic Reviews* (ed. F. Taylor). Chichester: John Wiley & Sons, Ltd https://doi.org/10.1002/14651858.CD004816.pub4.
21. Kim, N.H. and Kim, S.G. (2020). Fibrates revisited: potential role in cardiovascular risk reduction. *Diabetes Metab. J.* 44: 213. https://doi.org/10.4093/dmj.2020.0001.
22. Weisfeldt, M.L. and Zieman, S.J. (2007). Advances in the prevention and treatment of cardiovascular disease. *Health Aff.* 26: 25–37. https://doi.org/10.1377/hlthaff.26.1.25.
23. Lim, S.Y. (2013). Role of statins in coronary artery disease. *Chonnam Med. J.* 49: 1. https://doi.org/10.4068/cmj.2013.49.1.1.
24. Keech, A. (2005). Effects of long-term fenofibrate therapy on cardiovascular events in 9795 people with type 2 diabetes mellitus (the FIELD study): randomised controlled trial. *Lancet* 366: 1849–1861. https://doi.org/10.1016/S0140-6736(05)67667-2.
25. Ross, S., D'Mello, M., Anand, S.S. et al. (2015). Effect of bile acid sequestrants on the risk of cardiovascular events. *Circ. Cardiovasc. Genet.* 8: 618–627. https://doi.org/10.1161/CIRCGENETICS.114.000952.
26. Joynt Maddox, K.E. (2024). Health economics of cardiovascular disease in the United States. *Circulation* 150: 419–421. https://doi.org/10.1161/CIRCULATIONAHA.124.068295.
27. Global Burden of Cardiovascular Diseases and Risks 2023 Collaborators (2025). Global, regional, and national burden of cardiovascular diseases and risk factors in 204 countries and territories, 1990–2023. *J. Am. Coll. Cardiol.* 86 (22): 2167–2243. https://doi.org/10.1016/j.jacc.2025.08.015.
28. Farhan, M., Hussein, G.A., Alom, T. et al. (2025). Evaluating the role of PCSK9 inhibitors in reducing cardiovascular events among statin-intolerant patients: a systematic review and meta-analysis. *Ann. Med. Surg.* 87: 891–899. https://doi.org/10.1097/MS9.0000000000002927.
29. Casula, M., Olmastroni, E., Boccalari, M.T. et al. (2019). Cardiovascular events with PCSK9 inhibitors: an updated meta-analysis of randomised controlled trials. *Pharmacol. Res.* 143: 143–150. https://doi.org/10.1016/j.phrs.2019.03.021.
30. Thomopoulos, C., Parati, G., and Zanchetti, A. (2014). Effects of blood pressure lowering on outcome incidence in hypertension. 1. Overview, meta-analyses, and meta-regression analyses of randomized trials. *J. Hypertens.* 32: 2285–2295. https://doi.org/10.1097/HJH.0000000000000378.
31. Bertrand, M.E. (2004). Provision of cardiovascular protection by ACE inhibitors: a review of recent trials. *Curr. Med. Res. Opin.* 20: 1559–1569. https://doi.org/10.1185/030079904X4185.
32. Khalil, M.E., Basher, A.W., Brown, E.J., and Alhaddad, I.A. (2001). A remarkable medical story: benefits of angiotensin-converting enzyme inhibitors in cardiac patients. *J. Am. Coll. Cardiol.* 37: 1757–1764. https://doi.org/10.1016/S0735-1097(01)01229-3.
33. Munger, M.A. (2011). Use of Angiotensin receptor blockers in cardiovascular protection: current evidence and future directions. *P T* 36: 22–40.
34. Swiderski, J., Gadanec, L.K., Apostolopoulos, V. et al. (2023). Role of Angiotensin II in cardiovascular diseases: introducing bisartans as a novel therapy for coronavirus 2019. *Biomolecules* 13: 787. https://doi.org/10.3390/biom13050787.
35. Ray, S., Nair, T., Sawhney, J. et al. (2023). Role of β-blockers in the cardiovascular disease continuum: a collaborative Delphi survey-based

consensus from Asia-Pacific. *Curr. Med. Res. Opin.* 39: 1671–1683. https://doi.org/10.1080/03007995.2023.2256218.
36. Chen, H., Chen, C., Fang, J. et al. (2019). Efficacy and safety of antiplatelet therapy plus Xa factor inhibitors in patients with coronary heart disease: a meta-analysis. *Med. Sci. Monit.* 25: 5473–5481. https://doi.org/10.12659/MSM.917774.
37. Sharifi-Rad, J., Sharopov, F., Ezzat, S.M. et al. (2023). An updated review on glycoprotein IIb/IIIa inhibitors as antiplatelet agents: basic and clinical perspectives. *High Blood Press. Cardiovasc. Prev.* 30: 93–107. https://doi.org/10.1007/s40292-023-00562-9.
38. Clarke, R.J., Mayo, G., Price, P. et al. (1991). Suppression of thromboxane A2 but not of systemic prostacyclin by controlled-release aspirin. *N. Engl. J. Med.* 325: 1137–1141. https://doi.org/10.1056/NEJM199110173251605.
39. Jørgensen, N.R., Schwarz, P., Iversen, H.K., and Vestergaard, P. (2017). P2Y12 receptor antagonist, clopidogrel, does not contribute to risk of osteoporotic fractures in stroke patients. *Front. Pharmacol.* 8: 821. https://doi.org/10.3389/fphar.2017.00821.
40. Chen, W. and Chen, G. (2018). Danshen (*Salvia miltiorrhiza* Bunge): a prospective healing sage for cardiovascular diseases. *Curr. Pharm. Des.* 23: 5125–5135. https://doi.org/10.2174/1381612823666170822101112.
41. Nowrouzi-Sohrabi, P., Tabrizi, R., Rezaei, S. et al. (2020). The effect of voglibose on metabolic profiles in patients with type 2 diabetes mellitus: a systematic review and meta-analysis of clinical trials. *Pharmacol. Res.* 159: 104988. https://doi.org/10.1016/j.phrs.2020.104988.
42. Sharma, D., Saroj, U.R., Upadhyay, A., and Singh, B.K. (2020). Ayurvedic review on diagnosis and management of hridroga with the special reference to cardiovascular disease. *Ayushdhara* 7: 2719–2724. https://doi.org/10.47070/ayushdhara.v7i3.570.
43. Ma, L., Tang, L., and Yi, Q. (2019). Salvianolic acids: potential source of natural drugs for the treatment of fibrosis disease and cancer. *Front. Pharmacol.* 10: 97. https://doi.org/10.3389/fphar.2019.00097.
44. Verma, P., Singh, B., Kumar, A. et al. (2020). *In-vitro* anti-inflammatory and antioxidant potential of *Triphala guggul* tablets. *J. Med. Herbs Ethnomed.* 45–47. https://doi.org/10.25081/jmhe.2020.v6.6238.
45. Suman, P., Sharma, R., Kumari, S. et al. (2025). Dashmoola in Stri roga: a review on its therapeutic benefits. *J. Ayurveda Integr. Med. Sci.* 10: 259–266. https://doi.org/10.21760/jaims.10.4.39.
46. Y.R, S.K., Selvam, N.T., Gaidhani, N.S. et al. (2025). Acute and sub-chronic oral toxicity study of classical ayurvedic formulation Yogaraja Guggulu. *Res. J. Pharm. Technol.* 18: 2175–2180. https://doi.org/10.52711/0974-360X.2025.00312.
47. Sadhupati, D.P., Lakshmisudha, R., Chakravarthy, K.N.K., and Naidana, P.S. (2024). A standardized combination of *Terminalia chebula* and *Withania somnifera* extracts enhances immune function in adults: a pilot randomized, double-blind, placebo-controlled clinical study. *Food Nutr. Res.* 29: 68. https://doi.org/10.29219/fnr.v68.10297.
48. Pundarikakshudu, K. and Bhatt, C. (2015). Design, development and rationalization of Sarpagandha Ghanvati. *Indian J. Pharm. Sci.* 77: 626. https://doi.org/10.4103/0250-474X.169029.
49. Liu, B., Du, Y., Cong, L. et al. (2016). Danshen (*Salvia miltiorrhiza*) compounds improve the biochemical indices of the patients with coronary heart disease. *Evid. Based Complement. Alternat. Med.* 2016: 9781715. https://doi.org/10.1155/2016/9781715.
50. Li, J., Liu, A., Li, H. et al. (2014). Buyang Huanwu decoction for healthcare: evidence-based theoretical interpretations of treating different diseases with the same method and target of vascularity. *Evid. Based Complement. Alternat. Med.* 2014: 506783. https://doi.org/10.1155/2014/506783.
51. Dong, J., Zhou, Z., Chen, Y. et al. (2025). Comprehensive characterization of the material basis and network pharmacology of Dan-Shen-Yin in the treatment of gastritis. *Eurasian J. Med. Oncol.* 9: 168. https://doi.org/10.36922/EJMO025160124.
52. Liang, Y., Zhou, Y., Zhang, J. et al. (2014). Pharmacokinetic compatibility of ginsenosides and schisandra lignans in Shengmai-san: from the perspective of P-Glycoprotein. *PLoS One* 9: e98717. https://doi.org/10.1371/journal.pone.0098717.
53. Dong, Y., Jiang, K., Li, Z. et al. (2024). Tongxinluo and functional outcomes among patients with acute ischemic stroke. *JAMA Netw. Open* 7: e2433463. https://doi.org/10.1001/jamanetworkopen.2024.33463.
54. Alidadi, M., Jamialahmadi, T., Cicero, A.F.G. et al. (2020). The potential role of plant-derived natural products in improving arterial stiffness: a review of dietary intervention studies. *Trends Food Sci. Technol.* 99: 426–440. https://doi.org/10.1016/j.tifs.2020.03.026.
55. Lv, M., Wu, S., Zhang, Z. et al. (2024). The predictive value of LGR for distant metastasis-free survival in locally advanced rectal cancer patients. *Heliyon* 10: e32045. https://doi.org/10.1016/j.heliyon.2024.e32045.
56. Woo, K.S., Yip, T.W.C., Chook, P. et al. (2013). Cardiovascular protective effects of adjunctive alternative medicine (*Salvia miltiorrhiza* and *Pueraria lobata*) in high-risk hypertension. *Evid. Based Complement. Alternat. Med.* 2013: 1–8. https://doi.org/10.1155/2013/132912.
57. Guo, R., Pittler, M.H., and Ernst, E. (2008). Hawthorn extract for treating chronic heart failure. *Cochrane Database Syst. Rev.* 2013: CD005312. https://doi.org/10.1002/14651858.CD005312.pub2.
58. Hartley, L., Flowers, N., Holmes, J. et al. (2013). Green and black tea for the primary prevention of cardiovascular disease. *Cochrane Database Syst. Rev.* 2013: CD009934. https://doi.org/10.1002/14651858.CD009934.pub2.
59. Vaduganathan, M., Mensah, G.A., Turco, J.V. et al. (2022). The global burden of cardiovascular diseases and risk. *J. Am. Coll. Cardiol.* 80: 2361–2371. https://doi.org/10.1016/j.jacc.2022.11.005.
60. Zhao, D., Wang, Y., Wong, N.D., and Wang, J. (2024). Impact of aging on cardiovascular diseases. *JACC Asia* 4: 345–358. https://doi.org/10.1016/j.jacasi.2024.02.002.
61. Nicolaï, S.P., Kruidenier, L.M., Bendermacher, B.L. et al. (2009). *Ginkgo biloba* for intermittent claudication. In: *Cochrane Database of Systematic Reviews* (ed. S.P. Nicolaï). Chichester: John Wiley & Sons, Ltd https://doi.org/10.1002/14651858.CD006888.pub2.
62. Xiang, Q., Li, C., Zhao, X., and Cui, Y.M. (2017). The influence of CYP3A5*3 and BCRPC421A genetic polymorphisms on the pharmacokinetics of felodipine in healthy Chinese volunteers. *J. Clin. Pharm. Ther.* 42: 345–349. https://doi.org/10.1111/jcpt.12505.
63. Jara-Quijada, E., Pérez-Won, M., Tabilo-Munizaga, G. et al. (2023). Liposomes loaded with green tea polyphenols-optimization, characterization, and release kinetics under conventional heating and pulsed electric fields. *Food Bioprocess Technol.* 1–13. https://doi.org/10.1007/s11947-023-03136-8.
64. Azizi, S., Mahdavi Shahri, M., Rahman, H. et al. (2017). Green synthesis palladium nanoparticles mediated by white tea (*Camellia sinensis*) extract with antioxidant, antibacterial, and antiproliferative activities toward the human leukemia (MOLT-4) cell line. *Int. J. Nanomed.* 12: 8841–8853. https://doi.org/10.2147/IJN.S149371.
65. Ahmadi, N., Ahranjani, P.J., and Rashidi, L. (2025). Encapsulation of green tea extract (GTE) in nanoliposome and assessment of its characterization and *in vitro* release study of GTE. *Food Sci. Nutr.* 13: e70781. https://doi.org/10.1002/fsn3.70781.
66. Dzulhi, S. (2018). Formulation, characterization and *in vitro* skin penetration of green tea (*Camellia sinensis L.*) leaves extract-loaded solid lipid nanoparticles. *J. Appl. Pharm. Sci.* 8: 57–62. https://doi.org/10.7324/JAPS.2018.8809.
67. Fasulo, R., Marzano, A., Caccamo, L. et al. (2014). Italian survey on HBV and liver transplantation in a cohort of 2260 patients. *Dig. Liver Dis.* 46: e8–e9. https://doi.org/10.1016/j.dld.2014.01.023.
68. Alqahtani, M.S., Alqahtani, A., Kazi, M. et al. (2020). Wound-healing potential of curcumin loaded lignin nanoparticles. *J. Drug Deliv. Sci. Technol.* 60: 102020. https://doi.org/10.1016/j.jddst.2020.102020.

69. Jourghanian, P., Ghaffari, S., Ardjmand, M. et al. (2016). Sustained release curcumin loaded solid lipid nanoparticles. *Adv. Pharm. Bull.* 6: 17–21. https://doi.org/10.15171/apb.2016.04.
70. Aydin, B., Sagiroglu, A., Ozturk Civelek, D. et al. (2024). Development of curcumin and turmerone loaded solid lipid nanoparticle for topical delivery: optimization, characterization and skin irritation evaluation with 3D tissue model. *Int. J. Nanomed.* 19: 1951–1966. https://doi.org/10.2147/IJN.S453347.
71. Wahyudiono, H.J., Hu, X., Machmudah, S. et al. (2022). Curcumin-loaded liposome preparation in ultrasound environment under pressurized carbon dioxide. *Foods* 11: 1469. https://doi.org/10.3390/foods11101469.
72. Gabriel, T., Vestine, A., Kim, K.D. et al. (2022). Antibacterial activity of nanoparticles of garlic (*Allium sativum*) extract against different bacteria such as *Streptococcus mutans* and *Poryphormonas gingivalis*. *Appl. Sci.* 12: 3491. https://doi.org/10.3390/app12073491.
73. Yang, F.-L., Li, X.-G., Zhu, F., and Lei, C.-L. (2009). Structural characterization of nanoparticles loaded with garlic essential oil and their insecticidal activity against *Tribolium castaneum* (Herbst) (Coleoptera: Tenebrionidae). *J. Agric. Food Chem.* 57: 10156–10162. https://doi.org/10.1021/jf9023118.
74. Pinilla, C.M.B., Noreña, C.P.Z., and Brandelli, A. (2017). Development and characterization of phosphatidylcholine nanovesicles, containing garlic extract, with antilisterial activity in milk. *Food Chem.* 220: 470–476. https://doi.org/10.1016/j.foodchem.2016.10.027.
75. Zhang, W.-L., Gu, X., Bai, H. et al. (2010). Nanostructured lipid carriers constituted from high-density lipoprotein components for delivery of a lipophilic cardiovascular drug. *Int. J. Pharm.* 391: 313–321. https://doi.org/10.1016/j.ijpharm.2010.03.011.
76. Ren, T., Wang, J., Ma, Y. et al. (2025). Preparation of pH-responsive tanshinone IIA-loaded calcium alginate nanoparticles and their anticancer mechanisms. *Pharmaceutics* 17: 66. https://doi.org/10.3390/pharmaceutics17010066.
77. Zhang, S., Xia, J., Zhu, Y. et al. (2024). Establishing *Salvia miltiorrhiza*-derived exosome-like nanoparticles and elucidating their role in angiogenesis. *Molecules* 29: 1599. https://doi.org/10.3390/molecules29071599.
78. Shanmugapriya, J., Reshma, C.A., Srinidhi, V. et al. (2022). Green synthesis of copper nanoparticles using *Withania somnifera* and its antioxidant and antibacterial activity. *J. Nanomater.* 2022: 967294. https://doi.org/10.1155/2022/7967294.
79. Asgharzadeh, F., Moradi Binabaj, M., Fanoudi, S. et al. (2024). Nanomedicine strategies utilizing lipid-based nanoparticles for liver cancer therapy: exploring signaling pathways and therapeutic modalities. *Adv. Pharm. Bull.* 14: 513–523. https://doi.org/10.34172/apb.2024.061.
80. Jiang, Q.-F., Huang, M.-Y., Wu, K.-Y. et al. (2017). Intervention effects of atorvastatin combined with *Panax notoginseng* saponins on rats with atherosclerosis complicated with hepatic injury. *Pharmacogn. Mag.* 13: 430. https://doi.org/10.4103/pm.pm_424_16.
81. Zheng, B., Teng, L., Xing, G. et al. (2015). Proliposomes containing a bile salt for oral delivery of *Ginkgo biloba* extract: formulation optimization, characterization, oral bioavailability and tissue distribution in rats. *Eur. J. Pharm. Sci.* 77: 254–264. https://doi.org/10.1016/j.ejps.2015.06.007.
82. Kim, J.-H. (2012). *Cardiovascular diseases and Panax ginseng*: a review on molecular mechanisms and medical applications. *J. Ginseng Res.* 36: 16–26. https://doi.org/10.5142/jgr.2012.36.1.16.
83. Sarhene, M., Ni, J.Y., Duncan, E.S. et al. (2021). Ginsenosides for cardiovascular diseases; update on pre-clinical and clinical evidence, pharmacological effects and the mechanisms of action. *Pharmacol. Res.* 166: 105481. https://doi.org/10.1016/j.phrs.2021.105481.
84. You, X., Liu, H., Chen, Y., and Zhao, G. (2024). Multifunctional liposomes co-modified with ginsenoside compound K and hyaluronic acid for tumor-targeted therapy. *Polymers (Basel)* 16: 405. https://doi.org/10.3390/polym16030405.
85. Dong, Y., Fu, R., Yang, J. et al. (2019). Folic acid-modified ginsenoside Rg5-loaded bovine serum albumin nanoparticles for targeted cancer therapy *in vitro* and *in vivo*. *Int. J. Nanomed.* 14: 6971–6988. https://doi.org/10.2147/IJN.S210882.
86. Gaur, P.K., Mishra, S., and Aeri, V. (2014). Formulation and evaluation of guggul lipid nanovesicles for transdermal delivery of aceclofenac. *Sci. World J.* 2014: 1–10. https://doi.org/10.1155/2014/534210.
87. Lin, T., Huang, X., Wang, Y. et al. (2017). Long circulation nanostructured lipid carriers for gambogenic acid: formulation design, characterization, and pharmacokinetic. *Xenobiotica* 47: 793–799. https://doi.org/10.1080/00498254.2016.1229084.

CHAPTER 4

# Glycosides, Flavonoids, Polyphenols: Natural Cardioprotective Agents

**Bondada N.B. Vaidehi[1], Rudolf Bauer[2], Akshintala Sree Gayatri[1], and Bodapati Raju[1]**

[1] *Department of Pharmaceutical Chemistry, Aditya College of Pharmacy, Surampalem, Andhra Pradesh, India*
[2] *Institute of Pharmaceutical Sciences, University of Graz, Austria*

## 4.1 INTRODUCTION

Cardiovascular diseases (CVDs), which contribute significantly to morbidity and death globally, include hypertension, myocardial infarction (MI), and atherosclerosis. These conditions continue to be major global health issues. Numerous interconnected processes, such as oxidative stress, inflammation, endothelial dysfunction, lipid imbalance, and apoptosis, are involved in the pathophysiology of CVDs. Because of their safety record, effectiveness, and multitarget therapeutic qualities, naturally occurring phytochemicals have drawn more interest in recent decades as possible cardioprotective agents. Among these, three types of bioactive substances with significant cardiovascular advantages are glycosides, flavonoids, and polyphenols. Because they can affect cellular and molecular processes related to cardiovascular health and are found in a wide variety of fruits, vegetables, and plant-based beverages, they are essential parts of preventive cardiology.

## 4.2 GLYCOSIDES

Glycosides are organic substances derived from plants or animals that catalyze the hydrolysis of an acid or an enzyme to produce one or more sugar moieties and a non-sugar moiety. The former is called glycine, and the latter is called glycone or genin. The sugars involved in glycosides are of different types, but most commonly they are beta-D-glucose. The other sugars found are galactose, mannose, rhamnose, digitoxose, cymarose, etc. The aglycone hydroxyl group may be derived from alcohol, phenol, or, in some cases, amines [1].

### 4.2.1 CLASSIFICATION OF GLYCOSIDES: (See Figure 4.1)

Glycosides can be grouped in different ways by looking at features like which sugar is present, what the non-sugar part is, and how the sugar is connected.

#### 4.2.1.1 By Sugar Component (Glycone) (See Figure 4.2)

**O-glycosides:** Compounds in which an oxygen atom connects a sugar molecule to a noncarbohydrate moiety. They play important roles in biological processes and have applications in drug development, biochemical research, and various industries [2, 3]. In nature, these are particularly prevalent in higher plants like frangula, rhubarb, and senna.

They are hydrolyzed by treatment with alkali (base) or acid into glycone and sugar [4].

Example: Rhein-8-glucoside

**N-glycosides:** In N-glycosides, a nitrogen atom joins the sugar and aglycone. The most common type of N-glycosides are nucleosides, which are produced when the corresponding amino group of the base eventually combines with the ribose/deoxyribose –OH group [5].

Examples: Adenosine is found in nature in large quantities, such as in yeast nucleic acid [6].

**C-glycosides:** C-glycosides are compounds in which sugar's anomeric carbon is directly joined to an aglycone's carbon atom (the non-sugar portion) [7]. These are also called aloin-type glycosides and are mainly found in members of the Liliaceae family, for example, aloe. They are hydrolyzed by oxidative hydrolysis with ferric chloride. Cochineal contains a C-glycoside in the form of a coloring matter called carminic acid.

Examples: *Aloe vera* [8], cochineal.

**S-glycosides:** A molecule known as S-glycoside is created when a sugar moiety forms a C–S glycosidic bond with a thiol group (–SH) via the anomeric carbon [9].

Example: Sinigrin in mustard seeds [10].

#### 4.2.1.2 By Aglycone Component (See Figure 4.3)

**A. Cardiac glycosides or steroidal glycosides:** The steroid is an aglycone. These are a type of natural chemical that has asteroid aglycone (non-sugar part) linked to a glycosidic link that connects with one or more sugar molecules (glycone). These compounds, which have cardiotonic action, increase the work performance of the heart and exert remarkable cardiotonic activity, especially in a failing heart [11]. Clinically, cardiac glycosides are used to manage cardiac arrhythmias and congestive heart failure. Numerous regions of the plant kingdom contain these substances, especially in families such as Apocynaceae, Liliaceae, Asparagaceae, and Solanaceae, and they are also found in some animals and marine organisms. The aglycone part contains C23 or C24 steroids. Based on the

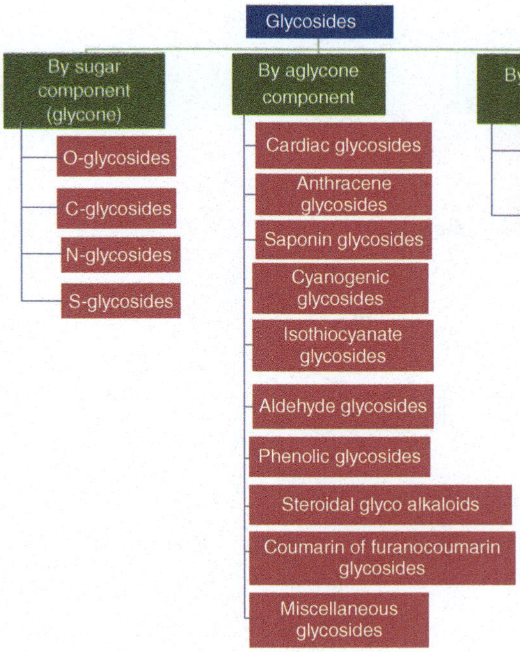


**FIGURE 4.1** Classification of glycosides.

number of carbons, the steroidal moiety is divided into cardenolides and bufadienolides [12]. The steroidal backbone gives these molecules their structural similarity to important biological steroids, such as hormones, while the sugar portion influences their solubility, absorption, and biological activity.

**Cardenolides** – These cardiac glycosides have a five-membered α, β-unsaturated lactone ring (butyrolactone ring), which is attached at the 17th position of the steroidal nucleus. *Digitalis* and *Strophanthus* species are naturally occurring cardenolides [13].

**Bufadienolides** – These cardiac glycosides have a six-membered lactone ring [14]. Bufadienolides are commonly called "toad poison" because they are also present in skin secretions of various toad species; e.g., toad venom contains bufotoxin.

Cardiac glycosides are steroidal glycosides that exert a strong effect on the heart, specifically by inhibiting the $Na^+$/$K^+$-ATPase enzyme, resulting in an increase in intracellular calcium levels. This strengthens myocardial contraction and is useful in treating cardiac arrhythmia and congestive heart failure. At the 17th position of the steroid nucleus, the cardiac glycosides aglycone part contains a 5- or 6-membered lactone ring, which is essential for their activity. Examples include

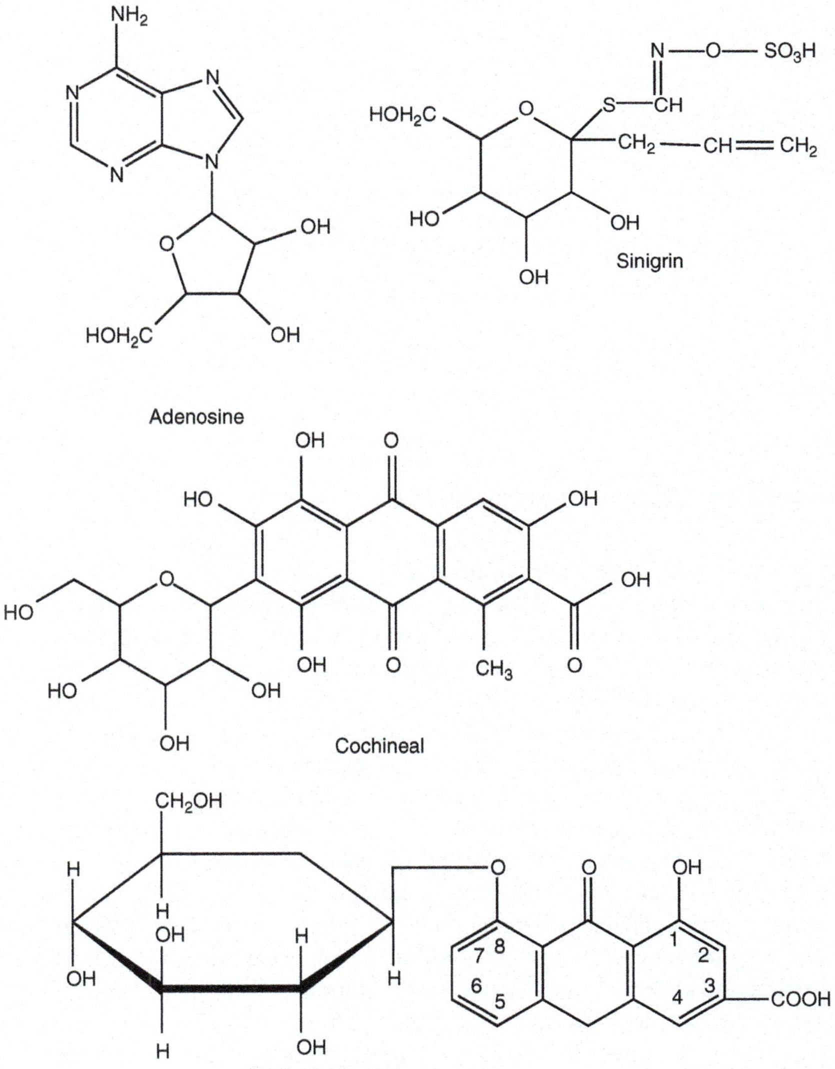


**FIGURE 4.2** Structures of glycosides.

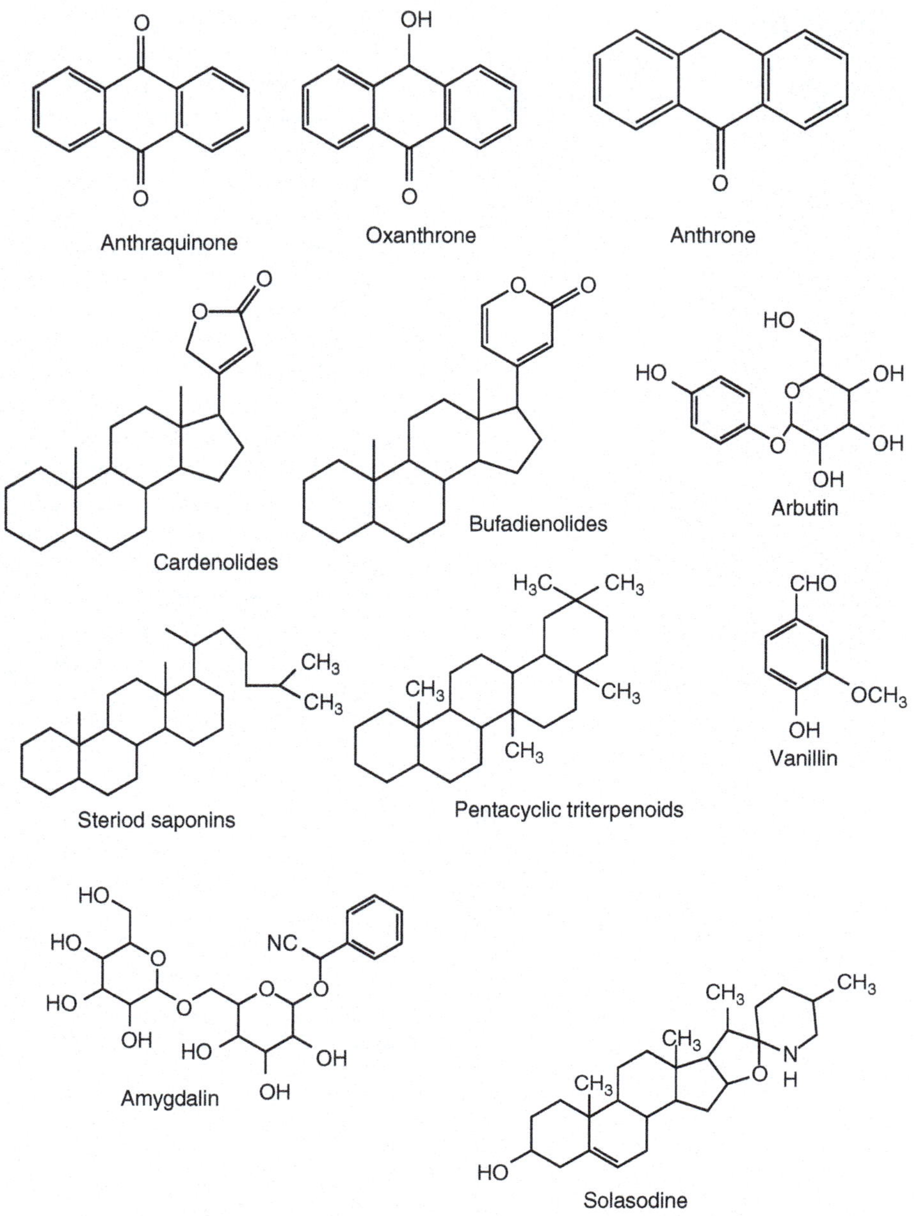


**FIGURE 4.3** Structures of glycosides.

digoxin and digitoxin from the plant *Digitalis purpurea* (foxglove), ouabain from *Strophanthus gratus*, and oleandrin from *Nerium oleander* [15]. These compounds are highly potent and must be used with caution due to their narrow therapeutic window and potential for toxicity.

**B. Anthracene glycosides:** The aglycone is an anthracene. Anthracene glycosides are another important category of glycosides. In dicot families such as the Euphorbiaceae, Ericaceae, Lythraceae, Rhamnaceae, etc., these are primarily found. It also indicates the presence of C-glycosides in the monocot family Liliaceae. Additionally, anthraquinone glycosides are found in certain lichens and fungi [16]. This group is naturally occurring substances composed of a glycone molecule linked to different aglycone moieties like anthraquinone, anthrone, dianthrol, oxaanthrone, and dianthrone. These glycosides are primarily found in medicinal plants such as senna (e.g., *Senna alexandrina*), aloe (*A. vera*, *Aloe ferox*), *rhubarb* (*Rheum palmatum*), cascara (*Rhamnus purshiana*), and buckthorn (*Rhamnus frangula*). The most important properties of anthraquinone glycosides are their stimulant laxative effect [17]. These then stimulate peristalsis (contractions of the intestinal muscles), increase water and electrolyte secretion into the colon, and reduce reabsorption, thus promoting bowel movements.

Common examples include **sennosides A and B** from senna leaves and pods.

**Aloin**, found in *A. vera*, is another well-known anthraquinone glycoside, used for similar laxative purposes. **Emodin glycoside**, present in rhubarb and buckthorn, not only acts as a laxative but also exhibits anti-inflammatory and antimicrobial properties.

**Frangulin A and B**, found in *Frangula* bark, are mild laxatives used in traditional medicine.

**C. Saponin glycosides:** The aglycone is a triterpenoid or steroid saponin. Many plants naturally contain saponin glycosides, which are defined by the structure of a sugar moiety (glycone) joined to a non-sugar component (aglycone or sapogenin), which may be a triterpenoid or a steroid. The word "saponin" comes from the Latin term "sapo," which means soap, and indicates the characteristic property of froth formation (foam formation) in aqueous solutions. These substances are frequently used in shampoos, soaps, and other personal care products. The biological activities of saponin glycosides are diverse and extend beyond their surfactant nature [18]. These activities include anti-inflammatory, antibacterial, antioxidant, and even anticancer capabilities [19]. An example of a saponin glycoside with anti-inflammatory and antiviral properties is glycyrrhizin, which is present in licorice root (*Glycyrrhiza glabra*). Another illustration is the steroidal saponin, dioscin, which is present in *Dioscorea* species (wild yam). Saponins are often classified according to the nature of the sapogenin (aglycone):

- **Steroidal saponins**: Mostly found in monocots (e.g., *Dioscorea*).
- **Pentacyclic triterpenoid saponins:** Common in dicots (e.g., *G. glabra*).

**Steroidal saponins** – Both monocot plants like the Liliaceae, Dioscoreaceae, and Amaryllidaceae, as well as dicot plants like Leguminosae, Solanaceae, and Apocynaceae contain steroidal saponins. Oral contraceptives like mestranol and norethisterone, sex hormones like progesterone and estradiol, corticoids like betamethasone and cortisone, and a variety of medicinally important steroids like vitamin D are all made from them.

**Pentacyclic triterpenoid saponins** – Sapogenins belonging to this group include pentacyclic triterpenoid saponins, which are linked to sugars or uronic acids. Several dicot plant families have them, including Umbelliferae, Polygalaceae, and Caryophyllaceae.

**D. Cyanogenic glycosides:** These are also known as cyanophoric glycosides because they contain hydrocyanic acid in the aglycone moiety. The liberated hydrogen cyanide (HCN) is responsible for its physiological activities as well as toxicity. One of the prominent glycosides from plants is amygdalin, which was isolated in 1830. According to reports, cyanogenic glycosides are found in about 110 plant groups. Among these are Leguminosae, Euphorbiaceae, Fabaceae, Rosaceae, Linaceae, and Gramineae. Chemically, these substances are made of a α-hydroxy nitrile type of aglycone moiety linked to glycine moieties, which can either be a monosaccharide or the disaccharide gentiobiose [20]. These glycosides yield HCN, an aldehyde, or a ketone on hydrolysis or when attacked by the enzyme β-glucosidase. Linamarin from linseed, prunasin from wild cherry bark, and amygdalin from bitter almonds, etc. Some of them are used as flavoring agents [21].

**E. Isothiocyanate glycosides:** They are also called glucosinolate compounds; the aglycone part of such glycosides contains isothiocyanate, as it contains sulfur along with nitrogen. In literature, more than 80 glucosinolate compounds have been isolated from various species of families like Capparidaceae, Brassicaceae, Resedaceae, and Moringaceae [22]. The most common examples containing these glycosides are cabbage, broccoli, horseradish, and mustard. These compounds impart a bitter taste and characteristic pungent flavor or odor [23].

Chemically, glucosinolates consist of a glycone moiety, β-D-thioglucose, with a thioester bond to an aglycone entity, which can either be an aromatic or aliphatic derivative in nature. These are generally anions and often found as potassium salts, which are soluble in water. Upon enzymatic hydrolysis, these glycosides yield isothiocyanate as the main product, along with other compounds like thiocyanate, nitrile, sulfate, and D-glucose. The enzyme myrosinase hydrolyzes isothiocyanate [24].

**F. Aldehyde glycosides:** The aglycone is an aldehyde. Aldehyde glycosides are a specialized class of glycosides characterized by having an aldehyde group in their aglycone (non-sugar) part. These substances are structurally made up of a sugar molecule, most commonly glucose, linked to an aldehyde-containing organic compound through a glycosidic link. This linkage generally renders the aldehyde moiety less reactive and often biologically inactive while bound, protecting the plant cells from potential toxicity [25]. Aldehyde glycosides play significant roles in plants, primarily in defense mechanisms and in contributing to characteristic aromas and flavors. Well-known examples of aldehyde glycosides include vanillin β-D-glucoside from vanilla beans, which, upon hydrolysis, releases vanillin, the primary compound responsible for the vanilla aroma. Another notable group includes cyanogenic aldehyde glycosides like amygdalin and prunasin, found in bitter almonds, apricot kernels, and cherry pits. These compounds release benzaldehyde and toxic HCN upon enzymatic hydrolysis, serving as potent defense chemicals [26].

**G. Phenolic glycosides:** Phenolic glycosides are naturally occurring plant compounds that consist of a sugar moiety, typically glucose, linked to a phenolic group. They are found in a wide range of plant species, especially in the family Salicaceae (such as willows and poplars). Phenolic glycosides are often stored in inactive forms and become biologically active when the plant is damaged, releasing toxic phenols that protect the plant. One well-known example is salicin, found in willow bark [27], which is metabolized into salicylic acid and has anti-inflammatory properties – serving as the basis for the development of aspirin. They also possess antioxidant, antimicrobial, and anti-inflammatory activities.

**Examples:** Arbutin, salicin

**H. Steroidal glycoalkaloids:** The families of Solanaceae and Liliaceae accumulate steroidal glycosides. These are nitrogenous analogs of steroidal saponins, which also have hemolytic activity. These compounds also have surface activity and are toxic in nature if ingested [28].

The commonly known examples are

i. Solasodine, present in *Solanum khasianum*

ii. α-Solanine, present in *Solanum tuberosum* (potato)

The sugar portion of steroidal glycoalkaloids contains one to four sugar moieties attached to the C-3 position of the steroidal nucleus. The commonly attached sugar moieties may be glucose, galactose, rhamnose, and xylose.

**I. Coumarin and furanocoumarin glycosides:** Coumarins are C3-C6 derivatives that belong to a group of compounds known as benzo-α-pyrones. In the kingdom of plants, coumarins are extensively dispersed and are commonly found in families like Umbelliferae, Oleaceae, Rubiaceae, and Caprifoliaceae [29]. Most of the coumarin compounds have anticoagulant activity. Coumarin compounds themselves are precursors for the drug warfarin, which is chemically used as an anticoagulant. Coumarins, present in umbelliferone, scopoletin, scopolin, etc., contain benzo-α-pyrones [30, 31].

Furanocoumarin: At either the 6- and 7- or the 7- and 8-positions, a furan can fuse with a coumarin to generate furanocoumarins. The common examples of such coumarins are psoralen and angelicin.

**J. Miscellaneous glycosides:** In nature, there are many secondary plant metabolites present as glycosides. These compounds do not belong to any single class. Some of these glycosides have bitter properties when taken before meals. Therefore, these bitter tonics help to improve appetite and are hence called bitter glycosides. Common examples are amarogentin from *Swertia chirata*, gentiopicroside from *Gentiana lutea*.

#### 4.2.1.3 By Glycosidic Linkage (See Figure 4.4)

**Alpha (α) glycosides** – These are a class of glycosidic compounds in which a sugar molecule is joined to another molecule (referred to as the aglycone) via an alpha-configured glycosidic bond. This suggests that the glycosidic bridge is created at the anomeric carbon beneath the plane of the sugar ring, in D-sugars in particular. Numerous structural and biological characteristics are determined by the direction of the glycosidic bond [32].

For example, maltose, an α-glycoside that is an essential step in the digestion of starch, is made up of two glucose units connected by an α (1→4) link. Sucrose, another significant α-glycoside, has an α (1→2) bond between fructose and glucose. Enzymes called alpha-glycosidases, which are unique to the alpha configuration of the bond, typically break down alpha glycosides. The difference between the alpha and beta configurations is biologically significant since it significantly impacts how enzymes recognize and interact with these molecules [33].

### 4.2.2 EXAMPLES OF α-GLYCOSIDES

**Maltose** – Two glucose units joined by an α (1→4) link form this disaccharide. It is created when starch is broken down.

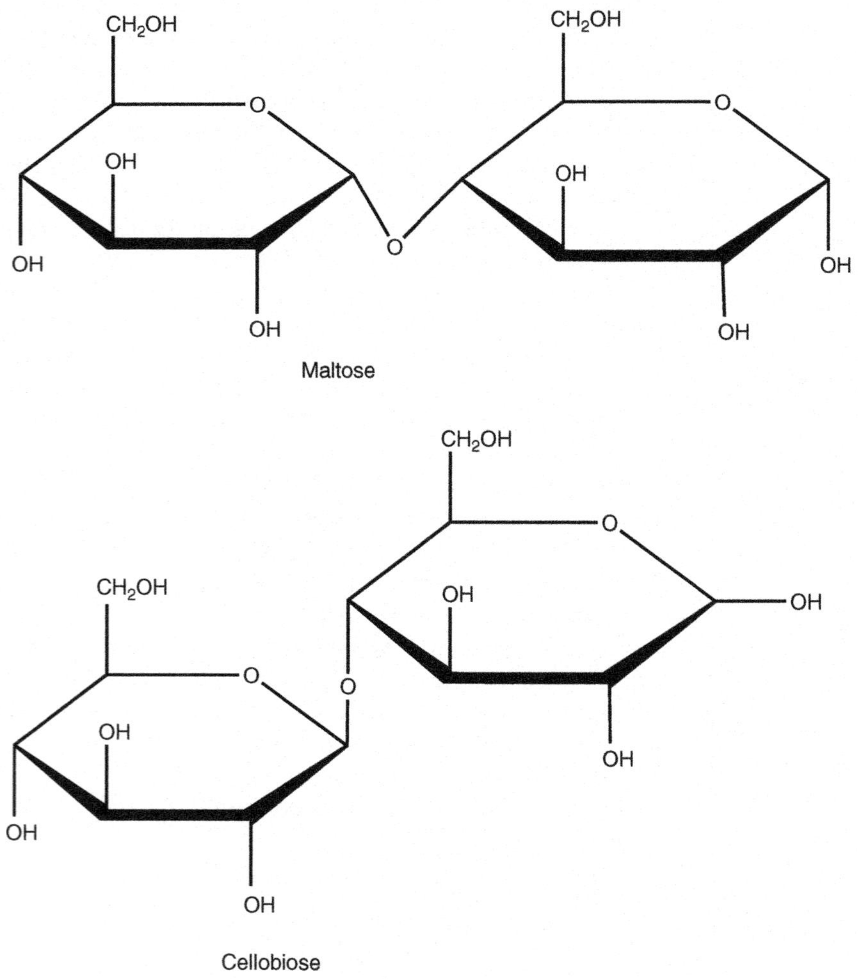


FIGURE 4.4 Structures of glycosides.

**Sucrose** – The glucose is in the alpha form, and the fructose and glucose disaccharide has an α (1→2) bond. This popular table sugar is present in a wide variety of plants.

**β-glycosides:** A sugar molecule is joined to another functional group or molecule by a β-configured glycosidic bond to form a β-glycoside, a type of glycosidic chemical. B-glycosides have a glycosidic bond above the plane of the sugar ring (in D-sugars) [34]. These substances are widely dispersed in nature, particularly in plants, where they perform a few biological functions, including defensive mechanisms for the plant or as building blocks for active substances that are released after hydrolysis. Cellobiose, a well-known example of a β-glycoside, is a building block of cellulose made up of two glucose units connected by a β (1→4) bond. Because of their stability and unique interactions with enzymes such as beta-glycosidases, which accelerate their hydrolysis, β-glycosides are also significant in biochemistry and pharmacology.

Examples: **Cellobiose** – this disaccharide contains a β (1→4) glycosidic bond joined by two glucose units. It is the repeating unit of cellulose, a key structural element of plant cell walls

### 4.2.3 GLYCOSIDES AS CARDIOPROTECTIVE AGENTS

Glycosides are a broad class of naturally occurring substances with a range of pharmacological actions, including significant cardioprotective properties. Among these, the most well known are the cardiac glycosides, which primarily act on the heart muscle to improve its function [35]. The most well known of these are cardiac glycosides, which mainly enhance the function of the heart muscle. These substances, which include ouabain (from *Strophanthus* species) and digoxin and digitoxin (from *Digitalis purpurea* or foxglove), function by blocking the sodium–potassium ATPase ($Na^+/K^+$-ATPase) pump in cardiac myocytes. This inhibition raises intracellular sodium levels, which reduces the activity of the sodium–calcium exchanger. As a result, calcium levels inside cells rise, boosting cardiac output and myocardial contractility (positive inotropic effect), especially in circumstances like congestive heart failure and atrial fibrillation. In addition to their inotropic effects, cardiac glycosides also have vagomimetic activity, which slows conduction through the atrioventricular (AV) node and helps control heart rate. Some newer plant-derived glycosides have shown promise in experimental studies for reducing oxidative stress, inflammation, and apoptosis in cardiac tissues, further supporting their role in protecting the heart [36]. For instance, ginsenosides, which are saponin glycosides from *Panax ginseng*, have demonstrated anti-apoptotic and antioxidant effects in ischemia–reperfusion injury models, offering cardioprotection at the cellular level. Thus, glycosides, through both classic and emerging mechanisms, play a valuable role in cardiovascular therapy and protection.

## 4.3 FLAVONOIDS

A common presence in fruits, vegetables, cereals, and medicinal plants is flavonoids, which are low-molecular-weight polyphenolic chemicals. The vivid hues of flowers, fruits, and fall foliage are mostly due to them. Through mechanisms like antioxidation, anti-inflammation, and cellular process modification, these essential compounds have numerous positive benefits, but they are especially effective in preventing CVDs. The precise functions of flavonoids in cardiovascular health, their modes of action, and possible clinical uses will be covered.

### 4.3.1 CLASSIFICATION (See Figure 4.5)

They can be classified into six main subgroups.

#### 4.3.1.1 Flavanones

Within the larger category of plant-derived flavonoids, flavanones are a class of chemicals distinguished by a particular chemical structure that consists of a chiral center at the C2 position and a dihydropyrone ring. They are commonly found as glycosides (sugars attached) and are abundantly found in citrus species like lemon and orange. They possess several biological properties, including antimycobacterial, antifungal, antiviral, anti-inflammatory, antioxidant, and potentially anti-neoplastic effects. Typical flavanones that give some citrus peels their distinctive bitter flavor are eriodictyol, naringenin, and hesperetin [37].

#### 4.3.1.2 Flavones

A subclass of flavonoids, flavones are one class of chemical molecules that exist naturally and are distinguished by their C6-C3-C6 carbon skeleton, which is present in plants, especially fruits and vegetables, and has the fundamental structure 2-phenyl-4H-1-benzopyran-4-one (also known as 2-phenylchromen-4-one). Because of their various biological properties, including anti-inflammatory, antioxidant, and possibly anticancer actions, they are ingested as part of the human diet. $C_{15}H_{10}O_2$ is the chemical formula for the fundamental flavone molecule. The sources of flavones are parsley and celery [38]. The flavones apigenin, luteolin, tangeretin, and chrysin are important examples.

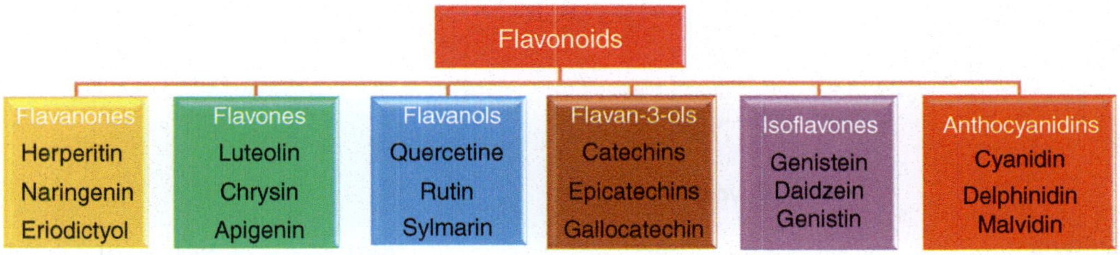


FIGURE 4.5 Classification of flavonoids.

#### 4.3.1.3 Flavanols

Many plant-based products, such as cocoa, green tea, red wine, berries, apples, and grapes, contain flavanols, sometimes referred to as flavan-3-ols, a family of natural substances. They are strong antioxidants that have several health advantages, including enhancing heart and brain function, reducing inflammation, and possibly assisting in the battle against other illnesses [39].

Examples: Quercetin, kaempferol, myricetin, rutin, sylmarin, etc.

#### 4.3.1.4 Flavan-3-ols

Plant-based foods, including cocoa, tea, berries, peaches, and pears, include a class of polyphenolic chemicals called flavan-3-ols, compounds renowned for their antioxidant, anti-inflammatory, and cardioprotective properties. They include flavanol monomers such as catechin and epicatechin, as well as oligomers and polymers like procyanidins. Their consumption is linked to improved vascular health, blood pressure (BP), and reduced risk of cardiometabolic disorders [40]. These are also known as dihydroflavanols.

Examples: Catechins, epicatechins, and gallocatechins.

#### 4.3.1.5 Isoflavones

Isoflavonoids are a class of advantageous polyphenolic substances that are mostly seen in leguminous family plants like lupin seeds, soybeans, and chickpeas. These are derivatives of Flavones. In addition to being crucial for human health, they are also essential for plants as defense compounds, signaling molecules, and symbiotic activities. They also have anti-inflammatory, anticancer, and antioxidant qualities. They can improve insulin function and increase the metabolism of carbohydrates, and reduce the risk of cardiac problems [41]. These are also called phytoestrogens because of their structural resemblance to estrogens.

Examples: Genistein, daidzein, genistin, biochanin A.

#### 4.3.1.6 Anthocyanidins

A class of sugar-free, water-soluble plant pigments called anthocyanidins are members of the flavonoids and are located in the outer layers of vegetables and fruits like purple potatoes and berries. They are the aglycone (sugar-free) version of anthocyanins, which are produced when a sugar molecule is added. Anthocyanidins are well known for their health advantages, which include antioxidant and anti-inflammatory qualities that promote metabolic, cardiovascular, and cognitive health [42] (see Figure 4.6).

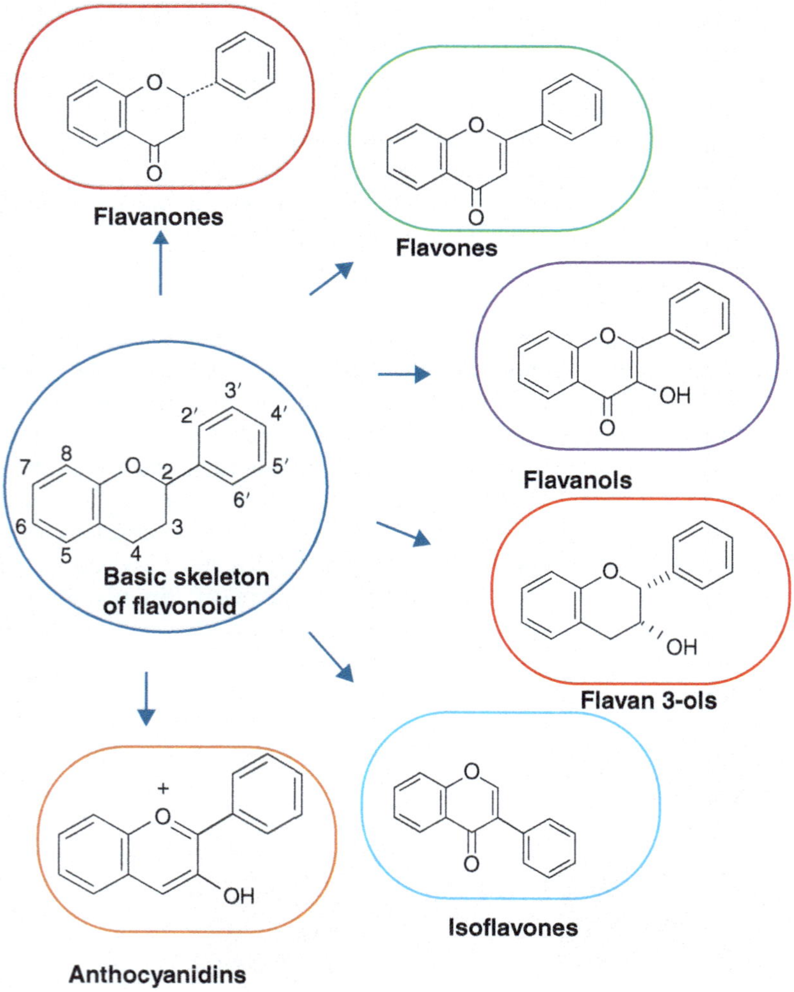


FIGURE 4.6 Structures of flavonoids.

Examples: Cyanidin, delphinidin, malvidin, petunidin, peonidin.

The existence of glycosidic linkages and the quantity and location of hydroxyl groups in these compounds are key factors that determine their biological activity. Enzyme interactions, antioxidant capacity, and cellular absorption are all impacted by structural variation.

## 4.3.2 CAUSES FOR CARDIOVASCULAR PROBLEMS

The following are the main causes of CVDs, which are complex conditions:

1. Atherosclerosis: Due to the development of plaque, endothelial dysfunction, and lipid buildup.
2. Includes both chronic inflammation and oxidative stress.
3. Elevated BP: Chronic hypertension causes vascular wall damage, which can lead to heart failure.
4. Stress and inflammation via oxidation: An overabundance of reactive oxygen species (ROS) in cardiac tissue damages the heart and promotes endothelial dysfunction by damaging DNA, proteins, and lipids.
5. Thrombosis and aggregation of platelets: Blood flow is blocked by increased platelet aggregation and clot formation, which can result in MI or stroke.
6. The condition of dyslipidemia: Reduced high-density lipoprotein (HDL) cholesterol and elevated low-density lipoprotein (LDL) cholesterol hasten atherosclerosis.
7. Damage from ischemia–reperfusion: Apoptosis, mitochondrial malfunction, and oxidative stress are brought on by the abrupt recovery of blood flow following ischemia.

## 4.3.3 MECHANISMS OF CARDIOPROTECTIVE ACTION

The cardioprotective actions of flavonoids and polyphenols are multifactorial and include:

### 4.3.3.1 Antioxidant Activity

Flavonoids neutralize ROS, reduce oxidative stress, and upregulate endogenous antioxidant enzymes such as superoxide dismutase (SOD), catalase, and glutathione peroxidase. The stress caused by oxidation is the major source for the development of CVDs, as it promotes oxidation of LDL cholesterol, endothelial dysfunction, and inflammation [43, 44].

### 4.3.3.2 Anti-inflammatory Effects

Persistent inflammation is one of the characteristics of CVDs. Pro-inflammatory transcription factors, such as nuclear factor kappa B (NF-κB), which regulate the expression of inflammatory genes, are inhibited by polyphenols and flavonoids. By preventing pro-inflammatory cytokine and chemokine production, these substances reduce the inflammatory reactions that underlie CVDs [45, 46].

### 4.3.3.3 Improvement of Endothelial Function

Flavonoids enhance vasodilation, reduce endothelial dysfunction, and boost nitric oxide (NO) production.

### 4.3.3.4 Lipid Profile Modulation

By raising HDL cholesterol levels and lowering total cholesterol, LDL, and triglyceride cholesterol, they help to enhance the lipid profile [47].

### 4.3.3.5 Antithrombotic and Antiplatelet Effects

By altering the cyclooxygenase and thromboxane pathways, flavonoids lessen thrombus formation, increase fibrinolytic activity, and limit platelet aggregation [48].

### 4.3.3.6 Blood Pressure Reduction

By vasodilating and altering the renin-angiotensin-aldosterone system (RAAS), flavonoids reduce BP at both the systolic and diastolic levels [49].

### 4.3.3.7 Anti-apoptotic and Anti-ferroptosis Effects

Ferroptosis, a non-apoptotic type of cell death, and apoptosis, or programmed cell death, are important causes of cardiac injury in diseases such as myocardial ischemia and reperfusion. By altering mitochondrial activity and iron metabolism, flavonoids and polyphenols have been demonstrated to prevent apoptosis and ferroptosis, thereby shielding cardiac cells from harm [50].

### 4.3.3.8 Modulation of Autophagy

A cellular mechanism called autophagy breaks down and recycles damaged proteins and organelles. Autophagy can be modulated by flavonoids and polyphenols to preserve cellular homeostasis and avoid heart problems. This process is especially significant in ischemic heart disease [51].

### 4.3.3.9 Inhibition of Adverse Cardiac Remodeling

One prevalent aspect of cardiovascular disorders is cardiac remodeling, which includes both anatomical and functional alterations in the heart. Polyphenols and flavonoids have been demonstrated to prevent detrimental cardiac remodeling by lowering fibrosis and enhancing ventricular function [52].

## 4.3.4 SPECIFIC FLAVONOIDS WITH CARDIOPROTECTIVE EFFECTS: (See Table 4.1)

### 4.3.4.1 Quercetin

One of the most researched flavonoids is quercetin. It can be found in tea, apples, and onions, among other foods. It has been demonstrated that quercetin reduces BP, prevents aggregation of platelets, and improves endothelial function, all of which lower the risk of cardiovascular illnesses.

**Table 4.1** Specific flavonoids with mechanisms of action (M.O.A).

| S. No | Flavonoid | Source | Cardioprotective effect |
|---|---|---|---|
| 1 | Quercetin | Apples, onions, tea | Reduces blood pressure, improves endothelial function, and inhibits platelet aggregation |
| 2 | Kaempferol | Broccoli, spinach, grapefruit | Reduces inflammation and oxidative stress, protects against myocardial ischemia |
| 3 | Hesperidin | Citrus fruits | Reduces inflammation, improves endothelial function, and lowers blood pressure |
| 4 | Anthocyanins | Berries, grapes, pomegranates | Improves lipid metabolism, reduces inflammation, and enhances antioxidant defenses |
| 5 | Catechins | Green tea | Improves endothelial function, reduces oxidative stress, and inhibits platelet aggregation |
| 6 | Luteolin | Oregano, celery, carrot | Anti-inflammatory, anti-apoptotic, and antioxidant qualities |

#### 4.3.4.2 Kaempferol

The flavonoid kaempferol also has important cardioprotective properties. It can be found in grapefruit, spinach, and broccoli. By reducing inflammation and oxidative stress, kaempferol has been shown to reduce myocardial ischemia and reperfusion injury.

#### 4.3.4.3 Hesperidin

A common flavanone found in citrus fruits is hesperidin. It has been demonstrated to enhance cardiovascular health by BP reduction, endothelial function improvement, and inflammation reduction [53, 54].

#### 4.3.4.4 The Anthocyanins

The red, purple, and blue hues of fruits and vegetables are caused by a subgroup of flavonoids called anthocyanins. It has been demonstrated that they lower the risk of cardiovascular illnesses by strengthening antioxidant defenses, decreasing inflammation, and improving lipid metabolism [55, 56].

#### 4.3.4.5 Catechins

High amounts of catechins, especially epigallocatechin gallate (EGCG), are present in green tea. They have been demonstrated to prevent cardiovascular illnesses by enhancing endothelial function, lowering oxidative stress, and preventing platelet aggregation [57, 58].

#### 4.3.4.6 Luteolin

Due to its anti-inflammatory, anti-apoptotic, and antioxidant qualities, luteolin, a naturally occurring flavonoid, has cardioprotective effects. It avoids cardiac damage, lowers oxidative stress, suppresses inflammatory cytokines, and enhances endothelial function. Furthermore, luteolin contributes to improved heart function and defense against ischemic damage by modulating signaling pathways such as nuclear factor kappa B (NF-κB) and phosphoinositide 3-kinase (PI3K/Akt) [46, 59–62].

## 4.4 POLYPHENOLS

A broad class of naturally occurring phytochemicals, polyphenols can be found in a variety of plant-based foods, including fruits, vegetables, tea, coffee, and wine. They are secondary metabolites that plants produce to protect themselves against oxidative stress, pathogens, and UV light. Because of their strong anti-inflammatory, cardioprotective, neuroprotective, antioxidant, and anticancer effects, polyphenols have drawn a lot of attention in the field of human health. The presence of one or more aromatic rings with many hydroxyl groups gives polyphenols their structural characteristics and allows them to scavenge free radicals and alter cellular signaling pathways. Nearly 100 mg of polyphenol can be found in a cup of tea, coffee, or a glass of red wine. Cereals, chocolate, and dry beans all raise polyphenol intake [63, 64]. Polyphenols are vital parts of defenses against UV radiation and the aggressiveness of pathogens [65].

Their degree of polymerization, bioavailability, and molecular structure all affect their biological action. A lower incidence of chronic diseases like diabetes, heart disease, and some types of cancer has been linked to dietary consumption of foods high in polyphenols [66, 67]. Due to these positive effects, polyphenols are regarded as essential nutraceutical ingredients that support overall health and disease prevention. Flavonoids, phenolic acids, lignans, tannins, stilbenes, and other polyphenols can be categorized based on their structural variations [68].

### 4.4.1 TYPES OF POLYPHENOLS

Numerous plant species have been shown to have over 8000 different types of polyphenolic chemicals. Phenolic compounds are derived either from phenylalanine, a common metabolic intermediate, or from shikimic acid, a closely related precursor. These compounds usually exist in conjugated forms, where one or more sugar residues, either monosaccharides or polysaccharides, are attached to hydroxyl groups, although they can also be directly bonded to an aromatic carbon. They often form complexes with other molecules such as lipids, amines, carboxylic acids, organic acids, and other phenolic compounds. Based on the number of phenolic rings and the structural linkages connecting them, polyphenols are classified into four major groups: flavonoids, phenolic acids, lignans, and stilbenes [64] (see Figures 4.7 and 4.8).

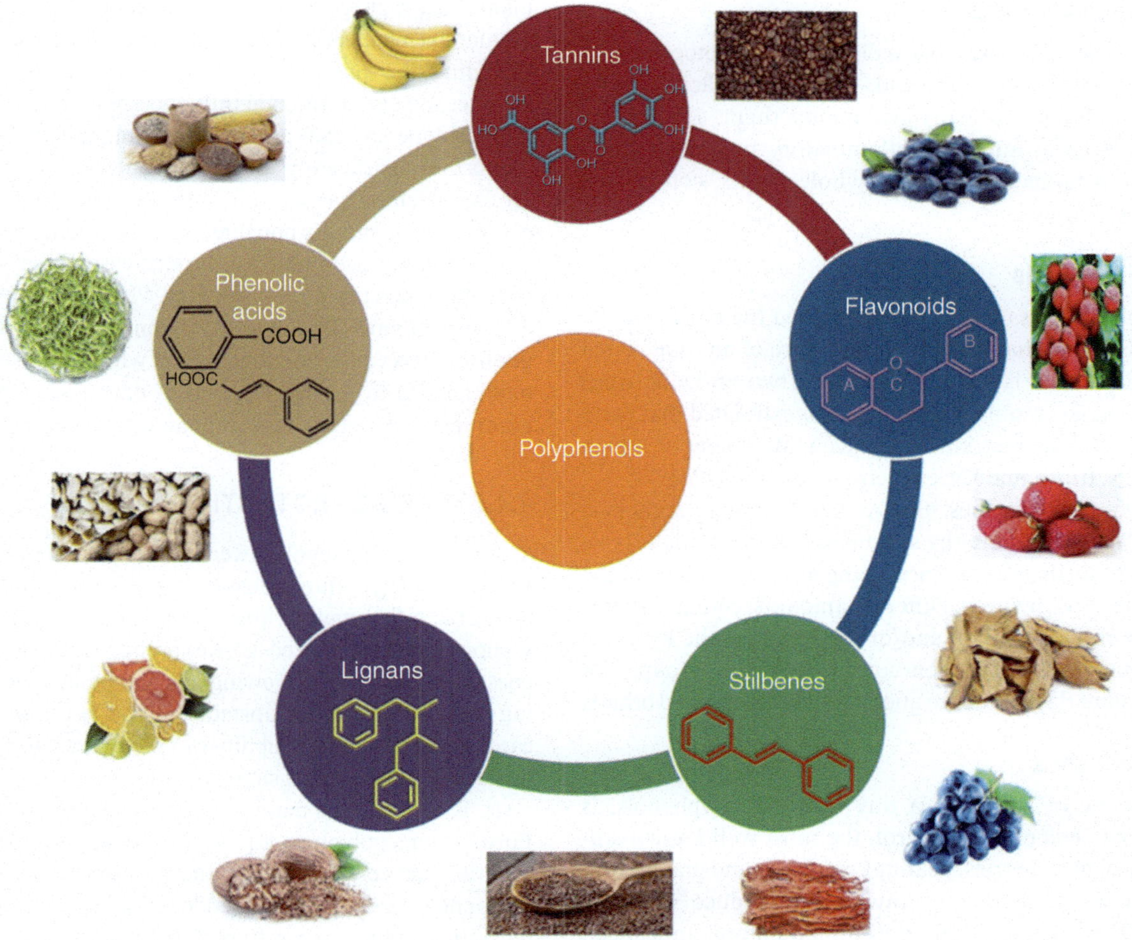


FIGURE 4.7 Occurrence and classification of polyphenols.

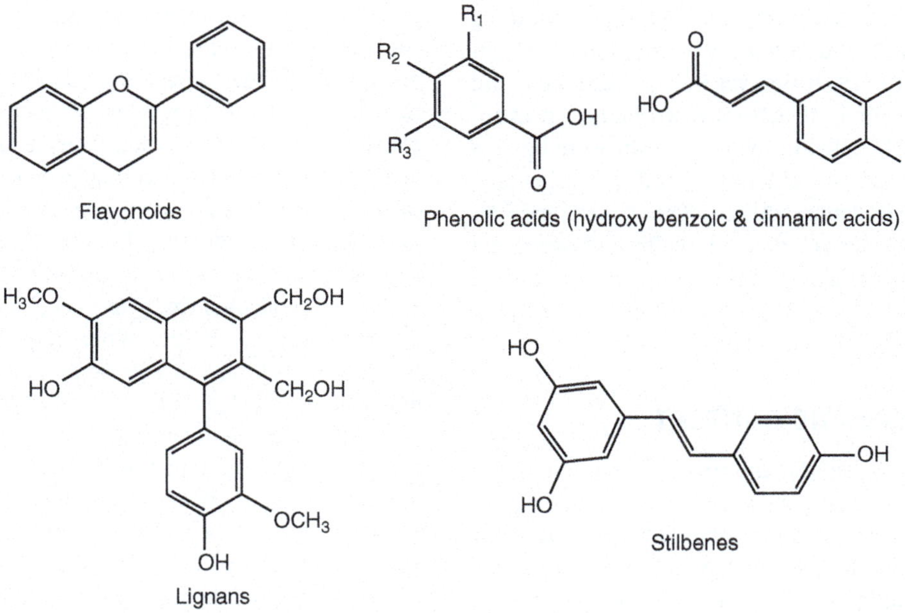


FIGURE 4.8 Structures of polyphenols.

#### 4.4.1.1 Phenolic Acids

The hydroxybenzoic acids (like gallic acid and protocatechuic acid) and hydroxycinnamic acids (like caffeic acid, ferulic acid, and chlorogenic acid) are among them. Known for their antibacterial and anti-inflammatory properties, they are found in large quantities in whole grains, coffee, and berries [69, 70].

#### 4.4.1.2 Flavonoids

The polyphenol class that has been studied the most is flavonoids. This group shares the basic structure of an oxygenated heterocycle, which is formed by joining two aromatic rings with three carbon atoms (Figure 4.2). It is estimated that there are about 4000 distinct kinds of flavonoids, many of which give flowers, fruits, and leaves their lovely colors [71].

Flavonoids, flavones, flavanones, flavanols, anthocyanins, and isoflavones are the six subclasses into which flavonoids can be further divided according to the variations in the heterocyclic type involved. Different amounts, configurations, and levels of glycosylation and/or alkylation of the hydroxyl groups cause individual alterations within each group. The most prevalent flavonoids are quercetin, catechins, and others.

#### 4.4.1.3 Stilbenes

The backbone of stilbenes, a tiny class of polyphenols, is 1,2-diphenylethylene. Resveratrol, the most well-known stilbene, is present in berries, peanuts, red wine, and grapes. Stilbenes modulate signaling pathways and reduce oxidative stress to demonstrate strong anti-inflammatory, anticancer, cardioprotective, and antioxidant activities.

#### 4.4.1.4 Lignans

Lignans are a unique family of polyphenols obtained from plants that are created when two phenylpropanoid units dimerize. They can be found in many different foods, including whole grains, legumes, fruits, vegetables, flaxseeds, and sesame seeds. Due to their structural resemblance to estrogens, intestinal bacteria in the human body transform lignans into enterolignans, such as enterodiol and enterolactone, which have phytoestrogenic activity. The significance of lignan-rich foods in preserving general health and hormonal balance is highlighted by the fact that regular consumption of these foods is linked to a lower risk of hormone-dependent cancer, CVDs, and metabolic disorders [72].

### 4.4.2 OCCURRENCE AND CONTENT

Plant tissue exhibits both cellular and subcellular anomalies in its phenolic distribution. Plant cell vacuoles have soluble phenolics, while cell walls have insoluble phenolics [73]. Although practically all foods include some polyphenols, such as quercetin, foods including cereals, fruits, vegetables, tea, wine, and fruit-based drinks and infusions contain flavanones and isoflavones that are exclusive to specific meals. Complex polyphenol combinations are typically seen in foods. The outer layers of plants have higher phenolic contents than the inner layers [74]. Numerous elements affect the plant's polyphenol content, including the plant's growth stage at harvest, processing, storage, and environmental influences. Rainfall, sun exposure, and soil type are examples of environmental and edaphic elements that significantly affect food's polyphenolic content. The level of ripeness has a major impact on the volumes and concentrations of various polyphenols [75]. Phenolic acid content has frequently been observed to decrease when anthocyanin concentrations rise during ripening. Plants' responses to different types of stress are directly influenced by a variety of polyphenols, especially phenolic acids, which have antibacterial qualities, aid in the lignification of damaged areas, and may become more concentrated after an infection [76].

### 4.4.3 CARDIOPROTECTIVE EFFECT

Consuming polyphenols lowers the risk of coronary heart disease, according to numerous studies [77–79]. Atherosclerosis is a chronic inflammatory illness that is normally manifested in sections of medium-sized arteries prone to lesions. It frequently goes decades without showing any symptoms before developing into conditions like unstable angina, acute MI, or sudden cardiac death [80]. The ability of polyphenols to prevent LDL oxidation, a crucial first step in the development of atherosclerosis, is one of their main anti-atherosclerotic functions [81]. Furthermore, polyphenols protect the cardiovascular system by a variety of complementary mechanisms, including raising HDL cholesterol, improving endothelial function, and exhibiting anti-inflammatory, antiplatelet, and antioxidant properties. Additionally, they might help stabilize preexisting atherosclerotic plaque. For instance, since it inhibits the metalloproteinase-1 (MMP1) expression and prevents plaque interference, quercetin, a polyphenol that is abundant in onions, has been found to have an inverse relationship with the death rate from coronary heart disease [82]. The vascular advantages of polyphenols are further supported by recent research, which shows that they reduce BP, prevent endothelial dysfunction, inhibit platelet aggregation, strengthen endogenous antioxidant defenses, and reduce inflammatory reactions. In particular, tea catechins prevent smooth muscle cells in the arterial wall from migrating and proliferating [83]. In addition, polyphenols have antithrombotic properties by inhibiting platelet aggregation. Red wine or alcohol-free wine consumption reduces platelet activity and bleeding time. When grape juice or red wine is injected into coronary artery stenosis models, thrombosis is reduced [84]. Polyphenols can also reduce the endothelial dysfunction linked to various atherosclerotic risk factors even before plaque formation; indeed, their utility as prognostic indicators for coronary heart disease has been suggested [85]. For example, consumption of 450 ml black tea leads to increased arterial dilation two hours post-ingestion, and administration of 240 ml red wine over 30 days counteracts high-fat diet-induced endothelial dysfunction [86]. Among 218 women over 70 who participated in a cross-sectional study, long-term frequent black tea consumption is connected with decreased

BP. Tea polyphenol biomarker 4-O-methylgallic acid (4OMGA) was excreted; a higher tea intake was linked to a lower BP because it increased 4OMGA excretion. This antihypertensive impact is linked to tea rich in polyphenols, possibly via their antioxidant properties, endothelial support, or estrogen-like activity [82]. Resveratrol, for instance, impedes aggregation of platelets by blocking cyclooxygenase 1 (COX-1) specifically, thereby reducing thromboxane $A_2$ production, platelet clumping, and vasoconstriction [87]. Moreover, resveratrol relaxes isolated arterial and aortic ring preparations; it activates $Ca^{2+}$-activated $K^+$ channels and enhances endothelial nitric oxide signaling, resulting in vasodilation. In summary, the protective actions of dietary polyphenols against CVD are multifaceted, and observational studies, including both case–control and cohort designs, consistently associate polyphenol-rich diets with a reduced risk of MI [88].

## 4.5 CONCLUSION

Natural cardioprotective substances like glycosides, flavonoids, and polyphenols have a great deal of promise to enhance cardiovascular health. They have anti-inflammatory, anti-apoptotic, and antioxidant qualities that make them valuable instruments for the treatment and prevention of cardiovascular diseases. Heart disease risk is lowered by eating a diet rich in flavonoids and polyphenols. Daily consumption of whole grains, nuts, seeds, fruits, and vegetables will maximize the intake of these beneficial compounds. Furthermore, the creation of phytopharmaceuticals and nutraceuticals based on glycosides, flavonoids, and polyphenols presents encouraging opportunities for the treatment and prevention of cardiovascular disorders, including heart failure, atherosclerosis, and hypertension.

## REFERENCES


1. Evans, W.C. (2009). *Trease and Evans Pharmacognosy*, 16e, 27. Edinburgh, New York: Saunders Elsevier.
2. Kokate, C.K., Purohit, A.P., and Gokhale, S.B. (2017). *Pharmacognosy*, 51e. Pune: Nirali Prakashan.
3. Hollman, P.C., Bijsman, M.N., Van Gameren, Y. et al. (1999). The sugar moiety is a major determinant of the absorption of dietary flavonoid glycosides in man. *Free Radic. Res.* 31 (6): 569–573.
4. Xie, L., Deng, Z., Zhang, J. et al. (2022). Comparison of flavonoid O-glycoside, C-glycoside and their aglycones on antioxidant capacity and metabolism during *in vitro* digestion and *in vivo*. *Foods* 11 (6): 882.
5. Wang, X., Zhang, L., and Zhao, Y. (2019). Enzymatic synthesis and application of nucleoside analogs: recent advances. *Front. Chem.* 7: 485.
6. Panova, N.G., Serebryakova, M.V., and Lavrik, O.I. (2022). Nucleoside modifications and their impact on RNA function and metabolism. *Int. J. Mol. Sci.* 23 (9): 5033.
7. Tian, Y., Li, Y., Zhang, S., and Liu, J. (2017). Structural diversity and biological activities of C-glycosides from natural sources. *Phytochem. Rev.* 16 (6): 1091–1115.
8. Dweck, A.C. (2009). The internal and external use of Aloe vera. *Phytother. Res.* 23 (9): 1234–1245.
9. Schwab, W., Fuchs, C., and Huang, F.C. (2018). Transformation of glucosinolates and their degradation products: mechanisms, functions, and applications. *Phytochem. Rev.* 17 (4): 1103–1123.
10. Hirt, H. and Shuman, J. (2019). The chemistry and biochemistry of sulfur-containing glycosides in plants. *Nat. Prod. Rep.* 36 (9): 1284–1303.
11. Klodos, I., Bloch, R., Eichler, J. et al. (2013). A structural view on the functional importance of the sugar moiety and steroid hydroxyls of cardiotonic steroids in binding to Na, K-ATPase. *J. Struct. Biol.* 183 (2): 223–230.
12. Seidel, H. (1997). Cardiac glycosides from plants as potential anticancer agents. *Phytochemistry* 46 (4): 535–543.
13. Ramu, S., Krishna, B.A., and Seshadri, V. (2016). Plant-derived cardiac glycosides: role in heart ailments and cancer management. *Clin. Med. Insights Cardiol.* 10: 1–10.
14. Mebs, D. (2002). Bufadienolides: toxic constituents of toad venoms and their pharmacological effects. *Toxicon* 40 (4): 331–343.
15. Prassas, I. and Diamandis, E.P. (2008). Novel therapeutic applications of cardiac glycosides. *Nat. Rev. Drug Discov.* 7 (11): 926–935.
16. Hostettmann, K. and Marston, A. (1995). *Saponins*. Cambridge: Cambridge University Press.
17. Harborne, J.B. and Baxter, H. (1993). *The Handbook of Natural Flavonoids and Anthraquinones*. Berlin: Springer.
18. Sparg, S.G., Light, M.E., and van Staden, J. (2004). Biological activities and distribution of plant saponins. *J. Ethnopharmacol.* 94 (2–3): 219–243.
19. Man, S., Gao, W., Zhang, Y. et al. (2010). Chemical study and medical application of saponins as anti-cancer agents. *Fitoterapia* 81 (7): 703–714.
20. Gleadow, R.M. and Møller, B.L. (2014). Cyanogenic glycosides: synthesis, physiology, and ecological roles. *Annu. Rev. Plant Biol.* 65: 155–185.
21. Conn, E.E. (1980). Cyanogenic glycosides. *Annu. Rev. Plant Physiol.* 31: 433–451.
22. Fahey, J.W., Zalcmann, A.T., and Talalay, P. (2001). The chemical diversity and distribution of glucosinolates and isothiocyanates among plants. *Phytochemistry* 56 (1): 5–51.
23. Mithen, R. (2001). Glucosinolates—biochemistry, genetics and biological activity. *Plant Growth Regul.* 34 (1): 91–103.
24. Bones, A.M. and Rossiter, J.T. (2006). The enzymic and chemical ecology of glucosinolates. *Plant Sci.* 172 (3): 165–184.
25. Brito-Arias, M. (2016). Glycosides, synthesis and characterization. In: *Synthesis and Characterization of Glycosides*, 1–79. Cham: Springer International Publishing.
26. Levy, D.E. and Tang, C. (ed.) (1995). *The Chemistry of C-Glycosides*, vol. 13. Amsterdam: Elsevier.
27. Mabry, T.J., Markham, K.R., and Thomas, M.B. (1970). *The Systematic Identification of Flavonoids*. New York: Springer-Verlag.
28. Wink, M. (2003). Evolution of secondary metabolites from an ecological and molecular phylogenetic perspective. *Phytochemistry* 64 (1): 3–19.

29. Venugopalan, P. and Jaiswal, R. (2018). Coumarins: chemistry, bioactivities and therapeutic potential. *Nat. Prod. Res.* 32 (22): 2660–2671.

30. Berenbaum, M. (1995). Furanocoumarins: ecological and chemical aspects. *Integr. Comp. Biol.* 35 (6): 234–242.

31. Yang, Y. and Yu, B. (2017). Recent advances in the chemical synthesis of C-glycosides. *Chem. Rev.* 117 (19): 12281–12356.

32. Liu, H.W. (2007). *Glycosidic Bonds and Carbohydrate Chemistry*. New York: Springer.

33. Chaplin, M. and Kennedy, J.F. (2000). *Carbohydrate Chemistry for Biochemists*, 2e. Boca Raton: CRC Press.

34. Voet, D., Voet, J.G., and Pratt, C.W. (2016). *Fundamentals of Biochemistry: Life at the Molecular Level*, 5e. Hoboken: Wiley.

35. Wang, T., Wu, S., Ibrahim, I.A.A., and Fan, L. (2023). Cardioprotective role of swertiamarin, a plant glycoside, against experimentally induced myocardial infarction via antioxidant and anti-inflammatory functions. *Appl. Biochem. Biotechnol.* 195 (9): 5394–5408.

36. Joubert, J.P.J. (2023). Cardiac glycosides. In: *Toxicants of Plant Origin*, 61–96. Boca Raton: CRC Press.

37. Barreca, D., Gattuso, G., Bellocco, E. et al. (2017). Flavanones: citrus phytochemical with health-promoting properties. *Biofactors* 43 (4): 495–506.

38. Hostetler, G.L., Ralston, R.A., and Schwartz, S.J. (2017). Flavones: food sources, bioavailability, metabolism, and bioactivity. *Adv. Nutr.* 8 (3): 423–435.

39. Rakha, A., Umar, N., Rabail, R. et al. (2022). Anti-inflammatory and anti-allergic potential of dietary flavonoids: a review. *Biomed. Pharmacother.* 1 (156): 113945.

40. Godos, J., Romano, G.L., Laudani, S. et al. (2024). Flavan-3-ols and vascular health: clinical evidence and mechanisms of action. *Nutrients* 16 (15): 2471.

41. Sajid, M., Stone, S., and Kaur, P. (2021). Recent advances in heterologous synthesis paving way for future green-modular bioindustries: a review with special reference to isoflavonoids. *Front. Bioeng. Biotechnol.* 9. 673270. http://doi.org/10.3389/fbioe.2021.673270

42. Khoo, H.E., Azlan, A., Tang, S.T., and Lim, S.M. (2017). Anthocyanidins and anthocyanins: colored pigments as food, pharmaceutical ingredients, and the potential health benefits. *Food Nutr. Res.* 61 (1): 1361779.

43. Xu, H., Yu, S., Lin, C. et al. (2024). Roles of flavonoids in ischemic heart disease: cardioprotective effects and mechanisms against myocardial ischemia and reperfusion injury. *Phytomed. Int. J. Phytother. Phytopharm.* 126: 155409.

44. Intharuksa, A., Kuljarusnont, S., Sasaki, Y., and Tungmunnithum, D. (2024). Flavonoids and other polyphenols: bioactive molecules from traditional medicine recipes/medicinal plants and their potential for phytopharmaceutical and medical application. *Molecules* 29(23), 5760. http://www.mdpi.com/1420-3049/29/23/5760.

45. Chibisov, S., Kharlitskaya, E., Singh, R.B. et al. (2022). Chapter 44 – Polyphenolics and flavonoids in health and diseases. In: *Functional Foods and Nutraceuticals in Metabolic and Non-Communicable Diseases* (ed. R.B. Singh, S. Watanabe, and A.A. Isaza), 671–689. Cambridge, MA: Academic Press http://www.sciencedirect.com/science/article/pii/B9780128198155000161.

46. Choy, K.W., Murugan, D., Leong, X.F. et al. (2019). Flavonoids as natural anti-inflammatory agents targeting nuclear factor-kappa B (NFκB) signaling in cardiovascular diseases: a mini review. *Front. Pharmacol.* 10: 1295. http://www.frontiersin.org/journals/pharmacology/articles/10.3389/fphar.2019.01295/full.

47. Schroeter, H., Heiss, C., Balzer, J. et al. (2006). (−)-Epicatechin mediates beneficial effects of flavanol-rich cocoa on vascular function in humans. *Proc. Natl. Acad. Sci. USA* 103 (4): 1024–1029.

48. Hooper, L., Kay, C., Abdelhamid, A. et al. (2021). Effects of chocolate, cocoa, and flavan-3-ols on cardiovascular health. *Am. J. Clin. Nutr.* 113 (6): 1365–1378.

49. Hubbard, G.P., Wolffram, S., Lovegrove, J.A., and Gibbins, J.M. (2004). Ingestion of quercetin inhibits platelet aggregation. *J. Thromb. Haemost.* 2 (12): 2138–2145.

50. Ried, K., Sullivan, T.R., Fakler, P. et al. (2012). Effect of cocoa on blood pressure. *Cochrane Database Syst. Rev.* 8: CD008893.

51. Intharuksa, A., Kuljarusnont, S., Sasaki, Y., and Tungmunnithum, D. (2024). Flavonoids and other polyphenols: bioactive molecules from traditional medicine recipes/medicinal plants and their potential for phytopharmaceutical and medical application. *Molecules* 29 (23): 5760. https://doi.org/10.3390/molecules29235760.

52. Y Liu, J Luo, L Peng, Q Zhang, X Rong, Y Luo, J Li, Flavonoids: potential therapeutic agents for cardiovascular disease, *Heliyon* 2024; 10 (12): 1–15. doi:https://doi.org/10.1016/j.heliyon.2024.e32563.

53. Ciumărnean L, Milaciu MV, Runcan O, Vesa ȘC, Răchișan AL, Negrean V, Perné MG, Donca VI, Alexescu TG, Para I, Dogaru G. The effects of flavonoids in cardiovascular diseases. *Molecules* 2020; 25 (18): 4320. doi:https://doi.org/10.3390/molecules25184320.

54. Mas-Capdevila A, Teichenne J, Domenech-Coca C, Caimari A, Del Bas JM, Escoté X, Crescenti A. Effect of hesperidin on cardiovascular disease risk factors: the role of intestinal microbiota on hesperidin bioavailability. *Nutrients* 2020; 12(5): 1488. doi:https://doi.org/10.3390/nu12051488.

55. Bhargava, P.; Arya, D.; Bhatia, J. Cardioprotective effect of hesperidin in an experimental model of cardiac hypertrophy. *J. Hypertens.* 2019; 37: e183–e184. doi:https://doi.org/10.1097/01.hjh.0000572356.32275.f4

56. Liobikas J., Skemiene K., Trumbeckaite S., Borutaite V., Anthocyanins in cardioprotection: a path through mitochondria, *Pharmacol. Res.* 2016, 113; (Pt B): 808–815. doi:https://doi.org/10.1016/j.phrs.2016.03.036.

57. P. Bharathy, P.V. Thanikachalam, Pharmacological relevance of anthocyanin derivative: a review. *Pharmacol. Res. Mod. Chin. Med.* 2025; 14; 100565. doi:https://doi.org/10.1016/j.prmcm.2024.100565.

58. Bhardwaj P, Khanna D. Green tea catechins: defensive role in cardiovascular disorders. *Chin. J. Nat. Med.* 2013; 11(4): 345–353. doi:https://doi.org/10.1016/S1875-5364(13)60051-5.

59. L. Rajan, A. Radhakrishnan, K.N. Alagarsamy, A. Srivastava, S. Dhingra, A. Booker, V. Rolfe, D. Palaniswamy, S.K. Mohankumar, Green tea polyphenols in cardiometabolic health: a critical appraisal on phytogenomics towards personalized green tea, *PharmaNutrition* 2022; 20, 100296 doi:https://doi.org/10.1016/j.phanu.2022.100296.

60. Armand, M., William, M., and Giulio, T. (2017). EEG differentiation analysis and stimulus set meaningfulness. *Front. Psychol.* 8: 1748. https://doi.org/10.3389/fpsyg.2017.01748.

61. Luo Y, Shang P, Li D. Luteolin: a flavonoid that has multiple cardioprotective effects and its molecular mechanisms. *Front. Pharmacol.* 2017, 6; 8: 692. doi:https://doi.org/10.3389/fphar.2017.00692.

62. Chen Z, Zhang SL. The role of flavonoids in the prevention and management of cardiovascular complications: a narrative review. *Ann. Palliat. Med.* 2021; 10(7): 8254–8263. doi:https://doi.org/10.21037/apm-21-1343.

63. Scalbert, A., Manach, C., Morand, C., and Remesy, C. (2005). Dietary polyphenols and the prevention of diseases. *Crit. Rev. Food Sci. Nutr.* 45: 287–306.

64. Spencer, J.P.E., Abd El Mohsen, M.M., Minihane, A.M., and Mathers, J.C. (2008). Biomarkers of the intake of dietary polyphenols: strengths, limitations and applications in nutrition research. *Br. J. Nutr.* 99 (1): 12–22.
65. Beckman, C.H. (2000). Phenolic-storing cells: keys to programmed cell death and periderm formation in wilt disease resistance and in general defence responses in plants? *Physiol. Mol. Plant Pathol.* 57 (3): 101–110.
66. Graf, B.A., Milbury, P.E., and Blumberg, J.B. (2005). Flavonols, flavones, flavanones and human health: epidemiological evidence. *J. Med. Food* 8 (3): 281–290.
67. Arts, I.C.W. and Hollman, P.C.H. (2005). Polyphenols and disease risk in epidemiologic studies. *Am. J. Clin. Nutr.* 81 (1): 317–325.
68. Grosso, G. (2018). Effects of polyphenol-rich foods on human health. *Nutrients* 10 (8): 1089.
69. Mattila, P., Pihlava, J.M., and Hellström, J. (2005). Contents of phenolic acids, alkyl- and alkenylresorcinols, and avenanthramides in commercial grain products. *J. Agric. Food Chem.* 53 (21): 8290–8295.
70. Shahidi, F. and Naczk, M. (1995). *Food Phenolics: Sources, Chemistry, Effects, Applications*. Lancaster, PA: Technomic Publishing Co Inc.
71. De Groot, H. and Rauen, U. (1998). Tissue injury by reactive oxygen species and the protective effects of flavonoids. *Fundam. Clin. Pharmacol.* 12 (3): 249–255.
72. Adlercreutz, H., Mazur, W., and Rauen, U. (1997). Phyto-oestrogens and western diseases. *Ann. Med.* 29 (2): 95–120.
73. Wink, M. (1997). Compartmentation of secondary metabolites and xenobiotics in plant vacuoles. *Adv. Bot. Res.* 25: 141–169.
74. Simon, B.F., Perez-Ilzarbe, J., Hernandez, T. et al. (1992). Importance of phenolic compounds for the characterization of fruit juices. *J. Agric. Food Sci.* 40: 1531–1535.
75. Manach, C., Scalbert, A., Morand, C. et al. (2004). Polyphenols: food sources and bioavailability. *Am. J. Clin. Nutr.* 70 (3): 727–749.
76. Sosulski, F.W., Krygier, K., and Hogge, L. (1982). Importance of phenolic compounds for the characterization of fruit juices. *J. Agric. Food Chem.* 30: 337–340.
77. Renaud, S. and de Lorgeril, M. (1992). Wine, alcohol, platelets, and the French paradox for coronary heart disease. *Lancet* 339: 1523–1526.
78. Dubick, M.A. and Omaye, S.T. (2001). Evidence for grape, wine, and tea polyphenols as modulators of atherosclerosis and ischemic heart disease in humans. *J. Nutraceut. Funct. Med. Foods* 3: 67–93.
79. Nardini, M., Natella, F., and Scaccini, C. (2007). Role of dietary polyphenols in platelet aggregation: a review of the supplementation studies. *Platelets* 18 (3): 224–243.
80. Vita, J.A. (2005). Polyphenols and cardiovascular disease: effects on endothelial and platelet function. *Am. J. Clin. Nutr.* 81 (1): 292–297.
81. Aviram, M., Dornfeld, L., Rosenblat, M. et al. (2000). Pomegranate juice consumption reduces oxidative stress, atherogenic modifications to LDL, and platelet aggregation: studies in humans and in atherosclerotic apolipoprotein E-deficient mice. *Am. J. Clin. Nutr.* 71 (5): 1062–1076.
82. Garcia-Lafuente, A., Guillamón, E., Villares, A. et al. (2009). Flavonoids as anti-inflammatory agents: implications in cancer and cardiovascular disease. *Inflamm. Res.* 58 (9): 537–552.
83. Maeda, K., Kuzuya, M., Cheng, X.W. et al. (2003). Green tea catechins inhibit the cultured smooth muscle cell invasion through the basement membrane. *Atherosclerosis* 166 (1): 23–30.
84. Demrow, H.S., Slane, P.R., and Folts, J.D. (1995). Administration of wine and grape juice inhibits *in vivo* platelet activity and thrombosis in stenosed canine coronary arteries. *Circulation* 91 (4): 1182–1188.
85. Schachinger, V., Britten, M.B., and Zeiher, A.M. (2002). Prognostic impact of coronary vasodilator dysfunction on adverse long-term outcome of coronary heart disease. *Circulation* 101 (16): 1899–1906.
86. Duffy, S.J., Keaney, J.F. Jr., Holbrook, M. et al. (2001). Short- and long-term black tea consumption reverses endothelial dysfunction in patients with coronary artery disease. *Circulation* 104 (2): 151–156.
87. Pirola, L. and Frojdo, S. (2008). Resveratrol: one molecule, many targets. *IUBMB Life* 60 (6): 323–332.
88. Harikumar, K.B. and Aggarwal, B.B. (2008). Resveratrol: a multi-targeted agent for age-associated chronic disease. *Cell Cycle* 7 (8): 1020–1035.
89. Kondratyuk, T.P. and Pezzuto, J.M. (2004). Natural product polyphenols of relevance to human health. *Pharm. Biol.* 42 (1): 46–63.

CHAPTER 5

# Herbal Antihypertensives: Mechanisms and Clinical Evidence

Garlanka Venkata Naga Kiranmayi[1], N. Harikrishnan[1], Long Chiau Ming[2], and Karumanchi Srikanth[3]

[1] *Department of Pharmacology, Faculty of Pharmacy, Dr. M.G.R. Educational and Research Institute, Chennai, Tamil Nadu, India*

[2] *School of Medical and Life Sciences, Sunway University, Sunway City, Malaysia*

[3] *Institute of Pharmaceutical Sciences and Research for Girls, Dattakala Shikshan Sanstha's Institute of Pharmaceutical Science & Research, Dr. Babasaheb Ambedkar Technical University, Pune, Maharashtra, India*

## 5.1 INTRODUCTION

### 5.1.1 GLOBAL BURDEN AND CLINICAL IMPORTANCE OF HYPERTENSION

Globally, it affects over one billion people, and its prevalence increases due to aging populations, urbanization, sedentary lifestyles, and dietary changes [1–3]. The disease is often asymptomatic, earning it the label "the silent killer," and is implicated in the pathogenesis of heart attacks, strokes, chronic kidney disease, and heart failure [4, 5].

### 5.1.2 CURRENT THERAPEUTIC APPROACHES AND THEIR CHALLENGES

These demonstrated effectiveness in lowering blood pressure and reducing cardiovascular risk (Table 5.1) [6, 7]. Despite this, optimal blood pressure control remains elusive for many patients. Factors such as drug intolerance, side effects, high treatment costs, and poor adherence contribute to therapeutic failure [8, 9]. Side effects such as chronic cough with angiotensin-converting enzyme (ACE) inhibitors, electrolyte imbalances with diuretics, and fatigue or sexual dysfunction with beta-blockers negatively impact quality of life and compliance [10]. Furthermore, in low-resource settings, limited access to medications and healthcare infrastructure complicate disease management [11]. These challenges necessitate exploring alternative and adjunct therapeutic options.

### 5.1.3 HISTORICAL AND CONTEMPORARY USE OF HERBAL ANTIHYPERTENSIVES

Traditional medicine systems across the world have long utilized medicinal plants for cardiovascular ailments, including hypertension [12]. Phytochemical constituents like flavonoids, phenolic acids, alkaloids, terpenoids, and saponins exhibit diverse pharmacodynamic properties [13]. Mechanistic studies show these compounds can induce vasodilation by enhancing nitric oxide bioavailability, inhibit ACE activity, exert diuretic effects, modulate calcium channels, and possess antioxidant and anti-inflammatory properties [14, 15].

### 5.1.4 INCREASING SCIENTIFIC VALIDATION AND INTEGRATION INTO MODERN THERAPY

In recent decades, scientific research has increasingly focused on validating the antihypertensive effects of medicinal plants through rigorous investigations. Randomized trials indicated blood pressure-lowering effects for garlic (*Allium sativum*), hibiscus (*Hibiscus sabdariffa*), arjuna (*Terminalia arjuna*), and rauwolfia (*Rauwolfia serpentina*) [16–18]. These findings have fueled interest in integrating herbal antihypertensives into mainstream medicine, particularly as adjuncts to conventional drugs or as accessible alternatives in resource-limited settings [19]. However, challenges remain regarding standardization, dosage optimization, herb–drug interactions, and regulatory oversight [20]. This chapter aims to comprehensively review the pharmacological mechanisms, clinical evidence, and future prospects of herbal antihypertensives to provide a scientific basis for their application in hypertension management.

## 5.2 PATHOPHYSIOLOGY OF HYPERTENSION

### 5.2.1 REGULATION OF BLOOD PRESSURE: AN INTEGRATED PHYSIOLOGICAL PERSPECTIVE

It is primarily governed by two closely linked parameters: cardiac output and systemic vascular resistance [21, 22]. Additionally, the kidneys serve a pivotal function in maintaining long-term blood pressure homeostasis. They achieve this by modulating glomerular filtration, tubular reabsorption, and secretion processes [23]. Endocrine systems operate synergistically that influence vasomotor tone and sodium retention, with hormones such as angiotensin II and aldosterone playing critical roles in vascular constriction and fluid balance [24].

**Table 5.1** Management of hypertension.

| Management of hypertension | Details |
|---|---|
| Lifestyle modifications | Diet changes, exercise, weight control, reduced salt intake |
| Pharmacological treatment | – |
| First-line drugs | Common classes of antihypertensive agents include diuretics, ACE inhibitors, angiotensin II receptor blockers (ARBs), calcium channel blockers, and beta-adrenergic antagonists |

### 5.2.2 PATHOGENIC MECHANISMS CONTRIBUTING TO HYPERTENSION

Hypertension develops when the finely tuned equilibrium between vasodilatory and vasoconstrictive forces becomes disrupted, resulting in sustained elevation of arterial pressure. This multifactorial condition involves several overlapping pathophysiological pathways.

**Endothelial dysfunction:** The blood vessel lining, called the endothelium, generates nitric oxide (NO), which helps relax the surrounding smooth muscle, leading to vessel widening and proper vascular function. In hypertension, excessive oxidative molecules interact with NO, lowering its levels by producing harmful peroxynitrite, which in turn damages the endothelial cells. This impairment leads to reduced vasodilatory capacity, increased vascular resistance, and promotes a pro-thrombotic and pro-inflammatory environment [25, 26].

### 5.2.3 RENIN-ANGIOTENSIN-ALDOSTERONE SYSTEM

It is an important cascade that monitors vascular tone and fluid homeostasis. It is triggered when blood flow to the kidneys diminishes or when there is increased sympathetic nervous activity (Figure 5.1) [27, 28].

**Sympathetic nervous system (SNS) overactivity:** Elevated sympathetic tone increases heart rate and peripheral vasoconstriction through α- and β-adrenergic receptor stimulation. Chronic sympathetic overactivity also induces structural vascular changes, contributing to arterial stiffness and sustained hypertension [29, 30].

**Oxidative stress and inflammatory processes:** Reactive oxygen species (ROS) interact with NO, reducing its vasodilatory effects and promoting inflammatory signaling cascades involving cytokines and adhesion molecules [31, 32].

**Disrupted calcium homeostasis in vascular smooth muscle:** Intracellular calcium ions serve as critical secondary messengers in vascular smooth muscle contraction. In hypertension, increased calcium leads to sustained contraction and increased vascular tone. Dysregulated

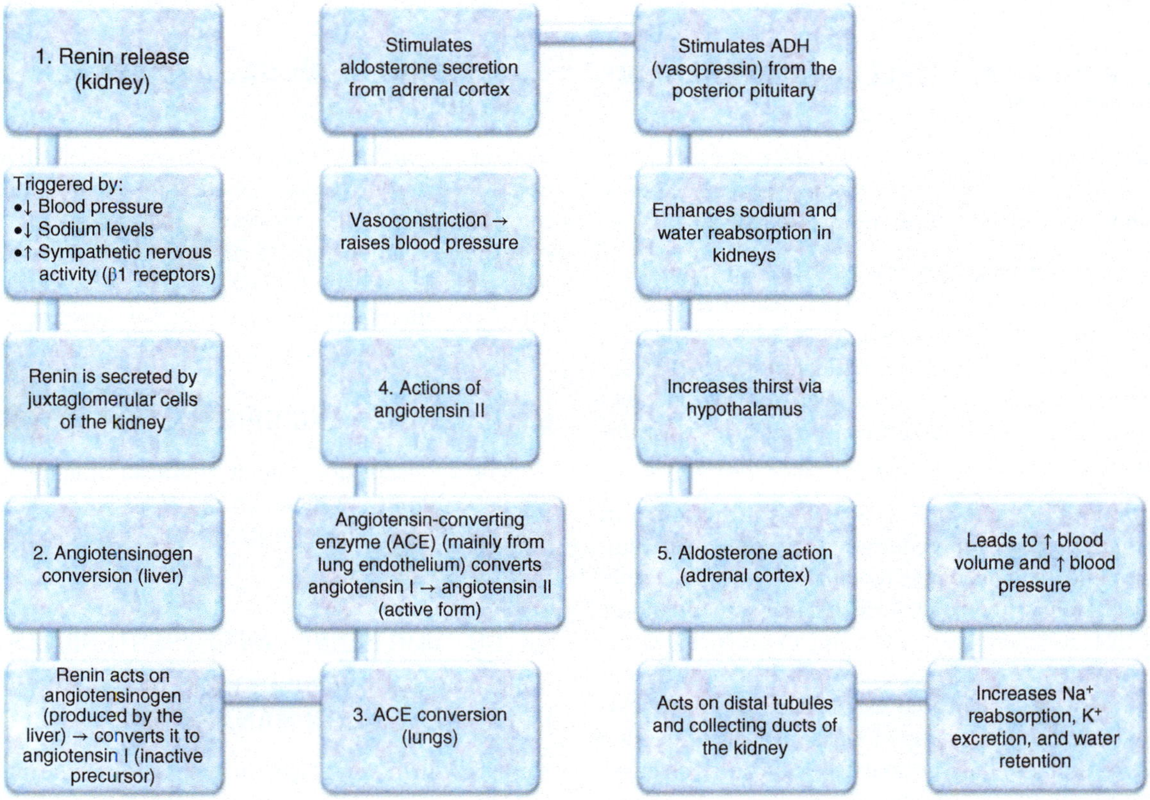


**FIGURE 5.1** Renin-angiotensin-aldosterone system (RAAS).

calcium signaling is therefore a key contributor to elevated peripheral resistance [33, 34].

**Genetic and environmental interactions:** Genetic predispositions influencing salt sensitivity, vascular reactivity, and neurohormonal regulation interact with factors such as excessive dietary salt, chronic stress, obesity, and lack of physical activity significantly contributing to the creation a complex etiological framework for hypertension [35, 36].

## 5.3 THERAPEUTIC IMPLICATIONS OF HYPERTENSION PATHOPHYSIOLOGY

The multifactorial nature of hypertension necessitates therapeutic strategies that can target multiple pathways simultaneously. Conventional drug classes exert their effects through modulation of distinct physiological mechanisms [37]. However, these agents often act on singular pathways, which may limit efficacy or cause compensatory mechanisms that undermine treatment.

Herbal antihypertensives frequently possess multiple bioactive constituents capable of interacting with diverse physiological targets. Their multifaceted modes of action include enhancing endothelial function, scavenging ROS, modulating renin-angiotensin-aldosterone system (RAAS) activity, promoting diuresis, and regulating calcium channels, thereby offering a holistic approach to blood pressure control with potentially fewer side effects [38, 39]. Such pleiotropic effects provide a rationale for their exploration and integration into hypertension management, especially in populations with limited access to conventional medicines.

### 5.3.1 MOLECULAR AND CELLULAR MECHANISMS IN HYPERTENSION

At the molecular level, hypertension involves complex alterations in cellular signaling pathways that govern vascular tone, inflammation, and structural remodeling.

**Endothelial cell dysfunction:** Besides decreased nitric oxide (NO) production, endothelial cells in hypertensive states exhibit reduced synthesis of other vasodilators such as prostacyclin and endothelium-derived hyperpolarizing factor (EDHF), coupled with increased secretion of vasoconstrictors like endothelin-1 [40–42]. The imbalance between these factors disrupts normal vascular relaxation and promotes vasoconstriction.

**Vascular smooth muscle cell (VSMC) dysfunction and remodeling:** VSMCs not only contract to regulate vessel diameter but also undergo phenotypic modulation in hypertension. When exposed to harmful conditions, vascular smooth muscle cells alter their function from contracting to producing structural components. This change promotes their growth and movement, as well as increased extracellular matrix (ECM) creation, which causes the arterial walls to thicken, develop fibrous tissue, and lose their normal elasticity. These changes, collectively referred to as vascular remodeling, help sustain high vascular resistance. Signaling molecules, including mitogen-activated protein kinases (MAPKs) and Rho kinase, assist in mediating these phenotypic alterations [43–45].

**Inflammation and immune system activation:** Infiltration of immune cells such as macrophages, T cells, and dendritic cells into vascular and renal tissues causes damage to the endothelium and enhances vasoconstriction [46, 47].

**Stress and redox signaling:** Free radicals in vascular tissues originate mainly from nicotinamide adenine dinucleotide phosphate (NADPH) oxidases, mitochondria, and uncoupled endothelial nitric oxide synthase (eNOS). ROS modulate signaling cascades that regulate vascular tone and remodeling, but excessive ROS cause oxidative damage to lipids, proteins, and DNA and impair NO bioavailability, which upregulates inflammatory genes [48, 49].

### 5.3.2 VASCULAR REMODELING AND ARTERIAL STIFFNESS

Chronic hypertension induces structural changes in blood vessels, collectively referred to as vascular remodeling. This process involves:

**Medial hypertrophy:** Thickening of the smooth muscle layer due to increased VSMC size and number.

**Reduced lumen diameter:** Narrowing of arteries increases resistance to blood flow.

These changes impair arterial compliance and contribute to increased pulse pressure and cardiac afterload, which exacerbate cardiac hypertrophy and heart failure risk [50, 51].

### 5.3.3 NEUROHORMONAL AND RENAL CONTRIBUTIONS

Enhanced sympathetic nerve activity stimulates renin release and directly promotes vasoconstriction. Additionally, kidneys may retain sodium excessively due to altered pressure–natriuresis relationships, further increasing plasma volume and systemic pressure [52]. Dysregulation of natriuretic peptides, endothelin, and other vasoactive substances also contributes to maladaptive blood pressure elevation [53].

### 5.3.4 GENETIC AND EPIGENETIC FACTORS

Genetic predisposition plays a significant role in an individual's susceptibility to hypertension [54]. These include genes coding for components of RAAS, ion channels, and vascular growth factors [55].

## 5.4 COMMON HERBAL ANTIHYPERTENSIVES

### 5.4.1 OVERVIEW OF HERBAL REMEDIES IN HYPERTENSION MANAGEMENT

Herbal medicine has played an integral role in the management of hypertension across various traditional healthcare systems globally. These systems employ an array of botanicals with

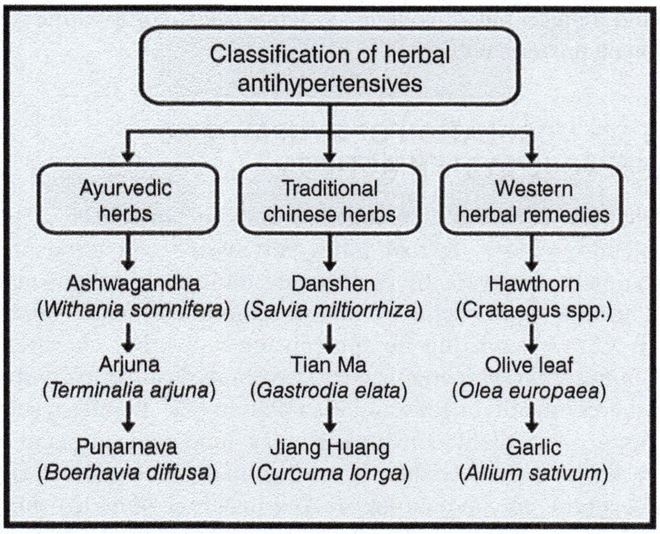


**FIGURE 5.2** Classification of herbal antihypertensives.

blood pressure-lowering properties, often used in combination to achieve synergistic effects. The resurgence of interest in herbal antihypertensives is fueled by their accessibility, cultural familiarity, lower cost, and the perception of a better safety profile compared to synthetic drugs [56, 57].

These phytochemicals, such as flavonoids, alkaloids, saponins, tannins, terpenoids, and phenolic acids, constitute the bioactive constituents and are believed to be the main contributors to the medicinal properties (Figure 5.2). These compounds modulate multiple targets, including endothelial function, oxidative stress pathways, neurohormonal systems, and vascular smooth muscle tone, thus offering a holistic approach to blood pressure regulation [58]. Understanding the specific herbs and their mechanistic actions lays the foundation for integrating traditional knowledge with modern pharmacotherapy.

***A. sativum*** **(garlic)**

Garlic is used to treat cardiovascular diseases, including hypertension. The bulb contains sulfur-containing compounds, primarily allicin, which is formed enzymatically when fresh garlic is crushed or chopped. Other active molecules include S-allyl cysteine and ajoene, which contribute to garlic's pharmacological properties [59].

The antihypertensive effect of garlic is multifactorial, causing NO release [60]. Additionally, garlic compounds exhibit ACE inhibitory activity, decreasing the generation of the potent vasoconstrictor [61]. Garlic's antioxidant properties help neutralize ROS, protect the endothelium from oxidative damage, and preserve its vasodilatory function [62].

The magnitude of BP reduction ranges approximately between 5 and 10 mmHg, which is clinically relevant and comparable to some conventional antihypertensive drugs. Furthermore, garlic exhibits antiplatelet and lipid-lowering effects, which may contribute to its overall cardiovascular protective profile.

***Hibiscus sabdariffa*** **(roselle)**

*H. sabdariffa*, commonly known as roselle or sour tea, is widely consumed as an herbal infusion. Its calyces are rich in bioactive anthocyanins, flavonoids, and organic acids such as hibiscus acid, which impart antioxidant and vasodilatory properties [63].

Mechanistic studies show that hibiscus extract improves endothelial function by increasing NO bioavailability and reducing oxidative stress. It also exhibits mild diuretic activity, facilitating sodium and water excretion, which contributes to reduced blood volume and pressure. Moreover, hibiscus compounds inhibit calcium influx in vascular smooth muscle, decreasing vasoconstriction.

***T. arjuna***

The bark contains flavonoids, tannins, glycosides, and triterpenoids, which contribute to its pharmacological actions [64].

The antihypertensive effect of *T. arjuna* is attributed to its antioxidant activity, which mitigates oxidative stress-induced endothelial dysfunction. It also modulates the RAAS by downregulating ACE activity. Furthermore, *T. arjuna* improves myocardial contractility and cardiac output, which may enhance overall cardiovascular function in hypertensive patients.

*T. arjuna* bark extract results in meaningful reductions in systolic and diastolic pressures, alongside improvements in lipid profiles and cardiac biomarkers, indicating its potential as a cardioprotective agent.

***R. serpentina***

Historically significant as one of the earliest plant sources of antihypertensive agents, *R. serpentina* contains the alkaloid reserpine. Reserpine acts by irreversibly blocking vesicular monoamine transporters (VMAT), leading to depletion of catecholamines such as norepinephrine from sympathetic nerve endings. This reduction in sympathetic tone results in decreased heart rate and vasodilation, lowering blood pressure [65].

Despite its proven efficacy, reserpine's use has declined due to side effects, including sedation and depression. Nevertheless, *R. serpentina* remains relevant in traditional medicine, and ongoing research explores its other alkaloids for safer therapeutic alternatives.

### 5.4.2 ADDITIONAL NOTEWORTHY HERBS

Several other herbs have garnered scientific interest for their antihypertensive potential:

**Olive leaf (*Olea europaea*):** Exhibits antioxidant and vasodilatory action by enhancing endothelial function and inhibiting ACE [66].

**Green tea (*Camellia sinensis*):** Green tea supports vascular health through antioxidant activity, improved nitric oxide production, and modulation of lipid metabolism [67].

**Celery seed (*Apium graveolens*):** Traditionally used as a mild diuretic and vasodilator, celery seed contains phthalides, which relax vascular smooth muscle and reduce peripheral resistance [68].

**Ginger (*Zingiber officinale*):** Exhibits calcium channel blocking effects, antioxidant properties, and inhibits platelet aggregation, contributing to its antihypertensive actions [69].

## 5.5 PHARMACOLOGICAL MECHANISMS OF HERBAL ANTIHYPERTENSIVES (Table 5.2)

### 5.5.1 ENHANCEMENT OF ENDOTHELIAL FUNCTION AND NITRIC OXIDE BIOAVAILABILITY

Many herbal antihypertensives exert their beneficial effects by restoring or enhancing endothelial function, primarily through the upregulation of eNOS activity and increased NO bioavailability.

Phytochemicals such as flavonoids and polyphenols present in plants like garlic (*A. sativum*), hibiscus (*H. sabdariffa*), and green tea (*C. sinensis*) have been shown to activate intracellular signaling pathways (e.g., Phosphoinositide 3-kinase [PI3K/Akt]) that stimulate eNOS phosphorylation, thereby boosting NO synthesis [70]. Additionally, these compounds protect NO from oxidative degradation by scavenging ROS [70]. This dual action of stimulating NO production and preventing its breakdown helps to restore vasodilation capacity in hypertensive patients, whose endothelial function is often impaired due to oxidative stress and inflammation [70].

### 5.5.2 INHIBITION OF RAAS

It acts as a cornerstone for the regulation of blood pressure, mediating vasoconstriction, sodium retention, and fluid balance [71]. For example, *T. arjuna* bark and olive leaf extracts contain bioactive molecules that inhibit ACE activity, leading to vasodilation and diuresis [71]. Additionally, hibiscus compounds interfere with angiotensin II receptor signaling, further dampening vasoconstrictive responses [71]. By modulating RAAS, these herbs alleviate vascular resistance and reduce blood volume, synergistically contributing to blood pressure reduction.

### 5.5.3 MODULATION OF SYMPATHETIC NERVOUS SYSTEM ACTIVITY

Heightened SNS activity contributes significantly to elevated blood pressure. Herbal antihypertensives can attenuate sympathetic overactivity through multiple mechanisms. The alkaloid reserpine from *R. serpentina* irreversibly binds to VMAT, depleting norepinephrine and other catecholamines from sympathetic nerve terminals, leading to diminished sympathetic tone and vasodilation [72]. Besides reserpine, other plant constituents may modulate adrenergic receptor activity, either by antagonizing beta-adrenergic receptors or modulating neurotransmitter release, thus reducing vasoconstriction and cardiac workload [72]. This mechanism is particularly useful in managing neurogenic hypertension.

### 5.5.4 CALCIUM CHANNEL BLOCKADE LEADING TO VASCULAR SMOOTH MUSCLE RELAXATION

Intracellular calcium levels in vascular smooth muscle cells directly regulate their contractile state. Voltage-gated calcium channels allow influx of extracellular calcium, triggering muscle contraction and vasoconstriction. Several herbal constituents act as natural calcium channel blockers, reducing calcium influx and promoting vasodilation [73]. Phytochemicals such as gingerols from *Z. officinale*, phthalides from celery seed (*A. graveolens*), and flavonoids from diverse plants inhibit calcium-related channels, mimicking the mechanism of conventional calcium channel blocker drugs [73]. This results in decreased intracellular calcium concentration, muscle relaxation, reduced peripheral resistance, and subsequent blood pressure lowering [73].

**Table 5.2** Mechanism of herbal antihypertensives.

| Herbal source | Proposed antihypertensive mechanism(s) | Key active compounds |
|---|---|---|
| Garlic (*Allium sativum*) | ACE inhibition, vasodilation, antioxidant effects | Allicin, S-allyl cysteine |
| Rauvolfia (*Rauvolfia serpentina*) | Central adrenergic inhibition, reduction in peripheral resistance | Reserpine |
| Hibiscus (*Hibiscus sabdariffa*) | Diuretic action, vasorelaxation via nitric oxide pathways | Anthocyanins, hibiscus acid |
| Olive leaf (*Olea europaea*) | Calcium channel blockade, antioxidant activity | Oleuropein, hydroxytyrosol |
| Green tea (*Camellia sinensis*) | Endothelial function improvement, ACE inhibition | Catechins (EGCG), theaflavins |
| Celery (*Apium graveolens*) | Diuretic action, vasodilation via calcium channel modulation | Phthalides |
| Indian snakeroot (*Rauvolfia tetraphylla*) | Sympathetic nerve inhibition, long-term blood pressure reduction | Ajmaline, rescinnamine |
| Turmeric (*Curcuma longa*) | Anti-inflammatory effects, modulation of endothelial function | Curcumin |
| Ginger (*Zingiber officinale*) | Calcium channel blockade, inhibition of angiotensin II | Gingerols, shogaols |
| Fenugreek (*Trigonella foenum-graecum*) | Diuretic action, insulin-sensitization, lipid-lowering effects | Saponins, 4-hydroxyisoleucine |

### 5.5.5 DIURETIC EFFECTS AND REGULATION OF FLUID BALANCE

Volume overload is a common contributor to hypertension, especially in salt-sensitive individuals. Herbal diuretics facilitate the excretion of excess sodium and water, reducing plasma volume and cardiac preload. Hibiscus and celery seed are notable for their mild diuretic properties. Their phytoconstituents enhance renal excretion of sodium by influencing tubular transport mechanisms, including inhibition of sodium reabsorption in the distal nephron [74]. Unlike potent synthetic diuretics, these herbal agents often maintain potassium balance by sparing potassium or promoting its retention, reducing the risk of electrolyte imbalances and associated side effects [74].

### 5.5.6 ANTI-INFLAMMATORY AND ANTIOXIDANT PROPERTIES

Many herbal antihypertensives are rich sources of antioxidants such as polyphenols, flavonoids, and phenolic acids that scavenge ROS and reduce oxidative damage [75].

For instance, green tea catechins, garlic sulfur compounds, and *T. arjuna* flavonoids enhance endogenous antioxidant enzyme activities, including superoxide dismutase (SOD), catalase, and glutathione peroxidase [75]. These actions not only neutralize ROS, thereby suppressing inflammatory cytokine production [75].

By attenuating oxidative stress and inflammation, these herbs preserve endothelial integrity, improve vasodilatory function, and inhibit maladaptive vascular remodeling, all of which contribute to blood pressure normalization.

### 5.5.7 MODULATION OF ION CHANNELS BEYOND CALCIUM

In addition to calcium channels, potassium and sodium ion channels regulate excitability and contractility. Stimulation of potassium channels causes hyperpolarization of the smooth muscle cell membrane.

Certain flavonoids and polyphenols found in herbs activate potassium channels, causing vasodilation and blood pressure reduction [76]. Additionally, inhibition of sodium channels or modulation of cyclic nucleotide signaling pathways (cyclic adenosine monophosphate [cAMP], cyclic guanosine monophosphate [cGMP]) by herbal compounds can further facilitate vascular smooth muscle relaxation and enhance antihypertensive effects [76].

### 5.5.8 SYNERGISTIC AND MULTI-TARGETED ACTIONS OF HERBAL ANTIHYPERTENSIVES

A distinctive feature of herbal antihypertensives is their ability to simultaneously modulate multiple molecular targets and physiological pathways involved in blood pressure regulation. This polypharmacology arises from the complex mixtures of bioactive compounds present in whole plant extracts, including alkaloids, flavonoids, terpenoids, phenolic acids, and glycosides [77].

The synergy among these constituents can potentiate antihypertensive effects through complementary mechanisms. For example, one compound may enhance endothelial NO production, while another may inhibit ACE activity, and a third may exert antioxidant effects. This combinatorial action often results in improved efficacy compared to isolated single compounds [77].

Such multi-targeted activity is especially advantageous in addressing the multifactorial nature of hypertension, which involves vascular, renal, neurohormonal, and inflammatory dysregulation. Moreover, these broad mechanisms may reduce the likelihood of drug resistance and adverse effects commonly seen with conventional monotherapy [77].

### 5.5.9 MODULATION OF VASCULAR REMODELING AND EXTRACELLULAR MATRIX

Chronic hypertension induces structural changes in blood vessels, termed vascular remodeling, which includes thickening of the vessel wall, fibrosis, and altered ECM composition. These changes increase vascular stiffness and perpetuate elevated blood pressure [78].

Certain herbal compounds modulate enzymes involved in ECM turnover, such as matrix metalloproteinases (MMPs), and inhibit profibrotic signaling pathways. For example, flavonoids from *T. arjuna* and polyphenols from olive leaf extract suppress MMP overexpression [78]. By attenuating remodeling, these herbs preserve arterial elasticity and improve long-term blood pressure control.

### 5.5.10 NEUROPROTECTIVE EFFECTS AND CENTRAL BLOOD PRESSURE REGULATION

Emerging evidence suggests that some herbal antihypertensives exert neuroprotective actions that influence blood pressure modulation. Oxidative stress and inflammation of brainstem areas controlling sympathetic outflow can exacerbate hypertension [79]. Herbs such as *R. serpentina* and *Withania somnifera* (Ashwagandha) contain neuroactive constituents that modulate neurotransmitter levels, reduce neuroinflammation, and promote neurogenesis [79]. Such central mechanisms complement peripheral vascular effects, providing a more holistic antihypertensive action.

### 5.5.11 SAFETY ASSESSMENT, TOXICOLOGICAL EVALUATION, AND INTERACTIONS BETWEEN HERBS AND MEDICATIONS (Table 5.3)

While herbal antihypertensives are generally perceived as safe due to their natural origin, it is critical to rigorously assess their safety profile, especially when used in combination with conventional antihypertensive drugs.

Some herbal agents, such as *R. serpentina*, may cause adverse effects, including sedation, depression, and bradycardia, limiting their clinical utility [80]. Other herbs may interact pharmacokinetically by affecting cytochrome P450 enzymes or

**Table 5.3** Safety and interaction chart of common herbal antihypertensives.

| Herbal antihypertensive | Active compounds | Potential benefits | Known or possible risks | Interactions with antihypertensive drugs |
|---|---|---|---|---|
| Garlic (*Allium sativum*) | Allicin, sulfur compounds | Vasodilation, ACE inhibition, antioxidant | Possible bleeding risk (antiplatelet effects) | Enhanced effect with anticoagulants and antihypertensives |
| *Ginkgo biloba* | Ginkgolides, flavonoids | Improved endothelial function, vasodilation | Risk of bleeding, gastrointestinal (GI) upset, allergic reactions | May potentiate effects of anticoagulants; caution with blood pressure meds due to additive effects |
| Olive leaf extract | Oleuropein, hydroxytyrosol | Antioxidant, ACE inhibition, vasodilation | Generally safe; mild GI discomfort possible | Possible additive hypotensive effects with standard drugs; monitor BP closely |
| Berberine | Isoquinoline alkaloids | Vasodilation, improved insulin sensitivity | GI upset, potential liver enzyme interactions | Can interact with CYP enzymes affecting metabolism of many drugs, including antihypertensives; caution advised |
| Hibiscus (*Hibiscus sabdariffa*) | Anthocyanins, flavonoids | Diuretic, vasodilatory effects | Generally well tolerated; possible GI upset | May potentiate antihypertensive drugs leading to hypotension |
| Licorice (*Glycyrrhiza glabra*) | Glycyrrhizic acid | Mild vasodilatory effects but also can cause sodium retention | Hypertension, hypokalemia, fluid retention (especially with chronic use) | Can antagonize antihypertensive drugs, may increase blood pressure; caution advised, especially with diuretics and ACE inhibitors |
| Hawthorn (*Crataegus* spp.) | Flavonoids, oligomeric proanthocyanidins | Positive inotropic, vasodilatory effects | GI upset, dizziness | Potential additive hypotensive effects; caution when combined with beta-blockers or calcium channel blockers |
| St. John's wort (*Hypericum perforatum*) | Hypericin, hyperforin | Limited evidence for BP effects; used more for depression | Induces CYP3A4 enzymes, reduces efficacy of many drugs | May reduce effectiveness of antihypertensive drugs by inducing metabolism; avoid concurrent use |

pharmacodynamically by potentiating hypotensive effects, increasing the risk of excessive blood pressure lowering, or electrolyte disturbances.

### 5.5.12 CHALLENGES IN HERBAL ANTIHYPERTENSIVE RESEARCH

One key issue is the variability in phytochemical composition due to differences in the types of plants, cultivation practices, timing of harvest, and methods of extraction contribute to variability in the reproducibility of both efficacy and safety outcomes [81].

Additionally, herbal extracts exhibit difficulties in identifying active ingredients and elucidating precise mechanisms of action.

Furthermore, clinical trials investigating herbal antihypertensives frequently suffer from small sample sizes, short durations, and heterogeneity in dosing and preparation, limiting the generalizability of results. Rigorous, large-scale, well-designed randomized controlled trials (RCTs) with standardized formulations are necessary.

## 5.6 CLINICAL TRIALS OF HERBAL ANTIHYPERTENSIVES

### 5.6.1 COMPREHENSIVE OVERVIEW OF CLINICAL RESEARCH ON HERBAL ANTIHYPERTENSIVES

Clinical research involving herbal medicines encounters distinct challenges. Variability in phytochemical content due to botanical source differences, extraction techniques, and dosage regimens complicates standardization efforts. Additionally, the placebo effect, patient adherence, and diverse population characteristics contribute to study heterogeneity, necessitating rigorous methodological designs [82].

Despite these obstacles, numerous clinical trials generated encouraging evidence supporting the blood pressure-lowering effects of select botanicals. These studies offer insights into optimal formulations, dosing schedules, and target patient populations, laying the groundwork for broader clinical integration.

### 5.6.2 RANDOMIZED CONTROLLED TRIALS: EVIDENCE FROM HIGH-QUALITY STUDIES

RCTs provide the highest level of evidence for clinical efficacy. In this domain, several herbal agents have demonstrated statistically significant reductions.

**Garlic (*A. sativum*)** Multiple RCTs and meta-analyses have reported that aged garlic extract can lower systolic blood pressure by approximately 8 to 12 mmHg and diastolic pressure by 5 to 9 mmHg in individuals with uncontrolled hypertension. The mechanisms proposed involve vasodilation through enhanced nitric oxide bioavailability, ACE inhibition, and antioxidant effects. Notably, garlic's tolerability profile is favorable, with few adverse events reported even at higher doses.

**Hibiscus (*H. sabdariffa*)** is another well-documented antihypertensive herb, commonly administered as an herbal tea. Controlled trials involving prehypertensive and stage 1 hypertensive subjects show consistent decreases in both systolic and diastolic pressures following daily consumption for several weeks. The hypotensive effect is attributed to hibiscus's mild diuretic properties, inhibition of ACE, and potent antioxidant activity.

**Olive leaf extract** trials have demonstrated reductions in blood pressure comparable to low-dose pharmacological agents, particularly in stage 1 hypertensive adults. Polyphenols such as oleuropein and hydroxytyrosol exert vasodilatory effects via modulation of RAAS and improved endothelial function.

Additional herbs, including ***T. arjuna***, ***Z. officinale*** (ginger), and ***A. graveolens*** (celery seed), have been examined in smaller-scale studies. While these trials often report modest but significant antihypertensive effects, variations in trial design and dosing limit definitive conclusions.

## 5.6.3 INSIGHTS FROM META-ANALYSES AND SYSTEMATIC REVIEWS

These reviews highlight the importance of extract standardization, as varying bioactive compound concentrations among preparations significantly influence clinical outcomes. Furthermore, they emphasize that the duration of intervention and baseline blood pressure levels are critical factors affecting efficacy [83].

Safety assessments within these meta-analyses indicate that, while most herbs are well tolerated, rigorous reporting of adverse events remains inconsistent. This gap underscores the need for standardized safety monitoring in future trials.

## 5.6.4 ADJUNCTIVE USE OF HERBAL AGENTS WITH CONVENTIONAL ANTIHYPERTENSIVES

A pragmatic approach in managing hypertension involves combining herbal supplements with conventional medications to achieve better blood pressure control, minimize doses of pharmaceuticals, and reduce side effects.

Clinical investigations demonstrate that garlic supplementation alongside antihypertensive drugs can enhance blood pressure reduction without significant herb–drug interactions or safety concerns. Similarly, hibiscus tea consumption as an adjunct has been linked to improved vascular function and greater reductions in blood pressure.

Nevertheless, these findings necessitate caution, as the potential for pharmacodynamic and pharmacokinetic interactions exists. Healthcare providers should closely monitor patients for hypotension or electrolyte imbalances when combining treatments.

## 5.6.5 LIMITATIONS AND FUTURE PERSPECTIVES IN CLINICAL RESEARCH

Despite promising data, current clinical research faces notable limitations. Many trials feature small sample sizes, limited durations, and heterogeneous patient populations, reducing the robustness and generalizability of results. Furthermore, the lack of universally accepted standards for herbal extract preparation hampers reproducibility.

Long-term studies assessing cardiovascular morbidity and mortality outcomes are scarce. Most clinical trials focus primarily on surrogate endpoints such as blood pressure reduction, without addressing effects on end-organ damage or quality of life.

Future research directions should emphasize large-scale, multicenter, RCTs employing standardized and well-characterized herbal preparations. Incorporating pharmacogenomic and metabolomic analyses may also elucidate individual variability in response, facilitating personalized herbal medicine approaches.

Furthermore, integrating rigorous safety monitoring and detailed adverse event reporting will enhance the clinical acceptance of herbal antihypertensives. Collaborations between conventional medical researchers and traditional medical practitioners could accelerate evidence generation and clinical integration.

## 5.6.6 SAFETY, TOXICOLOGY, AND REGULATORY ASPECTS OF HERBAL ANTIHYPERTENSIVES

### 5.6.6.1 Comprehensive Safety Profile Assessment

While herbal medicines are often considered safe based on historical usage, safety in modern clinical contexts should be evaluated. The therapeutic window, dose-dependent toxicity, and safety outcomes are influenced by individual patient variables, including age, existing comorbid conditions, and the use of concomitant medications [84]. For example, compounds like reserpine from *R. serpentina* have well-documented adverse neuropsychiatric effects, including depression and sedation, highlighting the necessity for careful dose optimization and monitoring.

Furthermore, hepatotoxicity has been reported with certain herbal preparations due to intrinsic toxicity or contamination with hepatotoxic agents. Renal toxicity is also a concern, particularly for patients with preexisting kidney conditions, as some herbs may exert nephrotoxic effects or alter renal hemodynamics. Emerging safety concerns also include immunomodulatory effects that may exacerbate or ameliorate autoimmune conditions, underscoring the complex systemic impacts of herbal constituents.

### 5.6.6.2 Herb–Drug Interaction Mechanisms and Clinical Implications

Herb–drug interactions are multifactorial, involving metabolic enzyme modulation, transporter effects, and additive or antagonistic pharmacodynamic interactions. Cytochrome P450 isoenzymes such as CYP3A4, CYP2D6, and CYP2C9 are commonly involved in drug metabolism and are susceptible to inhibition or induction by herbal compounds. For instance, St. John's wort is a well-known CYP3A4 inducer, although not primarily an antihypertensive, illustrating the relevance of such interactions.

Pharmacodynamic interactions may also involve synergistic blood pressure-lowering effects, raising risks of hypotension and electrolyte imbalances when combined with diuretics or

ACE inhibitors [85]. Clinicians must obtain detailed patient histories, including herbal supplement use, and provide guidance to avoid potentially harmful combinations. Development of interaction databases and decision support tools can facilitate safer integration of herbal therapies.

#### 5.6.6.3 Rigorous Toxicological Evaluations

Preclinical toxicological assessment involves acute, subacute, and chronic toxicity studies in animal models to determine no-observed-adverse-effect levels (NOAEL), 50 % lethal doses ($LD_{50}$), and target organ toxicities. Genotoxicity tests, such as the Ames test, micronucleus assay, and chromosomal aberration tests, evaluate potential mutagenic risks.

For many herbal antihypertensive preparations, comprehensive toxicology data remain limited. This gap necessitates systematic toxicological investigations employing standardized extracts with defined phytochemical profiles to ensure reproducibility and safety. Furthermore, evaluating herb metabolite profiles and their toxicodynamics can elucidate safety margins and identify biomarkers predictive of adverse effects.

#### 5.6.6.4 Regulatory Frameworks: Challenges and Progress

Herbal antihypertensives occupy a complex regulatory space globally. In some countries, herbal medicine is deeply integrated into healthcare systems, and regulatory frameworks reflect a hybrid model combining traditional usage evidence with modern scientific validation.

Challenges in regulatory oversight include ensuring product quality, standardization of active ingredients, preventing adulteration, and enforcing good manufacturing practices (GMP). International efforts such as the WHO's guidelines for assessing herbal medicines provide a framework for harmonizing standards, though global implementation remains uneven [86].

### 5.6.7 FUTURE PERSPECTIVES AND CHALLENGES IN HERBAL ANTIHYPERTENSIVE RESEARCH AND APPLICATION

#### 5.6.7.1 Collaborative Fusion of Ancestral Wisdom and Contemporary Scientific Understanding

The rich heritage of ethnomedicine offers a vast repository of botanical candidates with antihypertensive potential. Harnessing this knowledge through rigorous scientific validation can identify novel therapeutic agents and optimize existing formulations. Interdisciplinary collaboration involving ethnobotanists, pharmacologists, molecular biologists, and clinicians is pivotal to developing evidence-based herbal therapies [87].

Advances in systems biology and network pharmacology provide innovative tools to unravel the complex interactions between multiple phytochemicals and human physiological pathways. These approaches can illuminate the molecular basis of herbal efficacy and facilitate rational design of combination therapies.

#### 5.6.7.2 Technological Advances in Standardization and Formulation

Quality control remains a cornerstone for clinical success of herbal medicines. Novel drug delivery technologies, including nanoparticle encapsulation, liposomes, and transdermal systems, are being investigated to overcome limitations associated with poor solubility or rapid metabolism, thereby improving therapeutic efficacy. Formulation strategies that leverage synergistic interactions between multiple compounds can optimize efficacy while minimizing adverse effects. This concept aligns with traditional polyherbal formulations but requires scientific validation for dose standardization and safety.

#### 5.6.7.3 Personalized Herbal Medicine: The Frontier of Pharmacogenomics

Interindividual variability in herbal medicine response is increasingly recognized as a key factor in clinical outcomes.

Pharmacogenomic profiling may enable tailoring herbal therapies based on genetic makeup, thereby enhancing safety and maximizing therapeutic benefits.

#### 5.6.7.4 Overcoming Challenges in Clinical Translation

Despite the promising potential of herbal antihypertensives, several barriers impede their widespread clinical adoption. Key challenges include:

- **Heterogeneity of clinical trials:** Differences in study designs, participant selection, herbal preparations, and outcome measures limit comparability and meta-analytic synthesis.
- **Lack of long-term safety data:** Chronic use studies assessing end-organ protection and cardiovascular morbidity/mortality are insufficient.
- **Physician awareness and education:** Limited training in herbal medicine reduces clinician confidence in recommending or managing herbal therapies.
- **Patient adherence and cultural perceptions:** Variability in patient acceptance influenced by cultural beliefs and access issues can affect outcomes.

Addressing these challenges requires coordinated efforts to establish robust clinical evidence, develop clear clinical guidelines, and enhance education for healthcare providers and patients alike [88].

### 5.6.8 DETAILED MECHANISMS OF ACTION OF HERBAL ANTIHYPERTENSIVES

Herbal antihypertensives exert their effects through diverse biological pathways, often targeting multiple physiological mechanisms simultaneously. This polypharmacological profile differentiates them from many synthetic drugs, which typically focus on a single target, and may contribute to their broader therapeutic effects and relatively lower side effect profiles.

#### 5.6.8.1 Vasodilation and Endothelial Function Modulation

A principal mechanism by which many herbs lower blood pressure is through promoting vasodilation, thereby reducing peripheral vascular resistance. Several herbal extracts enhance endothelial function by increasing nitric oxide bioavailability. Polyphenols from green tea (*C. sinensis*) and olive leaf (*O. europaea*) scavenge ROS that degrade NO, thus preserving its vasodilatory effect. This antioxidative protection supports sustained endothelial health, crucial in preventing hypertension progression.

#### 5.6.8.2 Renin-Angiotensin-Aldosterone System Inhibition

By controlling sodium balance, vascular tone, and fluid volume, blood pressure is regulated. Overactivation of this system leads to vasoconstriction, sodium retention, and increased blood pressure.

Certain herbs contain phytochemicals capable of inhibiting key RAAS components. For instance, hibiscus (*H. sabdariffa*) calyces contain anthocyanins that help control high blood pressure. This mechanism parallels that of pharmaceutical ACE inhibitors but with generally milder effects and fewer side effects.

Other herbs, such as *T. arjuna*, have been reported to modulate aldosterone secretion, thereby influencing salt and water retention and contributing to blood pressure reduction.

#### 5.6.8.3 Diuretic and Natriuretic Effects

Increased excretion of sodium and water lowers blood volume and cardiac output, effectively reducing blood pressure. Several herbs act as mild natural diuretics, promoting renal elimination of excess fluids.

Celery seed (*A. graveolens*) contains compounds that stimulate diuresis, which can help manage hypertension linked to fluid overload. This diuretic effect also reduces the workload on the heart and blood vessels, mitigating hypertensive damage.

Other botanicals like dandelion (*Taraxacum officinale*) similarly increase urinary output, though their effects are generally less potent than synthetic diuretics, allowing for safer long-term use.

#### 5.6.8.4 Anti-inflammatory and Antioxidant Actions

Stress and low-grade inflammation contribute significantly to endothelial dysfunction, arterial stiffness, and the development of hypertension. Herbal antihypertensives often possess robust antioxidant and anti-inflammatory properties that protect vascular integrity.

Flavonoids, tannins, and phenolic acids found in numerous herbs neutralize free radicals and reduce oxidative damage to blood vessels. For example, extracts from *C. sinensis*, *Curcuma longa* (turmeric), and *Punica granatum* (pomegranate) have demonstrated potent antioxidant capacity in experimental and clinical studies [89].

By suppressing pro-inflammatory cytokines and adhesion molecules, these botanicals also reduce vascular inflammation, improving endothelial function and preventing hypertension-associated vascular remodeling.

#### 5.6.8.5 Calcium Channel Blockade and Sympatholytic Effects

Certain phytochemicals mimic the action of conventional calcium channel blockers. For example, compounds from *Z. officinale* (ginger) have been shown to modulate calcium channels, contributing to blood pressure lowering.

Additionally, some herbs exhibit sympatholytic properties, reducing SNS activity, which is often elevated in hypertensive patients. *R. serpentina*, through its active alkaloid reserpine, depletes catecholamines such as norepinephrine, lowering heart rate and peripheral resistance. However, its use requires caution due to central nervous system side effects.

### 5.6.9 PROMINENT HERBAL AGENTS WITH CLINICAL EVIDENCE IN HYPERTENSION MANAGEMENT

**Garlic (*A. sativum*)**

Garlic's cardiovascular benefits are well documented, supported by numerous clinical trials. Its active compounds contribute to vasodilation, antiplatelet effects, and lipid-lowering properties [90]. Clinical studies reveal that standardized aged garlic extracts can reduce uncontrolled hypertension.

**Hibiscus (*H. sabdariffa*)**

Widely consumed as an herbal tea, hibiscus exhibits mild ACE inhibitory activity and antioxidant effects that translate into significant blood pressure reductions in clinical settings. Its favorable safety profile and accessibility make it a popular adjunct in hypertension management.

**Olive leaf (*O. europaea*)**

Randomized clinical studies have demonstrated that extracts from olive leaves, abundant in polyphenolic compounds like oleuropein, can reduce blood pressure and promote better endothelial health. Its anti-inflammatory and antioxidative mechanisms also confer cardioprotective benefits.

***T. arjuna***

Traditionally used in Ayurveda for cardiovascular ailments, *T. arjuna* has demonstrated cardiotonic and vasodilatory effects.

**Other Notable Botanicals**

- *Z. officinale* (ginger): Exhibits calcium channel blockade and antioxidant activities contributing to vascular relaxation.
- *A. graveolens* (celery): It is a diuretic and also reduces hypertension.
- *Crataegus* spp. (hawthorn): Traditionally used for heart conditions, hawthorn extracts possess vasodilatory and antioxidative properties supporting hypertension management.

## 5.6.10 PHYTOCHEMICAL CONSTITUENTS UNDERLYING ANTIHYPERTENSIVE EFFECTS

The therapeutic efficacy of herbal antihypertensives largely depends on their complex mixtures of bioactive phytochemicals. These naturally occurring compounds interact with multiple molecular targets, producing synergistic effects that may enhance overall blood pressure control.

**Alkaloids**
Alkaloids are nitrogen-containing compounds with significant physiological activities. Reserpine, derived from *R. serpentina*, is a classic example that irreversibly binds to storage vesicles of catecholamines, causing depletion of norepinephrine and serotonin in peripheral and central neurons. This leads to reduced sympathetic tone, vasodilation, and lowered cardiac output.

**Flavonoids and Polyphenols**
Flavonoids represent a large group of polyphenolic compounds abundant in fruits, vegetables, and many medicinal plants. They contribute to antihypertensive effects primarily through antioxidant activity, ACE inhibition, and modulation of eNOS. Examples include quercetin and kaempferol, which have demonstrated blood pressure-lowering effects by improving endothelial function and reducing oxidative stress.

**Terpenoids**
Terpenoids, including monoterpenes and diterpenes, exhibit vasodilatory and diuretic properties. For instance, ginkgolides from *Ginkgo biloba* enhance cerebral blood flow and exhibit antioxidant effects, though their role in systemic hypertension management is still under investigation.

**Saponins**
Saponins, glycosides with surfactant properties, are reported to exert vasodilatory and diuretic effects. It has been suggested that these regulate the RAAS and contribute to improved cardiac function, though additional clinical studies are necessary.

**Other Bioactive Compounds**
Phenolic acids, tannins, and alk(en)yl sulfides also contribute to the antihypertensive action of herbal medicines. For example, ferulic acid, found in several herbs, reduces arterial stiffness and oxidative stress, contributing to vascular protection.

## 5.6.11 CLINICAL EVIDENCE AND TRIAL INSIGHTS

Clinical evaluation of herbal antihypertensives has expanded in recent decades, with numerous RCTs, observational studies, and meta-analyses contributing to the evidence base.

**Methodological Considerations**
Many clinical trials face challenges, including variability in herbal preparation standardization, dosing regimens, participant selection, and duration of therapy. Despite this heterogeneity, consistent findings of modest but significant blood pressure reductions have been observed for several herbal agents.

**Notable Clinical Trials**

- **Garlic**: Meta-analyses of RCTs report systolic blood pressure reductions ranging from 8 to 12 mmHg and diastolic reductions of 5 to 8 mmHg in hypertensive subjects using standardized aged garlic extracts.
- **Hibiscus**: Clinical trials have demonstrated that daily consumption of hibiscus tea reduces systolic blood pressure by approximately 7 mmHg in prehypertensive and stage 1 hypertensive patients.
- **Olive leaf extract**: Controlled trials show significant improvements in blood pressure and lipid profiles with olive leaf supplementation, comparable to standard antihypertensive medications in mild cases [91].

**Safety and Tolerability in Trials**
Herbal interventions generally exhibit good tolerability, with adverse events typically mild and transient. Safety data remain limited and warrant further study.

## 5.6.12 INTEGRATION OF HERBAL ANTIHYPERTENSIVES IN MODERN THERAPEUTIC STRATEGIES

**Nonconventional Therapies for Hypertension**
Increasing patient interest in herbal remedies has prompted integration efforts within conventional hypertension management. Evidence-based herbal therapies can complement pharmacologic regimens, potentially enhancing blood pressure control and improving patient adherence.

**Polypharmacy and Herb–Drug Interaction Management**
With the complexity of hypertensive patients often requiring multiple medications, careful assessment of herb–drug interactions is essential. Collaborative care models involving physicians, pharmacists, and herbalists optimize safety and efficacy.

**Patient Education and Healthcare Provider Training**
Effective communication of herbal antihypertensives is critical. Healthcare providers require training to counsel patients appropriately and to recognize signs of adverse effects or interactions [81].

## 5.6.13 PHARMACOKINETICS AND BIOAVAILABILITY OF HERBAL ANTIHYPERTENSIVES

Pharmacokinetics involves the absorption, distribution, metabolism, and excretion (ADME) of active compounds, which differ based on the chemical nature of phytochemicals and formulation.

**Absorption and Bioavailability Challenges**
Many phytochemicals in herbal antihypertensives exhibit poor oral bioavailability due to limited solubility, instability in gastrointestinal (GI) conditions, and extensive first-pass metabolism. For example, polyphenols such as quercetin and

curcumin have low water solubility and rapid metabolism, leading to reduced systemic concentrations after oral intake. The matrix of whole plant extracts may also affect absorption, with certain components enhancing or inhibiting uptake of active molecules. For instance, the presence of piperine in black pepper has been shown to increase bioavailability of curcumin by inhibiting metabolic enzymes [92].

**Metabolism and Biotransformation**
Herbal compounds are subjected to extensive metabolic transformation, primarily via hepatic cytochrome P450 enzymes and intestinal microbiota. These processes can generate active or inactive metabolites, influencing overall pharmacological effects.

Gut microbiota play a pivotal role by converting glycosides to aglycones, modulating absorption and activity. Variation in microbiota composition among individuals contributes to interpatient variability in response to herbal treatments.

**Distribution and Tissue Targeting**
After absorption, phytochemicals are distributed via the bloodstream to target organs, including the vasculature, heart, and kidneys. Lipophilicity and protein-binding affinity determine tissue penetration and residence time.

Strategies to improve tissue targeting, such as nanoparticle encapsulation and conjugation with targeting ligands, are under investigation to enhance efficacy and reduce off-target effects.

**Excretion and Elimination**
Herbal compounds and their metabolites are eliminated through renal and biliary pathways. Understanding elimination kinetics is essential to design appropriate dosing schedules and avoid accumulation that could lead to toxicity.

## 5.6.14 CHALLENGES IN STANDARDIZATION AND QUALITY CONTROL (Figure 5.3)

Ensuring consistency, potency, and purity of herbal antihypertensive preparations is a significant challenge that affects clinical efficacy and safety.

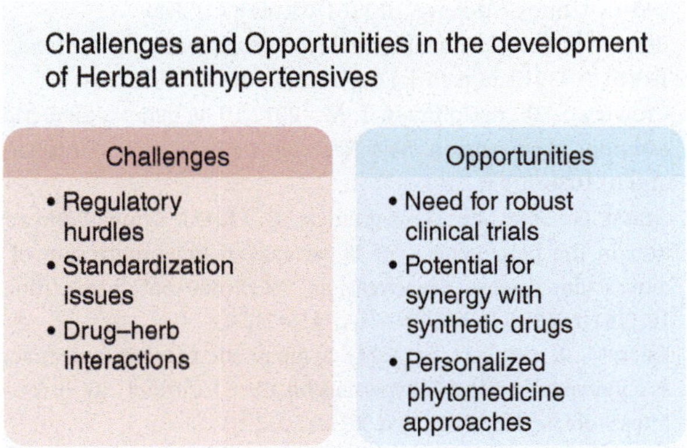


**FIGURE 5.3** Challenges and opportunities in the development of herbal antihypertensives.

**Variability in Raw Material**
The chemical composition of medicinal plants varies based on species, geographic origin, harvesting time, cultivation conditions, and postharvest processing. Such variability impacts the concentration of bioactive constituents.

**Extraction and Formulation Methods**
Differences in extraction solvents, temperatures, and durations lead to inconsistent phytochemical profiles. Standardized extraction protocols and quantification of marker compounds are vital for reproducible product quality.

**Adulteration and Contamination**
Adulteration with synthetic drugs or substitution with inferior species poses serious health risks. Heavy metals, pesticides, and microbial contamination also threaten safety, highlighting the need for stringent quality assurance protocols.

**Regulatory and Industry Initiatives**
Adherence to pharmacopeial standards contributes to improved product quality. Advances in chromatographic fingerprinting and DNA barcoding are powerful tools for authentication and quality control [93].

## 5.6.15 EMERGING RESEARCH TRENDS AND FUTURE DIRECTIONS

**Systems Biology and Network Pharmacology**
Herbal medicines contain multiple bioactive compounds acting on various molecular targets. Systems biology approaches integrate genomics, proteomics, and metabolomics data to elucidate complex herb–host interactions, paving the way for mechanistic understanding and novel therapeutic insights [94].

Network pharmacology maps interactions between phytochemicals and disease-related genes/proteins, guiding rational polyherbal formulation development with optimized efficacy and minimized toxicity [95].

**Nanotechnology and Novel Delivery Systems**
Advanced nanotechnology techniques enable improved dissolution, preservation, and targeted transport of bioactive compounds from plants. Delivery systems like nanosized particles, liposomal carriers, and nanoemulsions can boost the absorption efficiency and allow controlled release, opening new possibilities for herbal treatments in managing high blood pressure [96].

**Personalized Medicine and Pharmacogenomics**
Integrating genetic and epigenetic profiling can help predict individual responses to herbal therapies, optimizing personalized treatment plans. Pharmacogenomic studies identify genetic variants influencing metabolism, transport, and receptor sensitivity to phytochemicals.

**Integration into Global Health Strategies**
Given the global burden of hypertension and limitations of conventional therapy, incorporating validated herbal antihypertensives into national and international hypertension management guidelines could expand accessible treatment options, especially in resource-limited settings [84].

### 5.6.16 CONCLUSION

Herbal antihypertensives present a multifaceted approach to blood pressure management, combining diverse phytochemicals acting on multiple physiological targets. Supported by traditional use and growing scientific evidence, these agents offer promise as adjunctive or alternative therapies with favorable safety profiles.

However, realizing their full potential necessitates overcoming challenges related to standardization, safety evaluation, clinical validation, and regulatory harmonization. Future research integrating advanced analytical technologies, systems pharmacology, and personalized medicine paradigms will pave the way for their effective and safe incorporation into mainstream cardiovascular care [97].

## REFERENCES


1. Whelton, P.K., Carey, R.M., Aronow, W.S. et al. (2018). 2017 ACC/AHA guideline for the prevention, detection, evaluation, and management of high blood pressure in adults. *J. Am. Coll. Cardiol.* 71 (19): e127–e248. https://doi.org/10.1016/j.jacc.2017.11.006.
2. Mills, K.T., Stefanescu, A., and He, J. (2020). The global epidemiology of hypertension. *Nat. Rev. Nephrol.* 16 (4): 223–237. https://doi.org/10.1038/s41581-019-0244-2.
3. Kearney, P.M., Whelton, M., Reynolds, K. et al. (2005). Global burden of hypertension: analysis of worldwide data. *Lancet* 365 (9455): 217–223. https://doi.org/10.1016/S0140-6736(05)17741-1.
4. Chobanian, A. V., Bakris, G. L., Black, H. R., et al. (2003). The seventh report of the joint national committee on prevention, detection, evaluation, and treatment of high blood pressure: the JNC 7 report. *JAMA*, 289 (19), 2560–2572. https://doi.org/10.1001/jama.289.19.2560
5. World Health Organization (2013). *A Global Brief on Hypertension: Silent Killer, Global Public Health Crisis.* Geneva: WHO Press.
6. James, P. A., Oparil, S., Carter, B. L., et al. (2014). 2014 evidence-based guideline for the management of high blood pressure in adults: report from the panel members appointed to the Eighth Joint National Committee (JNC 8). *JAMA*, 311(5), 507–520. https://doi.org/10.1001/jama.2013.284427
7. Law, M. R., Morris, J. K., & Wald, N. J. (2009). Use of blood pressure lowering drugs in the prevention of cardiovascular disease: meta-analysis of 147 randomised trials in the context of expectations from prospective epidemiological studies. *BMJ*, 338, 1665. https://doi.org/10.1136/bmj.b1665
8. Burnier, M., & Egan, B. M. (2019). Adherence in hypertension. *Circ. Res.*, 124(7), 1124–1140. https://doi.org/10.1161/CIRCRESAHA.118.313220
9. Vrijens, B., Vincze, G., Kristanto, P., Urquhart, J., & Burnier, M. (2008). Adherence to prescribed antihypertensive drug treatments: longitudinal study of electronically compiled dosing histories. BMJ, 336 (7653), 1114–1117. https://doi.org/10.1136/bmj.39553.670231.25
10. Mancia, G., Fagard, R., Narkiewicz, K., et al. (2013). 2013 ESH/ESC guidelines for the management of arterial hypertension. *Eur. Heart J.*, 34 (28), 2159–2219. https://doi.org/10.1093/eurheartj/eht151
11. Mills, K. T., Bundy, J. D., Kelly, T. N., et al. (2016). Global disparities of hypertension prevalence and control: a systematic analysis of population-based studies from 90 countries. *Circulation*, 134(6), 441–450. https://doi.org/10.1161/CIRCULATIONAHA.115.018912
12. Tiwari, P. and Kumar, A. (2018). Herbal medicine in the management of hypertension: a review. *Int. J. Pharm. Pharm. Sci.* 10 (2): 10–18.
13. Panche, A. N., Diwan, A. D., & Chandra, S. R. (2016). Flavonoids: an overview. *J. Nutr. Sci.*, 5, e47. https://doi.org/10.1017/jns.2016.41
14. Momin, S., Malpathak, N., & Trivedi, P. (2010). Antioxidant and antihypertensive potential of herbal extracts: a review. *Pharmacogn. Rev.*, 4(8), 122–131. https://doi.org/10.4103/0973-7847.70902
15. Wang, J., & Jin, Z. (2016). The pharmacological activities of saponins from medicinal plants in hypertension management. *Front. Pharmacol.*, 7, 457. https://doi.org/10.3389/fphar.2016.00457
16. Ried, K., Fakler, P., & Stocks, N. P. (2013). Effect of garlic on blood pressure: a systematic review and meta-analysis. *BMC Cardiovasc. Disord.*, 13, 7. https://doi.org/10.1186/1471-2261-13-7
17. Liang, C., Lin, S., & Liu, Y. (2016). *Hibiscus sabdariffa* in the treatment of hypertension: a meta-analysis of randomized controlled trials. *Phytother. Res.*, 30 (11), 1754–1764. https://doi.org/10.1002/ptr.5676
18. Dwivedi, S. and Singh, P. (2012). *Terminalia arjuna*: cardioprotective effects and clinical significance. *Int. J. Pharmacol.* 8 (6): 435–443.
19. Ong, K. W., & Khoo, B. Y. (2014). Herbal medicines as adjunct therapies in hypertension: evidence and safety considerations. *Integr. Med. Res.*, 3(2), 63–68. https://doi.org/10.1016/j.imr.2014.04.002
20. Ernst, E. (2005). Herb-drug interactions: potential dangers. *Am. J. Med.* 118 (9): 945–946.
21. Guyton, A.C. and Hall, J.E. (2011). *Textbook of Medical Physiology*, 12e. Philadelphia: Saunders Elsevier.
22. Esler, M. (2010). The sympathetic nervous system through the ages: from Thomas Willis to resistant hypertension. *Exp. Physiol.*, 95(1), 14–19. https://doi.org/10.1113/expphysiol.2009.049730
23. Navar, L. G., Nishiyama, A., Imig, J., & Mitchell, K. D. (2011). Intrarenal renin-angiotensin system: locally synthesized or taken up from the circulation? *Kidney Int.*, 79(1), 22–26. https://doi.org/10.1038/ki.2010.427
24. Paul, M., Poyan Mehr, A., & Kreutz, R. (2006). Physiology of local renin-angiotensin systems. *Physiol. Rev.*, 86(3), 747–803. https://doi.org/10.1152/physrev.00036.2005
25. Vanhoutte, P. M., Shimokawa, H., Feletou, M., & Tang, E. H. (2017). Endothelial dysfunction and vascular disease. *Acta Physiol.*, 219(1), 22–35. https://doi.org/10.1111/apha.12646
26. Cai, H., & Harrison, D. G. (2000). Endothelial dysfunction in cardiovascular diseases: the role of oxidant stress. *Circ. Res.*, 87 (10), 840–844. https://doi.org/10.1161/01.res.87.10.840
27. Burnier, M. (2001). Angiotensin II type 1 receptor blockers. *Circulation*, 103(6), 904–912. https://doi.org/10.1161/01.CIR.103.6.904
28. Crowley, S. D., & Coffman, T. M. (2012). The genetic dissection of essential hypertension. *Nat. Rev. Genet.*, 13(1), 45–56. https://doi.org/10.1038/nrg3122
29. Grassi, G., Seravalle, G., & Mancia, G. (2015). Sympathetic activation in the pathogenesis of hypertension and progression of cardiovascular disease. *Hypertension*, 56(3), 660–667. https://doi.org/10.1161/HYPERTENSIONAHA.115.05823
30. Esler, M., & Lambert, E. (2014). Sympathetic nervous system activity as a therapeutic target in hypertension. *Can. J. Cardiol.*, 30(5), 506–514. https://doi.org/10.1016/j.cjca.2013.12.022
31. Touyz, R. M., & Schiffrin, E. L. (2004). Reactive oxygen species in vascular biology: implications in hypertension. *Histochem. Cell Biol.*, 122(4), 339–352. https://doi.org/10.1007/s00418-004-0667-0

32. Rodrigo, R., Libuy, M., Feliú, F., & Hasson, D. (2011). Oxidative stress-related biomarkers in essential hypertension and ischemia-reperfusion myocardial damage. *Int. J. Hypertens.*, 2011, 1–14. https://doi.org/10.4061/2011/567543
33. Félétou, M., & Vanhoutte, P. M. (2006). Endothelium-dependent hyperpolarization: a magic bullet or more complex? *Br. J. Pharmacol.*, 149(7), 843–856. https://doi.org/10.1038/sj.bjp.0706933
34. Ghosh, S., & Cokic, I. (2015). Calcium channels and hypertension. *Curr. Hypertens. Rep.*, 17(3), 16. https://doi.org/10.1007/s11906-015-0547-7
35. Lifton, R. P., Gharavi, A. G., & Geller, D. S. (2001). Molecular mechanisms of human hypertension. *Cell*, 104(4), 545–556. https://doi.org/10.1016/S0092-8674(01)00241-0
36. Chobanian, A. V. (2009). The hypertension paradox—more uncontrolled disease despite improved therapy. *N. Engl. J. Med.*, 361(9), 878–887. https://doi.org/10.1056/NEJMp0904410
37. Messerli, F. H., Bangalore, S., & Bavishi, C. (2018). Angiotensin-converting enzyme inhibitors in hypertension: to use or not to use? *J. Am. Coll. Cardiol.*, 71 (13), 1474–1482. https://doi.org/10.1016/j.jacc.2018.01.035
38. Patocka, J., Nepovimova, E., & Kuca, K. (2019). Herbal drugs in the treatment of hypertension. *Pharmaceuticals*, 12(3), 114. https://doi.org/10.3390/ph12030114
39. Choudhary, M. I., Azizuddin, K., & Chaudhary, M. I. (2015). Role of medicinal plants as antioxidant, anti-inflammatory, and anti-hypertensive agents in cardiovascular diseases. *Phytother. Res.*, 29(7), 995–1003. https://doi.org/10.1002/ptr.5323
40. Vanhoutte, P. M., & Shimokawa, H. (2015). Endothelium-dependent contractions and dysfunction in hypertension. *Curr. Hypertens. Rep.*, 17(4), 29. https://doi.org/10.1007/s11906-015-0545-9
41. Taddei, S., Virdis, A., Ghiadoni, L. et al. (2006). Endothelial dysfunction in hypertension. *J. Nephrol.* 19 (Suppl 9): S31–S34.
42. Hansson, G. K. (2005). Inflammation, atherosclerosis, and coronary artery disease. *N. Engl. J. Med.*, 352 (16), 1685–1695.https://doi.org/10.1056/NEJMra043430
43. Rzucidlo, E. M., Martin, K. A., & Powell, R. J. (2007). Regulation of vascular smooth muscle cell differentiation. *J. Vasc. Surg.*, 45 (Suppl A), A25–A32. https://doi.org/10.1016/j.jvs.2007.02.005
44. Intengan, H. D., & Schiffrin, E. L. (2001). Vascular remodeling in hypertension: roles of apoptosis, inflammation, and fibrosis. *Hypertension*, 38 (3 Pt 2), 581–587. https://doi.org/10.1161/hy1101.092422
45. Shimizu, T., Ishikawa, Kensuke L.; Takahashi, Hiroshi; Noma, Satoshi; Shimokawa, Hiroaki (2016). Role of mitogen-activated protein kinase and Rho-kinase pathways in vascular smooth muscle cell proliferation and migration. *Curr. Vasc. Pharmacol.*, 14(4), 357–367. https://doi.org/10.2174/1570161114666160318151532
46. Madhur, M. S., Lob, Alison L.; McCann, Lisa A.; Iwakura, Yoichiro; Blinder, Mark J.; Guzik, Harrison B.; Harrison, David G. (2010). Interleukin 17 promotes angiotensin II–induced hypertension and vascular dysfunction. *Hypertension*, 55(2), 500–507. https://doi.org/10.1161/HYPERTENSIONAHA.109.141598
47. Rodriguez-Iturbe, B., Johnson, Richard J. (2017). Role of the immune system in hypertension. *Physiol. Rev.*, 97(3), 1127–1164. https://doi.org/10.1152/physrev.00026.2016
48. Cai, H. (2005). Hydrogen peroxide regulation of endothelial function: origins, mechanisms, and consequences. *Cardiovasc. Res.*, 68(1), 26–36. https://doi.org/10.1016/j.cardiores.2005.06.022
49. Förstermann, U., & Münzel, T. (2006). Endothelial nitric oxide synthase in vascular disease: from marvel to menace. *Circulation*, 113 (13), 1708–1714. https://doi.org/10.1161/CIRCULATIONAHA.105.602532
50. Laurent, S., Boutouyrie P., Asmar R., et al. (2001). Aortic stiffness is an independent predictor of all-cause and cardiovascular mortality in hypertensive patients. *Hypertension*, 37(5), 1236–1241. https://doi.org/10.1161/01.HYP.37.5.1236
51. Schiffrin, E. L. (2012). Vascular remodeling in hypertension: mechanisms and treatment. *Hypertension*, 59(2), 367–374. https://doi.org/10.1161/HYPERTENSIONAHA.111.189141
52. Esler, M., Lambert, E., & Schlaich, M. (2010). Chronic activation of the sympathetic nervous system is the dominant contributor to systemic hypertension. *J. Appl. Physiol.*, 109(6), 1996–1998. https://doi.org/10.1152/japplphysiol.00558.2010
53. Danziger, R. S. (2008). The role of endothelin and endothelin receptor antagonists in the regulation of blood pressure and renal function. *Curr. Opin. Nephrol. Hypertens.*, 17(1), 43–48. https://doi.org/10.1097/MNH.0b013e3282f09a55
54. Ehret, G. B., & Caulfield, M. (2013). Genes for blood pressure: an opportunity to understand hypertension. *Eur. Heart J.*, 34 (13), 951–961. https://doi.org/10.1093/eurheartj/ehs337
55. Bell, C. G., Walley, A. J., & Froguel, P. (2011). The genetics of human obesity. *Nat. Rev. Genet.*, 12(4), 281–292. https://doi.org/10.1038/nrg2958
56. Ernst, E. (2006). Herbal medicines for hypertension: a systematic review. *Am. J. Hypertens.*, 19(3), 300–308. https://doi.org/10.1016/j.amjhyper.2005.10.011
57. Modak, M., Dixit, Prasad; Londhe, Jayant; Ghaskadbi, Thomas (2016). Traditional and herbal medicines in hypertension management: an overview. *J. Herb. Med.*, 6(2), 59–73. https://doi.org/10.1016/j.hermed.2016.04.001
58. Li, X., Zhang, Ying; Wang, Jianping; Zhao, Xiaohui (2015). Phytochemicals targeting vascular function for blood pressure control. *Phytother. Res.*, 29 (11), 1695–1706. https://doi.org/10.1002/ptr.5444
59. Rahman, K., & Lowe, G. M. (2006). Garlic and cardiovascular disease: a critical review. *J. Nutr.*, 136(3), 736S–740S. https://doi.org/10.1093/jn/136.3.736S
60. Ried, K., Frank, Oliver R.; Stocks, Nigel P. (2016). Effect of garlic on blood pressure: a systematic review and meta-analysis. *BMC Cardiovasc. Disord.*, 16, 129. https://doi.org/10.1186/s12872-016-0313-8
61. Banerjee, S. K., & Maulik, S. K. (2002). Effect of garlic on cardiovascular disorders: a review. *Nutr. J.*, 1, 4. https://doi.org/10.1186/1475-2891-1-4
62. Bayan, L., Koulivand, P.H., and Gorji, A. (2014). Garlic: a review of potential therapeutic effects. *Avicenna J. Phytomed.* 4 (1): 1–14.
63. Ojeda, D., Jiménez-Ferrer, M., Zamilpa, Z. et al. (2010). *Hibiscus sabdariffa* extract reduces blood pressure and improves endothelial function. *Phytomedicine* 17 (5): 388–393.
64. Dwivedi, S. (2007). *Terminalia arjuna* Wight & Arn.—a useful drug for cardiovascular disorders. *J. Ethnopharmacol.* 114 (2): 114–129.
65. de Bock, M., Thorstensen, E.B., Derraik, J.G.B. et al. (2013). Human absorption and metabolism of oleuropein and hydroxytyrosol: a randomized, double-blind, crossover trial. *Mol. Nutr. Food Res.* 57 (11): 2039–2045.
66. Hodgson, J.M. and Croft, K.D. (2010). Tea flavonoids and cardiovascular health. *Mol. Asp. Med.* 31 (6): 495–502.
67. Yao, X., Zhu, Y., Ren, Y. et al. (2013). Antihypertensive effect of celery seed extract in spontaneously hypertensive rats. *Phytother. Res.* 27 (4): 568–573.
68. Ghayur, M.N. and Gilani, A.H. (2005). Ginger lowers blood pressure through blockade of voltage-dependent calcium channels. *J. Cardiovasc. Pharmacol.* 45 (1): 74–80.

69. Houston, M. (2010). The role of vascular nitric oxide in health and disease. *J. Clin. Hypertens.* 12 (6): 357–364.
70. Houston, M. (2010). The role of cellular micronutrient analysis, nutraceuticals, vitamins, antioxidants, and minerals in the prevention and treatment of hypertension. *Ther. Adv. Cardiovasc. Dis.* 4 (3): 165–183.
71. Ojeda, D., Jiménez-Ferrer, E., Zamilpa, A. et al. (2010). Inhibition of angiotensin converting enzyme (ACE) activity by the aqueous extract of *Hibiscus sabdariffa*. *J. Ethnopharmacol.* 127 (1): 7–10.
72. Bhattacharya, S.K. and Ghosal, S. (2002). Antihypertensive effects of reserpine and other plant-derived alkaloids. *Indian J Pharmacol.* 34 (6): 418–425.
73. Li, P., Wang, F., Zheng, Y., and Hu, C.P. (2016). Natural calcium antagonists and hypertension: a new frontier. *J. Cardiovasc. Pharmacol.* 67 (6): 503–512.
74. Herrera-Arellano, A., Flores-Romero, S., Chávez-Soto, M.A., and Tortoriello, J. (2004). Effectiveness and tolerability of a standardized extract from *Hibiscus sabdariffa* in patients with mild to moderate hypertension: a controlled and randomized clinical trial. *Phytomedicine* 11 (5): 375–382.
75. Gupta, R.K., Patel, A.K., Shah, N. et al. (2014). Oxidative stress and antioxidants in disease and cancer: a review. *Asian Pac. J. Cancer Prev.* 15 (11): 4405–4409.
76. Tsioufis, C., Kasiakogias, A., and Thomopoulos, C. (2015). The role of potassium channels in the regulation of vascular tone. *Curr. Hypertens. Rep.* 17 (5): 37.
77. Yuan, H., Ma, Q., Ye, L., and Piao, G. (2016). The traditional medicine and modern medicine from natural products. *Molecules* 21 (5): 559.
78. Wu, J., Xia, S., Kalionis, B. et al. (2014). The role of oxidative stress and inflammation in cardiovascular aging. *Biomed. Res. Int.* 2014: 615312.
79. Kulkarni, S.K. and Dhir, A. (2008). *Withania somnifera*: an Indian ginseng with multiple neuroprotective and cardioprotective actions. *J. Ethnopharmacol.* 120 (2): 225–234.
80. Mahfoud, F. and Böhm, M. (2005). *Rauwolfia serpentina*: reappraisal of an ancient antihypertensive. *J. Hypertens.* 23 (2): 237–238.
81. Bent, S. (2008). Herbal medicine in the United States: review of efficacy, safety, and regulation. *J. Gen. Intern. Med.* 23 (6): 854–859.
82. Posadzki, P., Watson, L.K., and Ernst, E. (2013). Herb-drug interactions: an overview of systematic reviews. *Br. J. Clin. Pharmacol.* 75 (3): 603–618.
83. Izzo, A.A. and Ernst, E. (2009). Interactions between herbal medicines and prescribed drugs: a systematic review. *Drugs* 69 (13): 1777–1798.
84. Ekor, M. (2014). The growing use of herbal medicines: issues relating to adverse reactions and challenges in monitoring safety. *Front. Pharmacol.* 4: 177.
85. Izzo, A.A. and Ernst, E. (2001). Interactions between herbal medicines and prescribed drugs: a systematic review. *Drugs* 61 (15): 2163–2175.
86. WHO (2004). *Guidelines on Safety Monitoring of Herbal Medicines in Pharmacovigilance Systems*. Geneva: World Health Organization.
87. Fabricant, D.S. and Farnsworth, N.R. (2001). The value of plants used in traditional medicine for drug discovery. *Environ. Health Perspect.* 109 (Suppl 1): 69–75.
88. Barnes, J., Anderson, L.A., and Phillipson, J.D. (2007). *Herbal Medicines: A Guide for Healthcare Professionals*, 3e. London: Pharmaceutical Press.
89. Scalbert, A., Johnson, I.T., and Saltmarsh, M. (2005). Polyphenols: antioxidants and beyond. *Am. J. Clin. Nutr.* 81 (1 Suppl): 215S–217S.
90. Ried, K. (2016). Garlic lowers blood pressure in hypertensive individuals: a meta-analysis and review. *J. Nutr.* 146 (2): 389S–396S.
91. Serban, C., Sahebkar, A., Zanchetti, A. et al. (2016). Effects of olive leaf extract on blood pressure: a meta-analysis. *Phytomedicine* 23 (4): 409–416.
92. Shoba, G., Joy, D., Joseph, T. et al. (1998). Influence of piperine on the pharmacokinetics of curcumin in animals and human volunteers. *Planta Med.* 64 (4): 353–356.
93. Li, S.L., Han, Q.B., Liang, Y.Z. et al. (2004). Chromatographic fingerprinting and quality control of herbal medicines. *J. Chromatogr. B* 812 (1–2): 53–70.
94. Hopkins, A.L. (2008). Network pharmacology: the next paradigm in drug discovery. *Nat. Chem. Biol.* 4 (11): 682–690.
95. Li, S. and Zhang, B. (2013). Traditional Chinese medicine network pharmacology: theory, methodology and application. *Chin. J. Nat. Med.* 11 (2): 110–120.
96. Patra, J.K., Das, G., Fraceto, L.F. et al. (2018). Nano based drug delivery systems: recent developments and future prospects. *J. Nanobiotechnol.* 16 (1): 71.
97. World Health Organization (2013). *WHO Traditional Medicine Strategy 2014–2023*. Geneva: WHO Press.

# Natural Lipid-Lowering Agents: Role in Dyslipidemia and Atherosclerosis

CHAPTER 6

**Evelyn Sharon Sukumaran[1], Garlanka Venkata Naga Kiranmayi[1], K. Ravi Shankar[2], and Nakkala Danamurthy[3]**

[1] *Department of Pharmacology, Faculty of Pharmacy, Dr. M.G.R. Educational and Research Institute, Chennai, Tamil Nadu, India*

[2] *Aditya College of Pharmacy, Aditya University, East-Godavari District, Andhra Pradesh, India*

[3] *QIS College of Pharmacy, Vengamukkapalem, Prakasam District, Ongole, Andhra Pradesh, India*

## 6.1 INTRODUCTION

Elevated levels of one or more plasma lipids are the hallmark of a medical disorder called hyperlipidemia. The main lipids that are associated with proteins and transported as lipid–protein complexes, or lipoproteins, include cholesterol, triglycerides, and phospholipids. According to traditional description, hyperlipidemia occurs when the number of lipoproteins that transport cholesterol or triglycerides in plasma is beyond the normal level (Figure 6.1). This is because some lipids are insoluble in plasma, where efficient transportation occurs [1]. The five primary lipoproteins that have similar functions are low-density lipoproteins (LDL), very low-density lipoproteins (VLDLs), intermediate-density lipoproteins (IDLs), high-density lipoproteins (HDLs), and chylomicrons. Triglycerides are mostly carried by VLDL [2] (Table 6.1). Lipid abnormalities increase the risk of peripheral vascular artery disease, coronary disease, and cerebrovascular sickness. Atherosclerotic cardiovascular disease (ASCVD), or cardiovascular disease (CVD), is the main reason of mortality and morbidity. Worldwide, cardiovascular illnesses claim the lives of almost 12 million people each year. A diet heavy in cholesterol and saturated fats, age, family history, hypertension, and lifestyle are important risk factors for these conditions. However, elevated levels of cholesterol, especially LDL cholesterol, are primarily responsible for the development of coronary heart disease [4].

Therapeutic lifestyle changes, including diet modification, regular exercise, and cessation of tobacco use, are the first-line treatment for any lipoprotein problem. It should be noted that consuming less cholesterol is a consequence of dieting. Concurrently, there is an increase in cholesterol synthesis, particularly from the liver. It is advised that fat consumption be limited to 25–35% of total calorie intake, that saturated fats account for less than 7% of total energy intake, and that daily consumption of cholesterol should not exceed 200 mg. It is recommended to consume soluble fiber and plant sterol esters [5]. If lifestyle modifications are insufficient, lipid-lowering medications may be chosen depending on which lipid is at undesired level and the degree to which it will likely increase the risk of ASCVD [1]. Synthetic lipid-lowering medications used to treat hyperlipidemia include fibrates, statins, and bile acid sequestrants (BASs). Despite their positive therapeutic advantages, they are frequently associated with certain major adverse effects, including myopathy, rhabdomyolysis, and an elevated risk of gallstones. New lipid-lowering medications with significant therapeutic benefits and negligible adverse effects are therefore desperately needed [6].

## 6.2 DYSLIPIDEMIA

Dyslipidemia is a condition related to lipoprotein metabolism characterized by either inadequate or insufficient levels of lipoproteins. These conditions may be indicated by reduced levels of HDL cholesterol and increased levels of total cholesterol, LDL cholesterol, and triglycerides [7]. This may be a result of both genetic abnormalities and environmental factors. There are two types of underlying causes of dyslipidemia:

i. Primary dyslipidemia: This can result from inherited genetic factors that increase lipid levels (Table 6.2).

ii. Secondary or acquired dyslipidemia: This can result from aberrant lipid levels caused by nutrition, drugs, lifestyle choices, and illnesses (Table 6.3) [8–10].

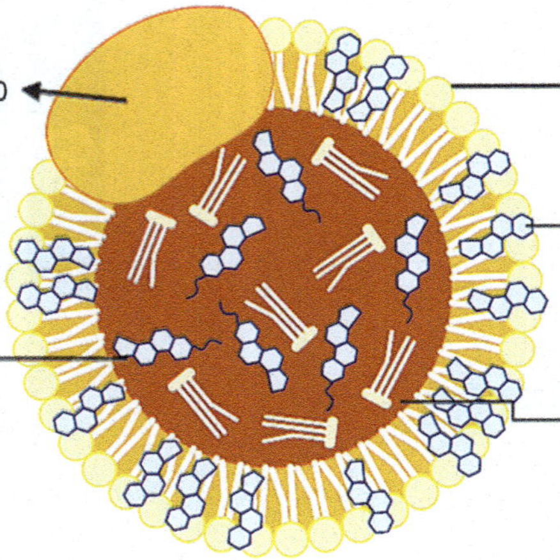


**FIGURE 6.1** Structure of lipoprotein.

**Table 6.1** Characteristics and functions of plasma lipoproteins.

| S. no. | Lipoprotein class | Diameter (mm) | Lipid content | Sources of lipid | Functions |
|---|---|---|---|---|---|
| 1 | Chylomicrons | 100–500 | TG>>CHE | Diet | Dietary TG transport |
| 2 | Chylomicron remnants | 30–50 | CHE>>TG | Diet | Dietary CH transport |
| 3 | VLDL | 40–80 | TG>>CHE | Liver | Endogenous TG transport |
| 4 | IDL | 30–35 | CHE≥TG | VLDL | Transport of CHE and TG to liver source of LDL |
| 5 | LDL | 20–25 | CHE | IDL | Transport of CH to tissue and liver |
| 6 | HDL | 5–10 | Phospholipids, CHE | Tissues, cell membrane | Removal of CH from tissues |

VLDL – very low-density lipoprotein, IDL – intermediate density lipoprotein, LDL – low density lipoprotein, HDL – high density lipoprotein, TG – triglycerides, CHE – cholesterol ester, CH – cholesterol [3].
*Source:* Data from Baumgartner et al. [3].

**Table 6.2** Primary dyslipidemia (Fredrickson classification).

| Type | Disorder | Cause | Occurrence | Description |
|---|---|---|---|---|
| Type I | Familial lipoprotein lipase deficiency | Genetic | Very rare | Elevated chylomicrons |
| Type II a | Familial hypercholesterolemia | Genetic | Less common | Elevated LDL only |
| Type II b | Polygenic hypercholesterolemia | Multifactorial | Common | Elevated LDL |
| Type III | Familial dysbetalipoproteinemia | Genetic | Rare | Increased IDL, chylomicrons, and chylomicron remnant |
| Type IV | Hypertriglyceridemia | Multifactorial, genetic | Common | Elevated VLDL |
| Type V | Familial combines hyperlipidemia | Genetic | Less common | Elevated VLDL, LDL |

*Source:* Data from Baumgartner et al. [3].

**Table 6.3** Secondary dyslipidemia.

| S.no | Causes | Cholesterol | Triglyceride |
|---|---|---|---|
| 1 | Hypothyroidism | Increase | – |
| 2 | Nephrotic syndrome | Increase | Increase |
| 3 | Chronic kidney disease | – | Increase |
| 4 | Primary biliary cholangitis | Increase | – |
| 5 | Obstructive jaundice | Increase | – |
| 6 | Diabetes | Increase | Increase |
| 7 | Cushing's syndrome | Increase | Increase |
| 8 | Obesity | – | Increase |
| 9 | Pheochromocytoma | Increase | Increase |

*Source:* Burčová et al. [8] / with permission of Elsevier.

## 6.3 ATHEROSCLEROSIS

The Greek word for "athero," which means "gruel" or "porridge," describes the fatty material found in the typical atheroma's core, and "sclerosis," which means "scarring," refers to the connective tissues in the plaques. This is where the name atherosclerosis originates [11]. Atherosclerosis, or "hardening of the arteries," is a complex chronic inflammation of the major and medium arteries that can be exacerbated by hyperlipidemia and/or other risk factors [12]. Chronic illness is conventionally understood to be the buildup of fibrofatty deposits in the intima of medium and large muscle arteries. Atherosclerotic plaques are distinguished by their complexity and accompanying instability. This complexity is shown in the thickness of the necrotic core, degree of inflammatory cell infiltration, lipid deposits, calcification, and blood vessels with intraplaque hemorrhages [13].

## 6.4 PATHOGENESIS OF ATHEROSCLEROSIS

Persistent inflammatory changes lead to the development of an atheromatous lesion in the innermost layer of blood vessels and endothelial cells in arteries, which causes triglycerides and pro-inflammatory cells to accumulate inside the intima of the vessels [14]. Both big and small-caliber arteries are affected by atherosclerosis, which can result in distal embolic disease, aneurysm development, high-grade stenosis that obstructs blood flow, and vascular rupture [15]. Atherosclerosis-related complications that endanger human health include acute coronary heart disease, angina, and myocardial infarction. Ross hypothesized in 1999 that atherosclerosis is an inflammatory condition [15]. The response-to-injury theory states that atherosclerosis is the arterial walls' long-term inflammatory and healing reaction to endothelial damage. Lesions are produced by the interaction of endothelial cells, smooth muscle cells of the arterial wall, T lymphocytes, macrophages, and modified lipoproteins. This schema describes how atherosclerosis develops [16], as shown in Figure 6.2.

- **Endothelial injury and dysfunction:** This process starts with damage or activation of the artery's endothelium, which is frequently brought on by risk factors such smoking, diabetes, high blood pressure, and high cholesterol. This malfunction encourages thrombosis, inflammatory cell adhesion, and increased vascular permeability [17].
- **Accumulation of lipoproteins:** After entering the subendothelial region, LDL cholesterol undergoes oxidation. Oxidized LDL, which is particularly atherogenic, draws circulating monocytes [18].
- **Inflammatory cell response:** After adhering to the endothelium, monocytes go into the vessel wall and undergo macrophage differentiation. Fatty streaks, a characteristic of early atherosclerosis lesions, are caused by these macrophages consuming oxidized LDL and turning into foam cells [16, 19].
- **Smooth muscle cell proliferation:** In general, pro-inflammatory stimuli that lead to endothelial dysfunction can disrupt the endothelial barrier or microtubules, increasing junctional permeability and facilitating the transendothelial migration of immune cells and atherogenic lipoproteins into the artery intima. Extracellular matrix (ECM) components are produced by smooth muscle cells when they move from the media to the intima and multiply [19].
- **Plaque progression:** By absorbing altered lipids and developing into the monocytes in the intima, foam cells are created, a characteristic of the early fatty streak lesion, when the resident macrophages are simultaneously stimulated by macrophage colony stimulating factor (M-CSF). Foam cell accumulation and smooth muscle cell migration and proliferation from the media to the intima result in the formation of a fibrous cap on top of a lipid-rich necrotic core. Plaques may also contain ECM components and calcifications [18].
- **Plaque complications:** Over time, plaques may become fragile. Although the exact reasons for plaque rupture are still unknown, the primary causes include high-shear stresss in the arterial region, macrophage calcification, iron accumulation, and the development of enzymes like myeloperoxidase and metalloproteinases (MMPs), which are generated by inflammatory cells and weaken the fibrous cap. When the fibrous cap bursts or erodes, thrombogenic material is exposed to the bloodstream, causing clot (thrombus) formation [13].

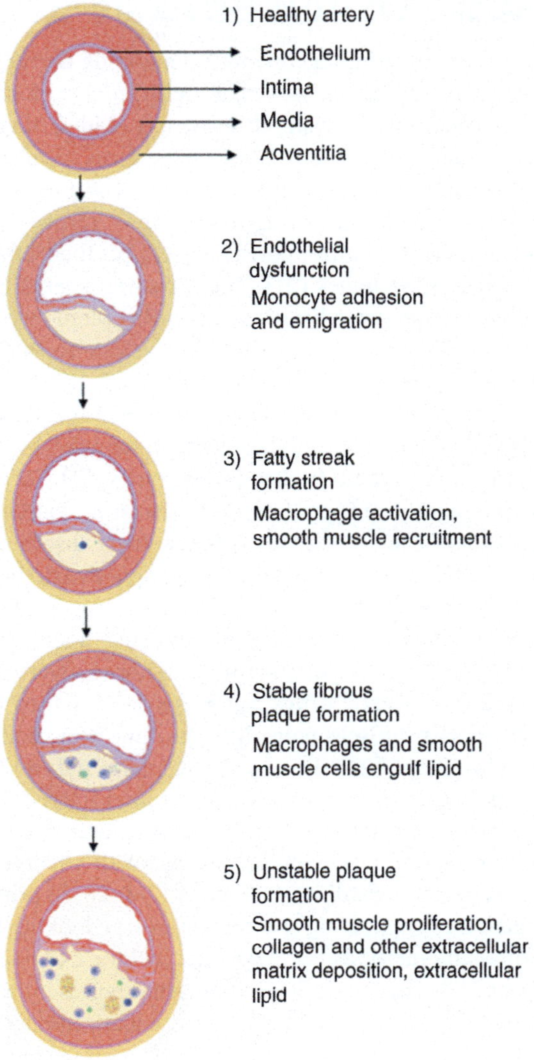


**FIGURE 6.2** Pathogenesis of atherosclerosis.

## 6.5 NATURAL LIPID-LOWERING AGENTS

Natural lipid-lowering agents are compounds derived from dietary or botanical sources that help reduce blood lipid levels, particularly cholesterol and triglycerides, through a variety of mechanisms [20]. These substances have drawn a lot of interest recently as supplements or substitutes for traditional synthetic lipid-lowering medications, mostly because of their accessible nature, positive safety profiles, and additional health advantages [21]. These natural agents encompass a broad range of substances, including plant sterols and stanols, soluble fibers, soy proteins, red yeast rice, berberine, artichoke leaf extract, and omega-3 fatty acids [20, 22]. Many of these compounds are found in common foods such as oats, nuts, fruits, vegetables, and fatty fish, or are available as dietary supplements and herbal preparations [21, 22]. They block the liver from producing cholesterol, increase the excretion of bile acids, stop the stomach from absorbing cholesterol, and promote the elimination of low-density lipoprotein cholesterol (LDL-C) from the bloodstream [23]. The growing interest in natural lipid-lowering agents is also driven by the search for treatments with fewer adverse effects compared to synthetic drugs, such as statins, which can be associated with muscle pain, liver enzyme elevations, and other side effects [24]. Furthermore, many natural agents offer pleiotropic advantages, such as cardioprotective, antioxidant, and anti-inflammatory qualities, which make them desirable options for individuals looking for all-encompassing strategies to lower cardiovascular risk [20]. These properties will make them appealing choices for anyone looking for all-encompassing methods for lowering cardiovascular risk [20, 21]. Overall, natural lipid-lowering agents represent a promising and multifaceted approach to dyslipidemia management, either as standalone interventions in mild cases or as complementary therapies alongside conventional medications in more severe or refractory cases [21, 23].

### 6.5.1 POLYPHENOLS

Plants create a wide range of secondary metabolites called natural polyphenols, which can be tiny molecules or complex polymeric substances. Polyphenols are a class of physiologically active substances that are vital to human nutrition and may be found in fruits, vegetables, cereals, coffee, and other foods [25]. Polyphenols are compounds that have at least one aromatic ring and one or more hydroxyl functional groups attached to it [26]. Phenolic acids and phenolic alcohols are the two primary categories into which they are frequently divided. Phenolic acids, flavonoids, lignans, phenolic alcohols, and stilbenes are the primary forms of polyphenols [27] (Figure 6.3). The six subclasses of flavonoids are flavanols, flavones, isoflavones, flavanones, and anthocyanidins. The most prevalent groups are flavones. Annually, approximately 12 million individuals worldwide succumb to CVDs. In addition to their ability to modify molecular targets and signaling pathways linked to angiogenesis, hormone activity, cell survival, proliferation, differentiation, migration, detoxification enzymes, immune responses, and more, natural polyphenols are widely recognized for their strong anti-inflammatory and antioxidant properties [26].

A wide range of fruits, vegetables, and drinks contain natural compounds known as polyphenols, which play a major role in reducing dyslipidemias and atherosclerosis through a number of different pathways. A key enzyme involved in cellular energy, AMP-activated protein kinase

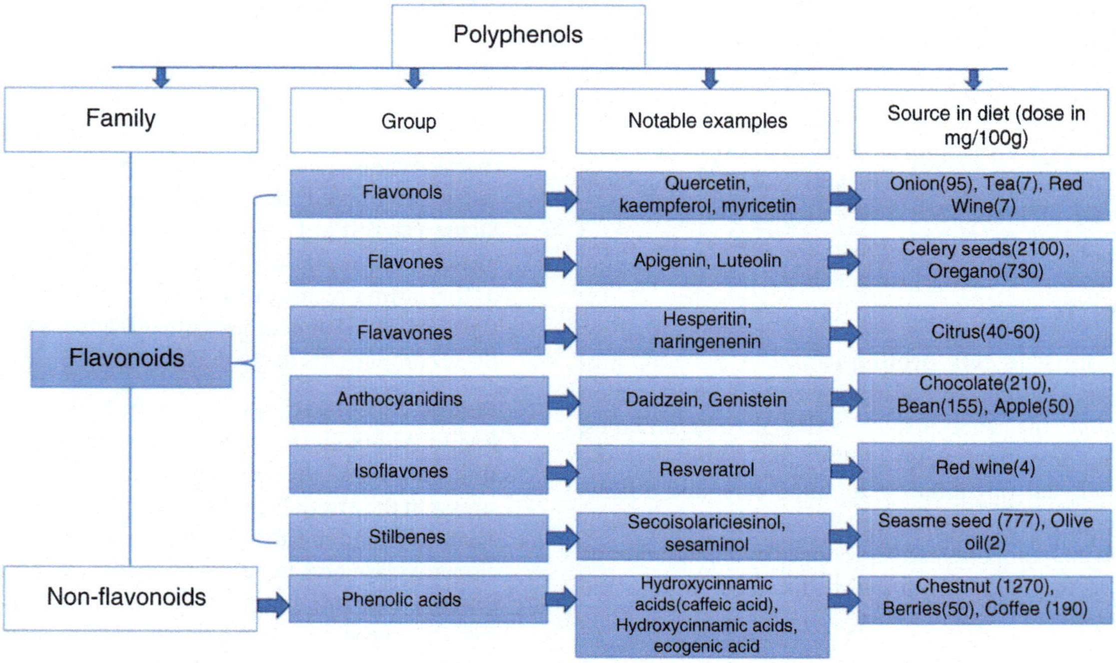


**FIGURE 6.3** Classification of polyphenols.

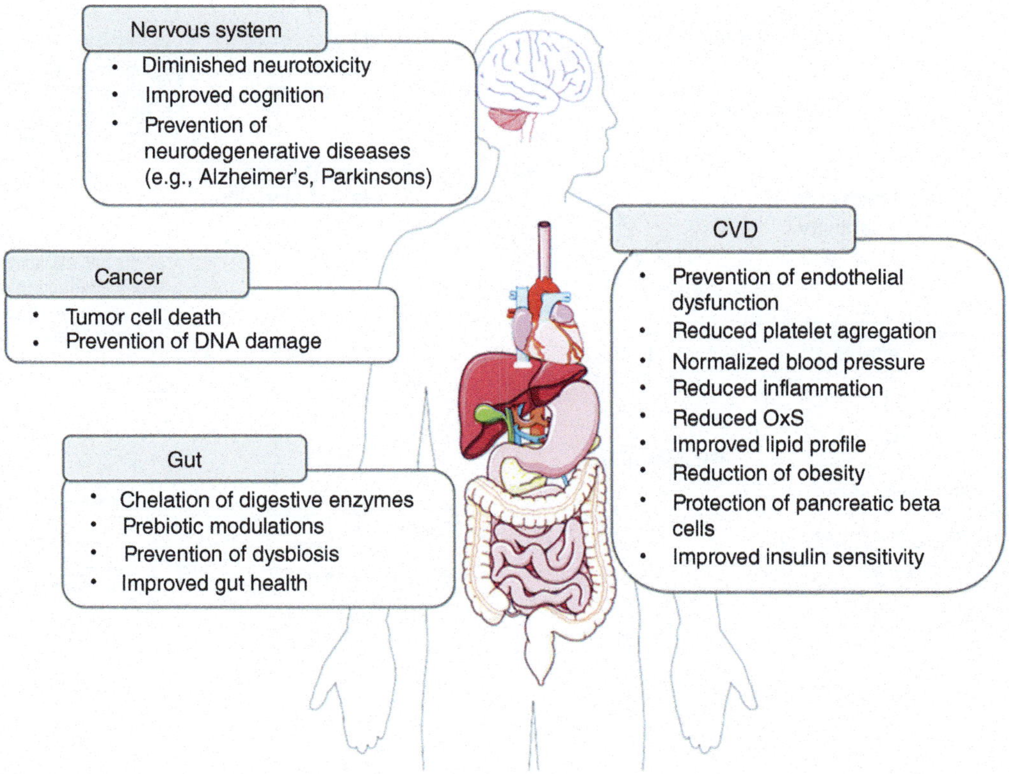


**FIGURE 6.4** Potential health benefits of dietary polyphenols in chronic diseases.

(AMPK), is activated. Research indicates that the phosphorylation and activity of AMPK and its downstream targets, such as acetyl-CoA carboxylase (ACC), can be markedly increased by polyphenols like resveratrol, apigenin, and synthetic versions. This activation leads to reduced lipid accumulation and improved lipid profiles, particularly in diabetic conditions, thus inhibiting the progression of atherosclerosis [28]. Polyphenols also enhance endothelial function and exhibit antioxidant and anti-inflammatory effects [68]. As a kind of polyphenol, flavonoids are especially good in lowering inflammation and oxidative stress, which enhances vascular health and lessens the development of atherosclerotic plaques (Figure 6.4). Flavonoids can change cholesterol levels and delay the onset of atherosclerosis by improving the function of HDL and reducing the oxidation of LDL [29]. Moreover, paraoxonase 1 (PON1), an enzyme associated with HDL, has been recognized for its role in preventing oxidative damage to lipids and has been linked to polyphenol activity. Polyphenols can improve PON1's resistance to oxidative stress and inflammation by modifying its activity, which may reduce the risk of atherosclerosis and CVDs [30]. Additionally, gut microbiota is essential for transforming dietary polyphenols into bioactive compounds that the body can absorb and use more efficiently [70]. Their anti-atherosclerotic qualities may be strengthened by this conversion, providing cardiovascular advantages associated with dietary practices [31].

### 6.5.2 PHYTOSTEROLS

"Phytosterols (PS)" refers to plant sterols and their corresponding unsaturated derivatives, known as plant stanols [32]. The three most prevalent forms of dietary sterols are stigmasterol, campesterol, and β-sitosterol. Stanols make up only a minor portion of the 200–400 mg of plant sterols that are often included in Western diets (up to 50 mg). Natural sources of plant sterols and stanols include sesame seeds, nuts, wheat germ oil, soybean oil, maize oil, and fruits like figs and oranges [33, 34]. The most common sterol in human cells has a similar structural function. In contrast to cholesterol, phytosterols have a side chain attached at position C-17 [35]. Plant sterols and stanols are structurally similar to cholesterol, which explains their lipid-lowering impact. Plant sterols in the colon reduce cholesterol absorption by binding to lipid-laden micelles, which are a key vehicle for cholesterol absorption and transport. Plant sterols have a higher hydrolysis rate than cholesterol. Their presence in the colon reduces cholesterol solubilization into micelles, leading to decreased absorption and increased fecal excretion [36]. By preventing the digestive system from absorbing cholesterol, phytosterols significantly lower LDL cholesterol. Plant sterols may interact with enterocyte ATP-binding cassette transport proteins to cause cholesterol to return to the intestinal lumen. Blood LDL cholesterol levels are lowered as a result of the unabsorbed cholesterol being expelled in the feces [37].

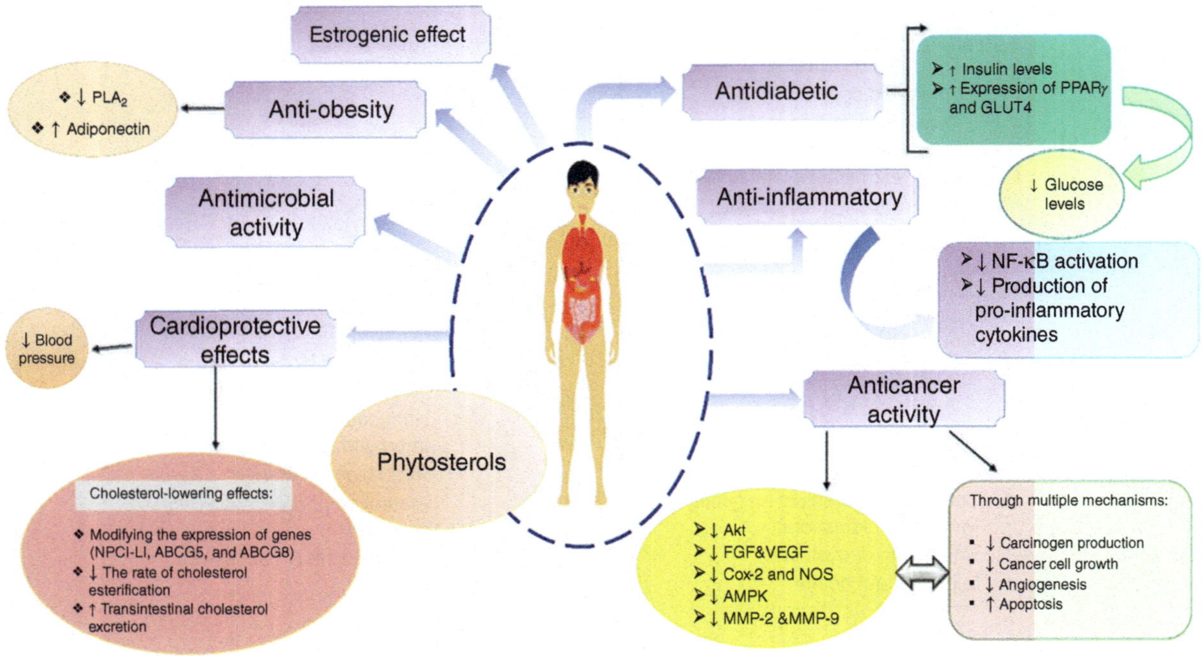


**FIGURE 6.5** Benefits of phytosterols for human health.

Other mechanisms consist of bile salt-formed micelles emulsify dietary lipids and transfer phytosterols to enterocytes through Niemann–Pick C1-Like 1 (NPC1L1), a well-known membrane transport protein. Phytosterols are mostly eliminated from the intestinal lumen by efflux transporters from the ABC family, such as ABCG5 and ABCG8. Phytosterols are mostly released into the bile by the ABCG5/G8 transporters found in the biliary pole of hepatocytes after being esterified in enterocytes, integrated into chylomicrons, and then collected by the liver [38, 39]. Because cholesterol (from food or bile) is absorbed from the stomach via the same mechanism as phytosterols, the two substances compete for inclusion in mixed micelles and subsequent absorption in enterocytes via the NPC1L1 transporter. As the intestine phytosterol level increases, the fractional absorption of cholesterol decreases. For daily doses of 300–400 mg (typical of most diets), phytosterols lower the absorption of cholesterol by around 5%. This inhibition reaches 35–40% at daily dosages of 1500–2000 mg, which is only achievable with enriched functional meals or supplements. By immediately co-crystallizing with cholesterol in the intestinal lumen and promoting its excretion through the fecal pathway, phytosterols can also reduce the absorption of cholesterol [36]. Phytosterols can be regarded as food preservatives because they have antibacterial properties. It has been demonstrated that ß-Sitosterol, which is extracted from the Brazilian plant *Cissus sicyoides*, has antibacterial properties against *Bacillus subtilis*. A study examined the antibacterial activity of β-sitosterol, one of the most significant antimicrobial elements in pre-extracts of sprue bark. The authors came to the conclusion that β-sitosterol might inhibit the growth of microbes. Although β-sitosterol's antibacterial activity was not verified, it did have a bacteriostatic effect on the bacteria [40]. This LDL-C-lowering activity reduces the risk of atherosclerotic CVD since LDL-C is a significant factor in the development of atherosclerotic plaques. Furthermore, there is mounting evidence that polysterols may exert mild anti-inflammatory effects by lowering systemic markers like interleukin 6 and C-reactive protein and by preventing the oxidation of LDL particles, a critical step in the development of plaque. Although polysterols are generally considered safe, individuals with sitosterolemia, a rare genetic condition characterized by excessive sterol absorption and accumulation, should avoid high doses of polysterols, as they may reduce the absorption of fat-soluble nutrients such as vitamin E and β-carotene. The use of polysterols as a non-pharmacological method of managing dyslipidemia is supported by health groups, including the National Lipid Association and the European Atherosclerosis Society. Polysterols, when included in a heart-healthy diet, are a useful tool for those who want to lower their cardiovascular risk, particularly when combined with lifestyle changes like consistent exercise and weight control (Figure 6.5) [41].

### 6.5.3 OMEGA 3 FATTY ACIDS

Polyunsaturated fatty acids (PUFAs) with at least one double bond between the third and fourth omega-end carbons are known as omega-3 fatty acids. The body cannot make these fats on its own, so it must acquire them from food sources such flaxseed, chia seeds, walnuts, fatty fish (tuna, mackerel, and salmon), and some vegetable oils. Alpha-linolenic acid (ALA), eicosapentaenoic acid (EPA), and docosahexaenoic acid (DHA) are the three main types of omega-3s that are mostly found in marine sources [42]. The rate at which the ethyl esters of EPA and DHA are absorbed depends on the amount of fat in the diet and needs further enzymatic processing [43]. Omega-3 fatty acids are effective as a standalone treatment or when combined with other triglyceride-lowering medications to manage extremely high triglyceride (TG) levels. They exert their effects by lowering TG, decreasing small dense LDL, increasing significant buoyant LDL, and raising HDL-C [43]. Omega-3 fatty acids have received a lot of attention in the prevention and treatment of dyslipidemia and atherosclerosis [44].

It is very well known that omega-3 fatty acids have hypotriglyceridemic effects when dyslipidemia is present. They help reduce blood triglyceride levels, which are a major risk factor for cardiovascular illnesses, including atherosclerosis. Mechanistically, they improve the removal of triglycerides from the circulation and reduce the production and secretion of VLDLs [45, 46]. Equally significant is the part that omega-3 fatty acids play in atherosclerosis. These fats have anti-inflammatory qualities that are essential for reducing inflammation, a necessary step in the formation of atherosclerotic plaques [47]. Because of decreased TG synthesis, omega-3 fatty acids suppress the hepatic VLDL-TG secretion rates, which in turn lowers blood TG levels in humans. Therefore, decreased production and release of VLDL will result from decreased hepatic TG synthesis [48]. The broad spectrum of physiological effects and the robust evidence base make omega-3 fatty acids a cornerstone of preventive nutrition and cardiovascular health. Clinical trials suggest high-dose omega-3s may reduce cardiovascular events in high-risk patients. Evidence shows that after one month of therapy, individuals taking EPA + DHA had a 22% lower P2Y12 receptor reactivity index (a measure of clopidogrel resistance) than those taking a placebo [49, 50].

### 6.5.4 ALKALOIDS

Alkaloids, a broad class of naturally occurring substances with basic nitrogen atoms, are becoming more widely acknowledged for their potential for treating atherosclerosis and dyslipidemia. Traditional Chinese medicine monomers have garnered interest because of their distinct structure, proven effectiveness, and exact mode of action. As a class of nitrogen-containing organic compounds, alkaloids have emerged as a research hotspot due to their numerous important biological actions. Alkaloid components found in natural products are primarily categorized into the following classes based on their various chemical structures: isoquinoline, organic amine, piperidine, pyrrolidine, terpene, pyridine, and indole.

According to research, several types of alkaloids are derived from plants, including berberine, nuciferine, coptisine, palmatine, and epiberberine, which significantly reduce cholesterol and prevent atherosclerosis through various mechanisms, as represented in Table 6.4 [51, 52]. In animal models of hyperlipidemias, the beneficial effects of natural alkaloids in delaying the onset of atherosclerosis have also been thoroughly investigated [51]. The main ways by which alkaloid compounds in natural products lower cholesterol include increasing hepatic cholesterol uptake, preventing hepatic cholesterol synthesis, increasing cholesterol conversion, preventing intestinal cholesterol absorption, encouraging fatty acid oxidation, preventing lipid synthesis, encouraging lipolysis, controlling bile acid metabolism, modifying intestinal flora, reducing lipid oxidation, reducing insulin resistance, and supporting additional research and development of novel lipid-lowering medications derived from alkaloids in natural products.

**Table 6.4** Mechanisms of different alkaloids in dyslipidemia and atherosclerosis.

| Mechanism | Alkaloids | Effects on lipids and atherosclerosis |
|---|---|---|
| Downregulation of lipid synthesis | Nuciferine, berberine | ↓ TC, ↓ TG, improved liver steatosis |
| Upregulation of LDLR | Berberine | ↑ LDL clearance, ↓ LDL-C |
| Inhibition of cholesterol synthesis | Berberine, coptisine | ↓ Endogenous cholesterol production |
| Inhibition of absorption | Piperine, berberine | ↓ Intestinal cholesterol uptake |
| Promotion of lipolysis | Various alkaloids | ↓ Triglyceride levels |
| Anti-atherogenic effects | Nuciferine | ↓ Foam cell formation, ↓ plaque development |
| Modulation of gut microbiota | Nuciferine | Improved lipid metabolism, ↓ fat accumulation |

Sterol regulatory element-binding protein 1 (SREBP-1), ATP citrate lyase (ACLY), acetyl-CoA carboxylase (ACC), and fatty acid synthase (FAS) are important enzymes associated with lipid formation in dyslipidemias that may be inhibited by alkaloids like nuciferine, which is present in lotus leaves. This results in improved hepatic steatosis, as well as lower levels of triglycerides (TG) and total cholesterol (TC). Additionally, it enhances serum lipid profiles by raising HDL-C and decreasing TG and LDL-C [52]. Nuciferine has been demonstrated to enhance lipid metabolism by controlling intestinal microbiota, lowering intestinal permeability, preventing weight gain and fat, buildup and reducing the risk of dyslipidemia [52].

In atherosclerosis, alkaloid therapy dramatically decreases the extent of aortic atherosclerotic lesions, according to meta-analyses of animal research, particularly in ApoE−/−mice [69]. Particularly useful are indole alkaloids and isoquinoline alkaloids (like berberine) [53, 54]. By modifying the phosphoinositide 3-kinase/protein kinase B (PI3K/Akt)/mechanistic target of rapamycin (mTOR) and peroxisome proliferator-activated receptor gamma (PPARγ)/liver X receptor alpha (LXRα)/ATP-binding cassette transporter A1 (ABCA1) signaling pathways, nuciferine and related alkaloids decrease lipid deposition by reducing the production of foam cells from macrophages, a crucial phase in atherogenesis [52, 55]. Additionally, alkaloids have antioxidative and anti-inflammatory qualities that assist stabilize plaques and stop them from rupturing or progressing [55].

In certain areas, alkaloids like berberine have received clinical approval for the treatment of atherosclerosis and dyslipidemia because of their strong lipid-lowering properties and good safety records. In animal models and clinical investigations, berberine, jatrorrhizine, coptisine, and palmatine (from *Rhizoma Coptidis*) have been demonstrated to increase HDL-C while decreasing blood TC, TG, and LDL-C. These effects are accomplished by boosting bile acid excretion, decreasing HMGCR, and upregulating low-density lipoprotein receptor (LDLR) [55]. The majority of the data is derived from meta-analyses and clinical trials; the steady improvement in lipid profiles and atherosclerotic load shows their potential as supplements or substitutes for traditional treatments [56].

### 6.5.5 PROBIOTICS

When ingested in appropriate quantities, probiotics – beneficial living microorganisms – offer health benefits to the host. They primarily enhance the growth of the body's natural digestive microflora. These beneficial properties have been identified in various microorganisms, particularly lactic acid bacteria (LAB). LAB belong to several families, such as *Leuconostoc*, *Pediococcus*, *Streptococcus*, *Lactobacillus*. Probiotic bacteria are nonpathogenic bacteria that are often present in the human gastrointestinal system and protect the intestines against harmful bacteria [57].

Probiotics, or live beneficial bacteria, are gaining increasing acceptance as complementary treatments for atherosclerosis and dyslipidemia. Probiotic supplements can enhance lipid profiles and modify cardiovascular risk factors, according to several clinical trials and mechanistic investigations [58].

In people with hyperlipidemia, probiotic use has been demonstrated to dramatically reduce blood triglycerides (TG), total cholesterol (TC), and LDL-C while raising high-density lipoprotein cholesterol (HDL-C) [59, 60]. Although the lipid-lowering effects of probiotics may be less pronounced than those of pharmacologic agents, they are comparable to the benefits achieved through lifestyle modification and can contribute to reduced cardiovascular risk [59].

Probiotics exert their lipid-lowering and anti-atherosclerotic effects through several key mechanisms (Figure 6.6):

- Many probiotic strains (especially *Lactobacillus* and *Bifidobacterium*) produce bile salt hydrolase, which deconjugates bile acids. This reduces cholesterol reabsorption and increases its excretion in feces [61]. Probiotics can assimilate cholesterol into their cell membranes or convert cholesterol to coprostanol, a nonabsorbable form excreted in feces [60].
- *Pediococcus pentosaceus* PP04 lowered blood LPS and tumor necrosis factor-alpha (TNF-α) levels, upregulated

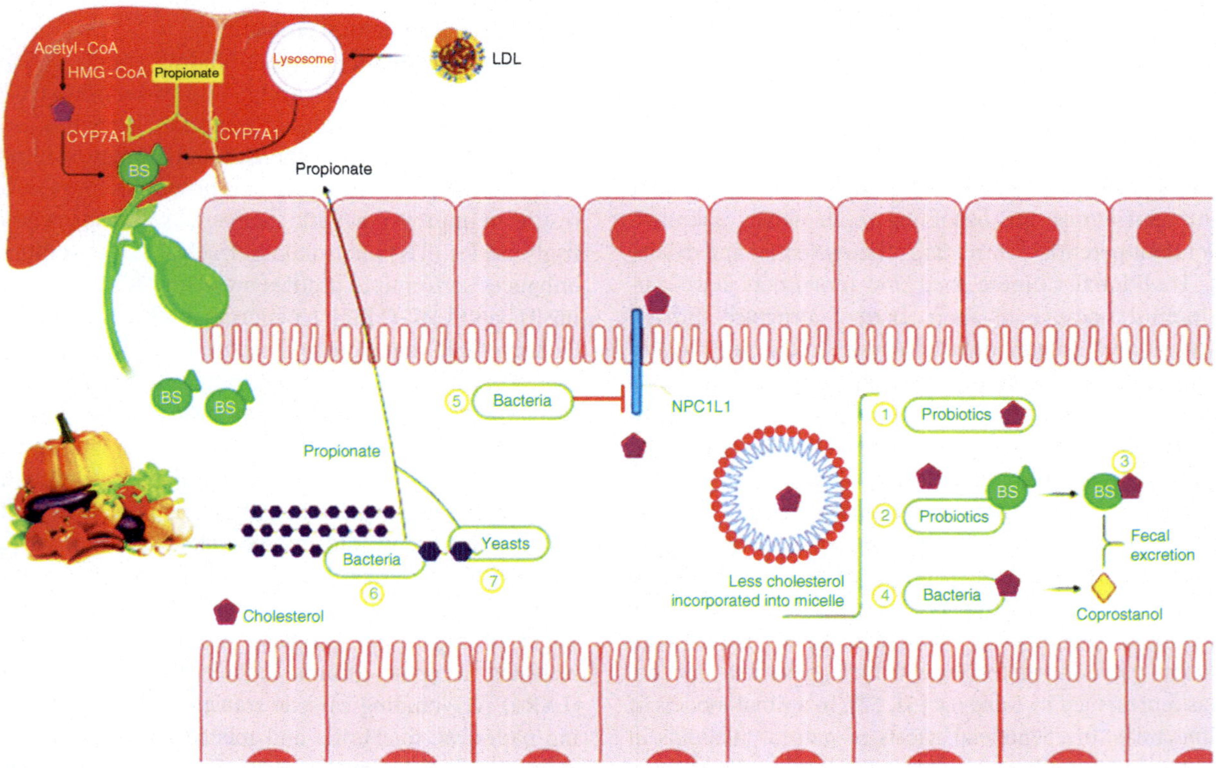


**FIGURE 6.6** Mechanism of probiotics.

PPARα to promote lipolysis, and downregulated FAS and stearoyl-CoA desaturase 1

- SCD1 to prevent lipogenesis, which in turn decreased TC, TG, LDL-C, and free FAs [62].
- Fermentation of dietary fibers by probiotics generates short-chain fatty acids (SCFAs), which can upregulate hepatic genes involved in HDL synthesis and downregulate cholesterol synthesis enzymes such as 3-hydroxy-3-methyl glutaryl-coenzyme A (HMG-CoA) reductase [63].
- Probiotics increase beneficial intestinal bacteria, such as *Lactiplantibacillus plantarum*, *Bifidobacterium animalis* subsp. *lactis,* which further support healthy lipid metabolism and reduce intestinal cholesterol absorption. Probiotics influence the gut–liver axis, modulating lipid metabolism and systemic inflammation, which are central to the pathogenesis of atherosclerosis [58, 64].
- Probiotics can downregulate genes involved in cholesterol synthesis (e.g., HMGCR) and upregulate those involved in cholesterol excretion and HDL formation [57].

Supplementing with strains like *Lactobacillus plantarum* L. has been confirmed by numerous studies and meta-analyses. Significant improvements in lipid profiles are produced by *Lactobacillus acidophilus* and *Bifidobacterium* species, which may also lower the incidence of metabolic syndrome and cardiovascular risk factors [60]. Probiotics offer a multifaceted approach to improving dyslipidemia and atherosclerosis by modulating gut microbiota, enhancing cholesterol excretion, regulating lipid metabolism-related genes, and reducing inflammation, as summarized in Table 6.5. Their safety profile and additional metabolic benefits make them a promising adjunct in cardiovascular risk management.

### 6.5.6 DIETARY FIBERS

Dietary fibers are a wide category of bioactive carbohydrate polymers. Natural edible carbohydrate polymers, as well as extracted or manufactured carbohydrate polymers, are included in current definitions of dietary fibers. Scientific research indicates that dietary fibers have physiological advantages for human health and are difficult for the body's own enzymes to hydrolyze in the small intestine [60]. Based on their chemical characteristics and physiological advantages, dietary fibers are categorized as soluble or insoluble, viscous or nonviscous, and properly or partially fermentable. Comprising many monosaccharide residues connected by glycosidic bonds, non-starch polysaccharides make up a significant portion of dietary fibers and are mostly found in plant cell walls. This category includes the cellulose and hemicelluloses found in fruits, vegetables, cereals, grains, nuts, legumes, and bran. It also includes yeast, bacteria, algae, mushrooms, alginates from seaweed, guar gum, locust bean gum, gum arabic and tragacanth from plant exudates, pectin's from citrus fruits and apples, β-glucans from cereal grains, particularly oats and barley, and mucilages (such as psyllium) (Figure 6.7).

Another kind of dietary fiber is resistant starch, which may be found in partially ground grains, seeds, legumes, potatoes, and bananas [65]. They undergo partial fermentation in the colon and are mostly insoluble. Usually fermentable and possessing prebiotic properties, resistant oligosaccharides, such as fructooligosaccharide, are made up of 3 to 10 monosaccharide molecules. Lignin is a polymer of phenylpropane units rather than a polysaccharide, despite its tight association with hemicellulose in plant cell walls. Usually categorized as dietary fiber, it is present in meals that include woody materials, like the outer layers of cereal grains [66].

Dietary fibers have been shown to produce hypocholesterolemic effects through various mechanisms.

- Dietary fibers cause the small intestine to absorb less bile salt, which increases the excretion of bile salt in the feces. Reduced enterohepatic bile salt circulation lowers hepatic cholesterol and promotes the liver to convert cholesterol into bile acids, which lowers plasma LDL-C-C and increases LDLR to absorb more cholesterol from plasma [67].
- Viscous dietary fibers, which similarly restrict intestinal digestion and absorption and postpone stomach emptying, may lessen the release of glucose into the bloodstream after a meal. Insulin levels may then decrease as a result.
- Hepatic production of cholesterol and fatty acids is attenuated by reduced insulin [71].
- The enhancement of the gut microbiota, the theory that fibers may boost the number of good bacteria and alter gene expression, and the lowering of blood pressure are some other processes that have been reported.

According to clinical research, meals high in water-soluble fiber, like beans or oat bran, can reduce blood total cholesterol by 19% and serum LDL cholesterol by 22%. Psyllium mucilloid and other soluble fiber-rich food supplements are well tolerated and have the potential to reduce blood cholesterol by 15%. Therefore, soluble fiber dietary supplements or high-fiber diets may reduce estimated risk for coronary heart disease by more than 30% and serum cholesterol by 15% to 19% [72].

**Table 6.5** Probiotic actions in dyslipidemia.

| Mechanism | Effects on lipids/CVD risk |
|---|---|
| Bile salt hydrolase activity | ↑ Cholesterol excretion, ↓ LDL-C |
| Cholesterol assimilation/ coprostanol | ↓ Absorption, ↑ fecal loss |
| SCFA production | ↑ HDL, ↓ cholesterol synthesis |
| Gut microbiota modulation | ↑ Beneficial bacteria, ↓ inflammation |
| Gene regulation | ↓ HMGCR expression, ↑ HDL synthesis |

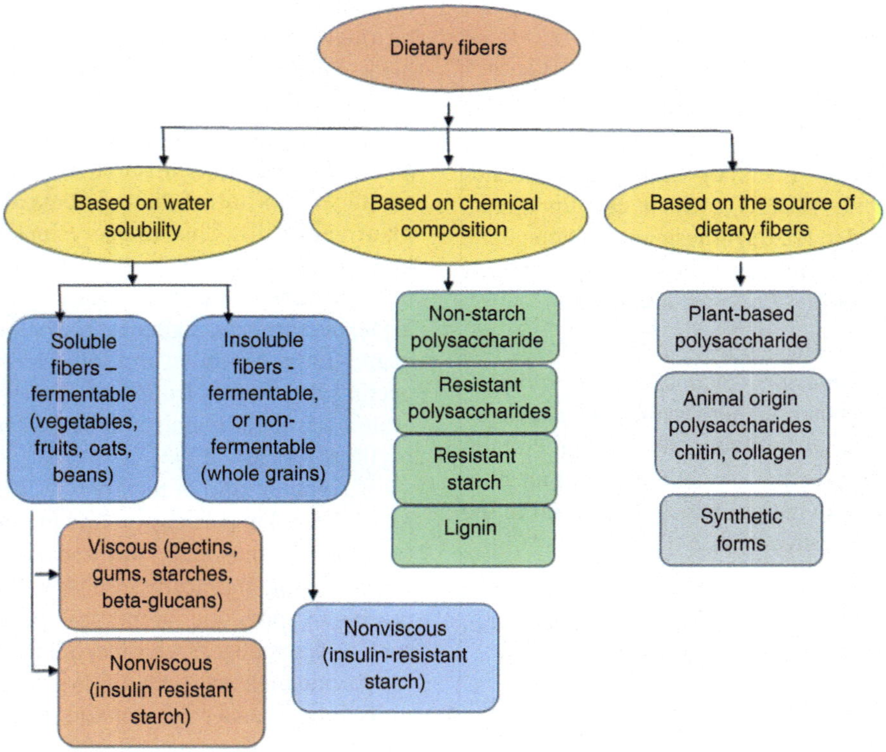


FIGURE 6.7 Classification of dietary fibers.

## 6.6 CONCLUSION

This review highlights the potential of natural lipid-lowering agents in managing dyslipidemia and atherosclerosis. It explores various compounds such as polyphenols, phytosterols, omega-3 fatty acids, alkaloids, terpenoids, and probiotics, detailing their mechanisms of action in modulating lipid profiles. These natural agents offer multiple benefits, including improved lipid profiles, reduced oxidative stress, and decreased inflammation, contributing to overall cardiovascular risk reduction. The integration of these natural remedies with lifestyle modifications provides a comprehensive approach to dyslipidemia management. While conventional pharmaceutical therapies remain effective, the growing interest in natural alternatives reflects concerns about the long-term safety of synthetic medications. This research underscores the potential of natural lipid-lowering agents in clinical practice, suggesting their role in reducing dependence on synthetic medications and contributing to global cardiovascular prevention efforts. Further research and clinical trials are needed to fully ascertain the efficacy and safety of these natural compounds in the long-term therapy of CVD.

## REFERENCES

1. Abbas, M., Saeed, F., Anjum, F. M., Afzaal, M., Tufail, T., Bashir, M. S., Ishtiaq, A., Hussain, S., & Suleria, H. A. R. (2017a). Natural polyphenols: an overview. *Int. J. Food Prop.*, 20(8), 1689–1699. https://doi.org/10.1080/10942912.2016.1220393

2. Abu Mweis, S. S., Marinangeli, C. P. F., Frohlich, J., & Jones, P. J. H. (2014). Implementing phytosterols into medical practice as a cholesterol-lowering strategy: overview of efficacy, effectiveness, and safety. *Can. J. Cardiol.*, 30 (10), 1225–1232. https://doi.org/10.1016/j.cjca.2014.04.022

3. Baumgartner, S., Mensink, R.P., & Plat, J. (2011). Plant sterols and stanols in the treatment of dyslipidemia: new insights into targets and mechanisms related to cardiovascular risk. *Curr. Pharm. Des.*, 17(9), 922–932. https://doi.org/10.2174/138161211795428795

4. Adkins, Y., & Kelley, D. S. (2010). Mechanisms underlying the cardioprotective effects of omega-3 polyunsaturated fatty acids. *J. Nutr. Biochem.*, 21(9), 781–792. https://doi.org/10.1016/j.jnutbio.2009.12.004

5. Anderson, J. W. (1987). Dietary fiber, lipids and atherosclerosis. *Am. J. Cardiol.*, 60 (12), G17–G22. https://doi.org/10.1016/0002-9149(87)90587-X

6. Barry, A. R., & Dixon, D. L. (2021). Omega-3 fatty acids for the prevention of atherosclerotic cardiovascular disease. *Pharmacotherapy*, 41 (12), 1056–1065. https://doi.org/10.1002/phar.2615

7. Bays, H. E., Tighe, A. P., Sadovsky, R., & Davidson, M. H. (2008). Prescription omega-3 fatty acids and their lipid effects: physiologic mechanisms of action and clinical implications. *Expert. Rev. Cardiovasc. Ther.*, 6(3), 391–409. https://doi.org/10.1586/14779072.6.3.391

8. Burčová, Z., Kreps, F., Greifová, M., Jablonský, M., Ház, A., Schmidt, Š., & Šurina, I. (2018). Antibacterial and antifungal activity of phytosterols and methyl dehydroabietate of Norway spruce bark extracts. *J. Biotechnol.*, 282, 18–24. https://doi.org/10.1016/j.jbiotec.2018.06.340

9. Berberich, A. J., & Hegele, R. A. (2022). A modern approach to dyslipidemia. *Endocr. Rev.*, 43(4), 611–653. https://doi.org/10.1210/endrev/bnab037

10. Bhat, S., Sarkar, S., Zaffar, D., Dandona, P., & Kalyani, R. R. (2023). Omega-3 fatty acids in cardiovascular disease and diabetes: a review of recent evidence. *Curr. Cardiol. Rep.*, 25(2), 51–65. https://doi.org/10.1007/s11886-022-01831-0
11. Cabral, C. E., & Klein, M. R. S. T. (2017). Phytosterols in the treatment of hypercholesterolemia and prevention of cardiovascular diseases. *Arq. Bras. Cardiol.*, 109, 475–482. https://doi.org/10.5935/abc.20170158
12. Carracedo, M., Artiach, G., Arnardottir, H., & Bäck, M. (2019). The resolution of inflammation through omega-3 fatty acids in atherosclerosis, intimal hyperplasia, and vascular calcification. *Semin. Immunopathol.*, 41(6), 757–766. https://doi.org/10.1007/s00281-019-00767-y
13. Chan, Y.-M., Varady, K. A., Lin, Y., Trautwein, E., Mensink, R. P., Plat, J., & Jones, P. J. H. (2006). Plasma concentrations of plant sterols: physiology and relationship with coronary heart disease. *Nutr. Rev.*, 64(9), 385–402. https://doi.org/10.1111/j.1753-4887.2006.tb00224.x
14. Chen, G., Wang, H., Zhang, X., & Yang, S.-T. (2014). Nutraceuticals and functional foods in the management of hyperlipidemia. *Crit. Rev. Food Sci. Nutr.*, 54(9), 1180–1201. https://doi.org/10.1080/10408398.2011.629354
15. Chen, Y., Duan, Y., Yang, X., Sun, L., Liu, M., Wang, Q., Ma, X., Zhang, W., Li, X., Hu, W., Miao, R. Q., Xiang, R., Hajjar, D. P., & Han, J. (2015). Inhibition of ERK1/2 and activation of LXR synergistically reduce atherosclerotic lesions in Apo E-deficient mice. *Arterioscler. Thromb. Vasc. Biol.*, 35(4), 948–959. https://doi.org/10.1161/ATVBAHA.114.305116
16. Cheung, B., Sikand, G., Dineen, E. H., Malik, S., & Barseghian El-Farra, A. (2023). Lipid-lowering nutraceuticals for an integrative approach to dyslipidemia. *J. Clin. Med.*, 12 (10), 3414. https://doi.org/10.3390/jcm12103414
17. Chi, L., Peng, L., Hu, X., Pan, N., & Zhang, Y. (2014). Berberine combined with atorvastatin downregulates LOX-1 expression through the ET-1 receptor in monocyte/macrophages. *Int. J. Mol. Med.*, 34(1), 283–290. https://doi.org/10.3892/ijmm.2014.1748
18. Cicero, A. F. G., Fogacci, F., Stoian, A. P., Vrablik, M., Al Rasadi, K., Banach, M., Toth, P. P., & Rizzo, M. (2021). Nutraceuticals in the management of dyslipidemia: Which, When, and for Whom? Could nutraceuticals help low-risk individuals with non-optimal lipid levels? *Curr. Atheroscler. Rep.*, 23 (10), 57. https://doi.org/10.1007/s11883-021-00955-y
19. Devaraj, S., & Jialal, I. (2006). The role of dietary supplementation with plant sterols and stanols in the prevention of cardiovascular disease. *Nutr. Rev.*, 64(7), 348–354. https://doi.org/10.1111/j.1753-4887.2006.tb00219.x
20. Farias, R. A. F., Neto, M. F. O., Viana, G. S. B., & Rao, V. S. N. (1996). Effects of *Croton cajucara* extract on serum lipids of rats fed a high fat diet. *Phytother. Res.*, 10(8), 697–699. https://doi.org/10.1002/(SICI)1099-1573(199612)10:8<697::AID-PTR925>3.0.CO;2-I
21. Feng, M., Zou, Z., Zhou, X., Hu, Y., Ma, H., Xiao, Y., Li, X., & Ye, X. (2017). Comparative effect of berberine and its derivative 8-cetylberberine on attenuating atherosclerosis in Apo E−/−mice. *Int. Immunopharmacol.*, 43, 195–202. https://doi.org/10.1016/j.intimp.2016.12.001
22. Grundy, S. M. (1999). Cholesterol lowering in the elderly population. *Arch. Intern. Med.*, 159 (15), 1670. https://doi.org/10.1001/archinte.159.15.1670
23. Gunness, P., & Gidley, M. J. (2010). Mechanisms underlying the cholesterol-lowering properties of soluble dietary fibre polysaccharides. *Food Funct.*, 1(2), 149–155. https://doi.org/10.1039/c0fo00080a
24. Gylling, H., Plat, J., Turley, S., Ginsberg, H. N., Ellegård, L., Jessup, W., Jones, P. J., Lütjohann, D., Maerz, W., Masana, L., Silbernagel, G., Staels, B., Borén, J., Catapano, A. L., De Backer, G., Deanfield, J., Descamps, O. S., Kovanen, P. T., Riccardi, G., . . . Chapman, M. J. (2014). Plant sterols and plant stanols in the management of dyslipidaemia and prevention of cardiovascular disease. *Atherosclerosis*, 232(2), 346–360. https://doi.org/10.1016/j.atherosclerosis.2013.11.043
25. Gylling, H., & Simonen, P. (2015). Phytosterols, phytostanols, and lipoprotein metabolism. *Nutrients*, 7(9), 7965–7977. https://doi.org/10.3390/nu7095374
26. Harris, W. S., Miller, M., Tighe, A. P., Davidson, M. H., & Schaefer, E. J. (2008). Omega-3 fatty acids and coronary heart disease risk: clinical and mechanistic perspectives. *Atherosclerosis*, 197(1), 12–24. https://doi.org/10.1016/j.atherosclerosis.2007.11.008
27. He, K., Kou, S., Zou, Z., Hu, Y., Feng, M., Han, B., Li, X., & Ye, X. (2016). Hypolipidemic effects of alkaloids from rhizoma coptidis in diet-induced hyperlipidemic hamsters. *Planta Med.*, 82 (08), 690–697. https://doi.org/10.1055/s-0035-1568261
28. Hegele, R. A., & Tsimikas, S. (2019). Lipid-lowering agents. *Circ. Res.*, 124(3), 386–404. https://doi.org/10.1161/CIRCRESAHA.118.313171
29. Hoskins, M., & Jacobson, T. (2006). Combination use of statins and omega-3 fatty acids: an emerging therapy for combined hyperlipidemia. *Futur. Lipidol.*, 1(5), 579–591. https://doi.org/10.2217/17460875.1.5.579
30. Hu, Y., Chen, X., Hu, M., Zhang, D., Yuan, S., Li, P., & Feng, L. (2022). Medicinal and edible plants in the treatment of dyslipidemia: advances and prospects. *Chin. Med.*, 17(1), 113. https://doi.org/10.1186/s13020-022-00666-9
31. Jebari-Benslaiman, S., Galicia-García, U., Larrea-Sebal, A., Olaetxea, J. R., Alloza, I., Vandenbroeck, K., Benito-Vicente, A., & Martín, C. (2022). Pathophysiology of atherosclerosis. *Int. J. Mol. Sci.*, 23(6), 3346. https://doi.org/10.3390/ijms23063346
32. Dipiro, J.T., Yee, G.C., Posey, M., and Stuart, T.H.T.D.N. (2020). *Pharmacotherapy – A Physiological Approach*, 11e (ed. M. Weitz and P.J. Boyle), McGraw Hill Education. p. 272.
33. Tripathi, K.D. (2019). *Essentials of Medical Pharmacology*, 8e. JP Brothers Medical Publishers.
34. Kriaa, A., Bourgin, M., Mkaouar, H., Jablaoui, A., Akermi, N., Soussou, S., Maguin, E., & Rhimi, M. (2019). Microbial reduction of cholesterol to coprostanol: an old concept and new insights. *Catalysts*, 9(2), 167. https://doi.org/10.3390/catal9020167
35. Laka, K., Makgoo, L., & Mbita, Z. (2022). Cholesterol-lowering phytochemicals: targeting the mevalonate pathway for anticancer interventions. *Front. Genet.*, 13. https://doi.org/10.3389/fgene.2022.841639
36. Li, C., & Uppal, M. (2010). Canadian diabetes association national nutrition committee clinical update on dietary fibre in diabetes: food sources to physiological effects. *Can. J. Diabetes*, 34(4), 355–361. https://doi.org/10.1016/S1499-2671(10)44010-1
37. Li, H., He, C., Wang, J., Li, X., Yang, Z., Sun, X., Fang, L., & Liu, N. (2016). Berberine activates peroxisome proliferator-activated receptor gamma to increase atherosclerotic plaque stability in Apoe −/− mice with hyperhomocysteinemia. *J. Diabetes Investig.*, 7(6), 824–832. https://doi.org/10.1111/jdi.12516
38. Libby, P., Buring, J. E., Badimon, L., Hansson, G. K., Deanfield, J., Bittencourt, M. S., Tokgözoğlu, L., & Lewis, E. F. (2019). Atherosclerosis. *Nat. Rev. Dis. Primers*, 5(1), 56. https://doi.org/10.1038/s41572-019-0106-z
39. Begley, M., Hill, C., and Gahan, C.G.M. (2006). Bile salt hydrolase activity in probiotics. *Appl. Environ. Microbiol.* 72 (3): 1729–1738.
40. Micallef, M. A., & Garg, M. L. (2009). Beyond blood lipids: phytosterols, statins and omega-3 polyunsaturated fatty acid therapy for hyperlipidemia. *J. Nutr. Biochem.*, 20 (12), 927–939. https://doi.org/10.1016/j.jnutbio.2009.06.009
41. Momin, E. S., Khan, A. A., Kashyap, T., Pervaiz, M. A., Akram, A., Mannan, V., Sanusi, M., & Elshaikh, A. O. (2023). The effects of

probiotics on cholesterol levels in patients with metabolic syndrome: a systematic review. *Cureus*, 15, e37567. https://doi.org/10.7759/cureus.37567

42. V. Neveu, J. Perez-Jiménez, F. Vos, V. Crespy, L. du Chaffaut, L. Mennen, C. Knox, R. Eisner, J. Cruz, D. Wishart, & A. Scalbert (2010). Phenol-explorer: an online comprehensive database on polyphenol contents in foods. *Database*, 2010, bap 024. https://doi.org/10.1093/database/bap024
43. Phillips, G. O., & Cui, S. W. (2011). An introduction: evolution and finalisation of the regulatory definition of dietary fibre. *Food Hydrocoll.*, 25(2), 139–143. https://doi.org/10.1016/j.foodhyd.2010.04.011
44. Pirillo, A., & Catapano, A. L. (2013). Omega-3 polyunsaturated fatty acids in the treatment of atherogenic dyslipidemia. *Atheroscler. Suppl.*, 14(2), 237–242. https://doi.org/10.1016/S1567-5688(13)70004-7
45. Poli, A., Marangoni, F., Corsini, A., Manzato, E., Marrocco, W., Martini, D., Medea, G., & Visioli, F. (2021). Phytosterols, cholesterol control, and cardiovascular disease. *Nutrients*, 13(8), 2810. https://doi.org/10.3390/nu13082810
46. Pongpirul, K., Janchot, K., and Dai, Y. (2019). Single strain probiotics for dyslipidemia, fatty liver, and obesity: a systematic review and meta-analysis. *World J. Meta-Anal.* 7 (6): 323–338. https://doi.org/10.13105/wjma.v7.i6.323.
47. Singh, R.B., Mengi, S.A., Xu, Y.-J. et al. (2002). Pathogenesis of atherosclerosis: a multifactorial process. *Exp. Clin. Cardiol.* 7 (1): 40–53.
48. Virmani, R. (2025). Atherosclerosis pathology. *Medspace*.
49. V. Kumar, A.K. Abbas, & J.C. Aster (2020). *Robbins and Cotran Pathologic Basis of Disease*. (M.K. Singh, 10e, 1, Elsevier Health Sciences. p. 450.
50. Ahmed, S.M., Clasen, M.E., and Donnelly, J.E. (1998). Management of dyslipidemia in adults. *Am. Fam. Physician* 57 (9): 2192–2204.
51. Saghir, S. A. M., Revadigar, V., & Murugaiyah, V. (2014). Natural lipid-lowering agents and their effects: an update. *Eur. Food Res. Technol.*, 238(5), 705–725. https://doi.org/10.1007/s00217-014-2194-z
52. Shattat, G.F. (2014). A review article on hyperlipidemia: types, treatments and new drug targets. *Biomed. Pharmacol. J.* 7 (2): 399–409. https://doi.org/10.13005/bpj/504.
53. Siasos, G., Tousoulis, D., Tsigkou, V., Kokkou, E., Oikonomou, E., Vavuranakis, M., Basdra, E. K., Papavassiliou, A. G., & Stefanadis, C. (2013). Flavonoids in atherosclerosis: an overview of their mechanisms of action. *Curr. Med. Chem.*, 20 (21), 2641–2660. https://doi.org/10.2174/0929867311320210003
54. Silverman, R.G. (2013). The natural approach to treatment of high cholesterol profiles. *Nutr. Perspect.* 36 (1): 15.
55. Singh, S. P., & Sashidhara, K. V. (2017). Lipid lowering agents of natural origin: an account of some promising chemotypes. *Eur. J. Med. Chem.*, 140, 331–348. https://doi.org/10.1016/j.ejmech.2017.09.020.
56. Song, X., Liu, Y., Zhang, X., Weng, P., Zhang, R., & Wu, Z. (2023). Role of intestinal probiotics in the modulation of lipid metabolism: implications for therapeutic treatments. *Food Sci. Human Wellness*, 12(5), 1439–1449. https://doi.org/10.1016/j.fshw.2023.02.005.
57. Susanti, I., Haryo Bimo Setiarto, R., Kahfi, J., Giarni, R., Muhamaludin, Putri Ramadhaningtyas, D., & Randy, A. (2023). The mechanism of probiotics in preventing the risk of hypercholesterolemia. *Rev. Agric. Sci.*, 11, 156–170. https://doi.org/10.7831/ras.11.0_156.
58. Theuwissen, E., & Mensink, R. P. (2008). Water-soluble dietary fibers and cardiovascular disease. *Physiol. Behav.*, 94(2), 285–292. https://doi.org/10.1016/j.physbeh.2008.01.001
59. Vander Laan, P. A., Reardon, C. A., & Getz, G. S. (2004). Site specificity of atherosclerosis. *Arterioscler. Thromb. Vasc. Biol.*, 24(1), 12–22. https://doi.org/10.1161/01.ATV.0000105054.43931.f0.
60. Wang, H., Ma, C., Li, Y., Zhang, L., Lima A., Yang, C., Zhao, F., Han, H., Shang, D., Yang, F., Zhang, Y., Zhang, H., Sun, Z., & Guo, R. (2023). Probio-X relieves symptoms of hyperlipidemia by regulating patients' gut microbiome, blood lipid metabolism, and lifestyle habits. *Microbiol. Spectrum*, 11(3). https://doi.org/10.1128/spectrum.04440-22.
61. Wang, T., & Butany, J. (2017). Pathogenesis of atherosclerosis. *Diagn. Histopathol.*, 23 (11), 473–478. https://doi.org/10.1016/j.mpdhp.2017.11.009.
62. Yanai, H. and Yoshida, H. (2021). Secondary dyslipidemia: its treatments and association with atherosclerosis. *Glob. Health Med.* 3 (1): 15–23. https://doi.org/10.35772/ghm.2020.01078.
63. Yashodhara, B. M., Umakanth, S., Pappachan, J. M., Bhat, S. K., Kamath, R., & Choo, B. H. (2009). Omega-3 fatty acids: a comprehensive review of their role in health and disease. *Postgrad. Med. J.*, 85 (1000), 84–90. https://doi.org/10.1136/pgmj.2008.073338.
64. You, M., Zhou, L., Wu, F., Zhang, L., Zhu, S., & Zhang, H. (2025). Probiotics for the treatment of hyperlipidemia: focus on gut-liver axis and lipid metabolism. *Pharmacol. Res.*, 214, 107694. https://doi.org/10.1016/j.phrs.2025.107694.
65. Zhang, Y., Li, M., Li, X., Zhang, T., Qin, M., & Ren, L. (2018). Isoquinoline alkaloids and indole alkaloids attenuate aortic atherosclerosis in apolipoprotein E deficient mice: a systematic review and meta-analysis. *Front. Pharmacol.*, 9: 602. https://doi.org/10.3389/fphar.2018.00602.
66. Zhou, Y., Zheng, J., Li, Y., Xu, D.-P., Li, S., Chen, Y.-M., & Li, H.-B. (2016). Natural polyphenols for prevention and treatment of cancer. *Nutrients*, 8(8): 515. https://doi.org/10.3390/nu8080515.
67. Ziółkiewicz, A., Kasprzak-Drozd, K., Rusinek, R., Markut-Miotła, E., & Oniszczuk, A. (2023). The influence of polyphenols on atherosclerosis development. *Int. J. Mol. Sci.*, 24(8), 7146. https://doi.org/10.3390/ijms24087146.
68. Sirca, T., Mureşan, M., Pallag, A., Marian, E., Jurca, T., Vicaş, L., Tunduc, I., Manole, F., & Ştefan, L. (2024). The role of polyphenols in modulating PON1 activity regarding endothelial dysfunction and atherosclerosis. *Int. J. Mol. Sci.*, 25(5), 2962. https://doi.org/10.3390/ijms25052962.
69. Wang, Y., You, Y., Tian, Y., Sun, H., Li, X., Wang, X., Wang, Y., & Liu, J. (2020). Pediococcuspentosaceus PP 04 ameliorates high-fat diet-induced hyperlipidemia by regulating lipid metabolism in C57BL/6N mice. *J. Agric. Food Chem.*, 68 (51), 15154–15163. https://doi.org/10.1021/acs.jafc.0c05060.
70. Zang, M., Xu, S., Maitland-Toolan, K. A., Zuccollo, A., Hou, X., Jiang, B., Wierzbicki, M., Verbeuren, T. J., & Cohen, R. A. (2006). Polyphenols stimulate AMP-activated protein kinase, lower lipids, and inhibit accelerated atherosclerosis in diabetic LDL receptor-deficient mice. *Diabetes*, 55(8), 2180–2191. https://doi.org/10.2337/db05-1188.
71. Ziółkiewicz, A., Kasprzak-Drozd, K., Rusinek, R., Markut-Miotła, E., & Oniszczuk, A.(2023). The influence of polyphenols on atherosclerosis development. *Int. J. Mol. Sci.*, 24(8), 7146. https://doi.org/10.3390/ijms24087146.
72. Anderson, J.W. (1987). Dietary fiber, lipids and atherosclerosis. *Am. J. Cardiol.*, 60(12),17G–22G. http://doi.org/10.1016/0002-9149(87)90587-X.

# Herbal Anticoagulants, Antiplatelets, and Thrombolytics for Cardiovascular Health

CHAPTER 7

**Sadhe Amala[1], Sarikonda Tripura Venkata Raghavamma[2], and Asapu Hema KIranmayi[1]**

[1] *Aditya College of Pharmacy, Jawaharlal Nehru Technological University, Surampalem, Andhra Pradesh, India*

[2] *Chalapathi Institute of Pharmaceutical Sciences, Acharya Nagarjuna University, Guntur, Andhra Pradesh, India*

## 7.1 INTRODUCTION

Cardiovascular disorder is a primary contributor to implications caused by noncommunicable diseases. The most familiar underlying pathology of thrombosis is the occurrence of three major cardiovascular disorders, namely acute coronary syndrome (ischemic heart disease), stroke, and thromboembolism (clots mostly at vein) [1]. An important pathogenic mechanism underlying these conditions is the imbalance between procoagulant and anticoagulant systems, leading to more "thrombus" formation [2]. Pharmacological anticoagulation, therefore, remains a cornerstone in preventing and managing cardiovascular complications. While synthetic drugs which inhibit thrombus are clinically established such as warfarin, prasugrel, streptokinase, and direct oral anticoagulants (DOACs) [3] (rivaroxaban, apixaban, dabigatran), they are not without limitations, which include varying pharmacokinetics, bleeding risks, dietary restrictions, and monitoring requirements. Hence, there has been growing interest in identifying safe and effective herbal alternatives that can modulate coagulation pathways through natural mechanisms. Traditional medicinal practices like Ayurveda, Siddha, Unani, and Traditional Chinese Medicine (TCM) and others have long employed plant-based formulations for blood purification and circulation enhancement. Current pharmacological studies have validated several of these herbs for antiplatelet, anticoagulant, or fibrinolytic activities. In fact, plants are rich in bioactive secondary metabolites with powerful anti-inflammatory and antioxidant properties and may also block the function of enzymes such as serine proteases in plasma. With all these effects, many herbs demonstrate antiplatelet and anticoagulant activities [4]. Natural compounds are important alternative drugs for the treatment of hemostatic disorders, owing to the nature of their inception, low cost, and safety compared with manufactured medicament. Some important plants distributed worldwide can interfere with coagulation, platelet function, fibrin plug formation. In order to assess their potential as novel therapies involving herbal anticoagulant and antithrombotic drugs for the treatment of hemostatic disabilities, it is necessary to describe their active ingredients and potential mechanisms. Furthermore, integrating these bioactive compounds into advanced drug delivery systems can improve their physicochemical characteristics, enhance bioavailability, and enable targeted delivery, thereby overcoming the limitations associated with crude extracts.

## 7.2 HEMOSTASIS

The body's natural processes for maintaining a stable internal balance within the blood vessels in a physiological state, and the development of thrombi to stop bleeding from injured vessels, define "Hemostasis" [5]. Procoagulant and anticoagulant substances must remain in balance for the hemostatic process to function properly. Any changes in the balance brought on by inherited and acquired disorders can cause hypercoagulability, which is characterized by an increased propensity for thrombus formation. According to Rudolf Virchow, endothelial damage to the vascular wall, decreased blood flow rate, and changes in blood composition are some of the factors that can cause hypercoagulability [6, 7]. Other factors like trauma to blood vessels and inflammation can also be the reason for endothelial injury. Blood flow rate can be reduced by patient restraint and blood composition can be altered by genetic and acquired conditions. Of all genetic disorders, the most significant ones are prothrombin gene mutation, factor V Leiden, antithrombin III (AT-III), protein C and protein S deficiencies, elevated fibrinogen and homocysteine levels, increased concentration of plasminogen activator inhibitor (PAI), and interference with the fibrinolytic system [8]. Blood composition can be altered by acquired conditions such as neoplasms, which alter the hemostatic system by influencing various mechanisms that regulate thrombin formation and factors that cause thrombotic events. This condition results in hypercoagulability and can cause venous thromboembolism (VTE) and pulmonary embolism (PE). Both

PE and deep vein thrombosis (DVT) are VTE diseases and are associated with a high morbidity and mortality worldwide [9, 10].

Hemostasis can be classified into two main types: primary hemostasis and secondary hemostasis, each one playing a crucial role in stopping bleeding.

- Primary hemostasis
- Secondary hemostasis and
- Fibrinolysis

## 7.2.1 PRIMARY HOMEOSTASIS

The vascular endothelium plays a central part in regulating hemostasis. While endothelial injury occurs, subendothelial components such as collagen, fibronectin, and von Willebrand factor (vWF) become exposed, initiating the platelet response. Primary hemostasis occurs sequence step of events as follows: (1) adhesion of platelets to the vessel wall, (2) activation of platelets, (3) aggregation of platelets at the site of vascular injury after exposure to collagen, and (4) platelet plug formation, which has as an objective to form a blood clot that seals a breach formed in the vessel wall.

i. Platelet adhesion is the initial step of primary hemostasis, in which circulating platelets attach to the exposed subendothelial surface of a damaged blood vessel. In an intact blood vessel, the endothelial lining acts as a barrier, preventing the contact of platelets with subendothelial matrix. When vascular injury occurs (due to trauma, inflammation, or rupture), the subendothelial structures such as collagen, fibronectin, laminin, and vWF are released from storage granules (Weibel–Palade bodies) of endothelial cells and alpha-granules of platelets become exposed [11]. Platelet adhesion occurs through a series of molecular interactions between platelet surface receptors and the exposed components of the damaged vessel wall. These molecules act as ligands for platelet receptors.

ii. Platelet activation is the second major step of primary hemostasis. Once platelets adhere to the damaged vascular endothelium, they undergo a series of biochemical and morphological changes that transform them from resting, inactive cells into active, adhesive, and aggregating cells. Adhesion triggers intracellular signaling pathways, leading to release of calcium ions ($Ca^{2+}$) from platelet stores, activation of phospholipase $A_2$, leading to synthesis of thromboxane $A_2$ ($TXA_2$), degranulation and release of serotonin, adenosine diphosphate (ADP), and fibrinogen, and also recruitment of plasma clotting factors [12] on the surface of platelets. Release of factor V and acid phospholipids further contributes to the augmentation of the process. This marks the transition from adhesion to activation, leading to platelet aggregation [13, 14].

iii. Platelet aggregation is the third major step of primary hemostasis. The released substances act as agonists for promoting glycoprotein IIb/IIIa (GpIIb/IIIa) and GpIIb/IIIa (integrin αIIbβ3) activation, which are the most abundant receptors present on the platelet surface. Upon activation, conformational changes expose the binding sites for fibrinogen and vWF, enabling platelet–platelet bridging [15].

iv. Platelet plug formation is the final and most important event of primary hemostasis. The aggregated platelets adhere tightly to the site of injury and to each other, forming the primary platelet plug. The plug is initially loose and reversible but becomes denser and more stable through the action of thrombin from the coagulation cascade. Thrombin converts fibrinogen into fibrin, which works through and around the platelet mass, anchoring and stabilizing the plug. This results in a firm, irreversible secondary hemostatic plug. The platelet membranes contain negatively charged phosphatidylserine, which causes localized coagulation through thrombin formation, resulting in secondary hemostasis [16, 17]. In addition to being a strong platelet activator for its particular receptor on the thrombocytic membrane, thrombin also influences its own production by triggering coagulation factors V, VIII, and XI, which contribute to the formation of fibrin clots [18]. Consequently, platelets are essential for hemostasis and thrombin production, which intensifies the blood coagulation cascade and results in secondary hemostasis [19]. Primary hemostasis is presented in Figure 7.1.

## 7.2.2 SECONDARY HEMOSTASIS

The second stage of the hemostatic process is "secondary hemostasis." Secondary hemostasis stabilizes a temporary platelet plug created by primary hemostasis by forming a fibrin mesh via the coagulation cascade [20]. A number of positive and negative feedback mechanisms, including intrinsic, extrinsic, and common pathways, balance secondary hemostasis, which primarily activate plasminogen coagulation proteins. Certain sequence of events, like activation of protein cofactors and zymogens (inert precursors of enzymes), are responsible for the blood coagulation cascade [21].

The coagulation cascade comprises three convergent pathways.

➢ **Intrinsic pathway:** This pathway commences when XII factor binds to a negatively charged surface and proceeds with a sequential activation of various factors like XI, IX, and VIII and connect with the extrinsic pathway at the stage of factor X activation [22].

➢ **Extrinsic pathway:** It is initiated by tissue factor (TF) exposure [23], and it is the cellular receptor for factor VII. Once factor VII binds to TF, it undergoes into an active

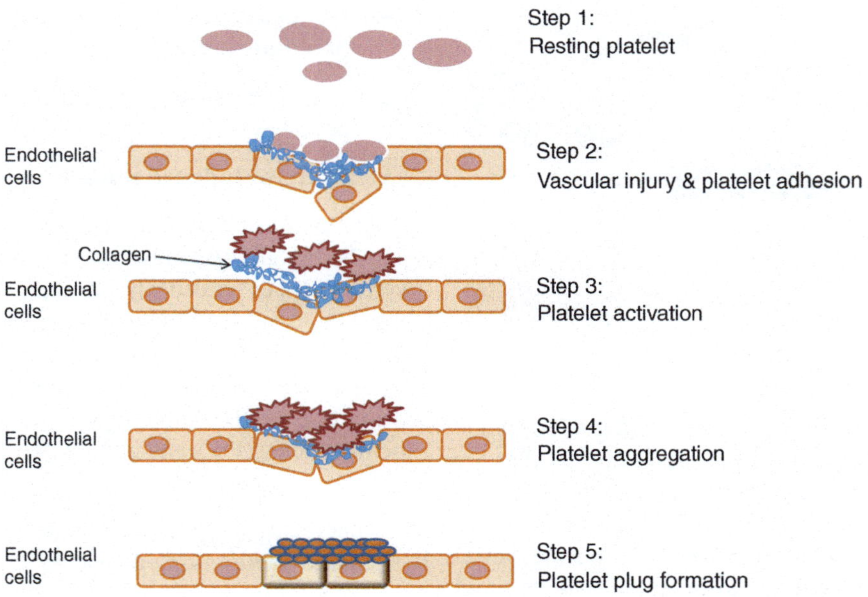


**FIGURE 7.1** Primary hemostasis.

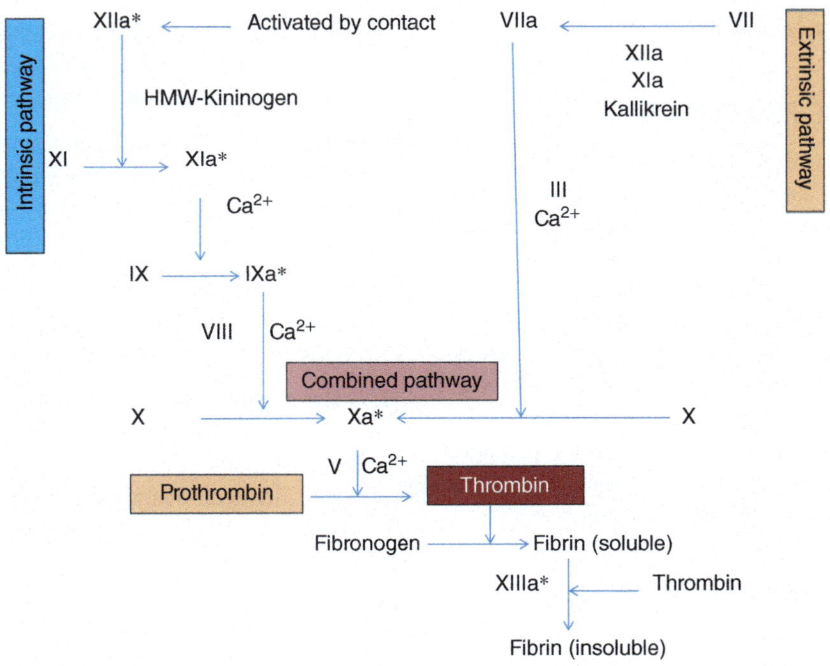


**FIGURE 7.2** Secondary hemostasis.

transition (from VII to VIIa*) in the presence of $Ca^{2+}$. The tissue factor–VII*a activates factors IX and X [24]. During platelet activation, acidic phospholipids are exposed, and, in turn, these activate various clotting factors.

- **Common pathway:** This pathway in blood coagulation is a critical step in the clotting cascade. It begins by the activation of factor X and concludes with fibrin clot formation. The common pathway is significant because it is the meeting point for both intrinsic and extrinsic pathways. Factor X is an important element of the common pathway. Factor X is activated by both intrinsic and extrinsic pathways. Activated factor Xa converts prothrombin (factor II) into thrombin (IIa). Factor IIa cleaves fibrinogen into fibrin monomers, which polymerize to produce a stable clot [25]. The complete coagulation cascade is represented in Figure 7.2.

### 7.2.3 FIBRINOLYSIS

The platelet plug is reinforced by fibrin deposition to form a "thrombus" at the site of blood vessel damage. The fibrinolytic system is triggered to eliminate fibrin clots after the repair is

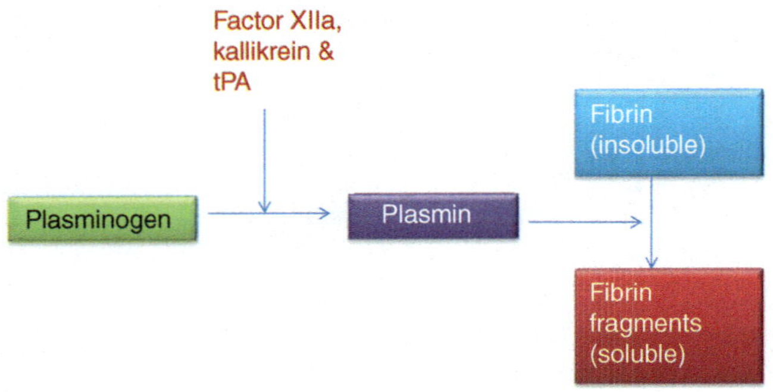


**FIGURE 7.3** Fibrinolysis.

complete. Trypsin-like serine proteases called t-PA (tissue type) and u-PA (urokinase type) are plasminogens that are naturally found in blood. They directly activate the plasminogen that causes thrombolysis [26]. Plasmin cleaves fibrin into soluble degradation products, restoring vessel patency. The balance between endogenous fibrinolytics and plasminogen activator inhibitor-1 (PAI-1) is crucial. Many herbal plants show fibrinolytic activity it helps to prevent or dissolve blood clots by amplifying the breakdown of fibrin. The process of fibrinolysis is indicated in Figure 7.3.

## 7.3 CARDIOVASCULAR PROTECTION

Synthetic anticoagulant, antiplatelet, and fibrinolytic agents are core pharmacological classes used in cardiovascular medicine to prevent and treat thrombotic diseases. Each class works through distinct mechanisms targeting various stages of hemostasis and thrombosis. The following are some of the examples of drugs that mainly act on the cardiovascular system (CVS) to provide protection against various CVS disorders.

Anticoagulants: Heparin, warfarin, low-molecular-weight heparins (LMWH), fondaparinux, rivaroxaban, apixaban.

Antiplatelets: Aspirin, clopidogrel, ticagrelor, prasugrel

Fibrinolytics: Streptokinase, alteplase (tissue-type plasminogen activator [tPA]), reteplase, tenecteplase.

### 7.3.1 MECHANISMS OF CARDIOVASCULAR PROTECTION

Cardiovascular protection mechanisms are the biological and physiological processes that maintain the health of the heart and blood vessels, preventing damage from stressors such as oxidative stress, ischemia, inflammation, and metabolic imbalance. These mechanisms can be classified into endogenous (natural) and induced (external) protective systems. Cardiovascular protection mechanisms function through antioxidant stabilization, mitochondrial preservation, ischemic and exercise-induced conditioning, and endothelial immune regulation. Together, these systems adaptively shield the CVS from oxidative, metabolic, and inflammatory stress. The following are the different types of mechanisms:

i. **Antioxidant defense mechanisms**
ii. **Mitochondrial protection and energy balance**
iii. **Ischemic conditioning and cellular preconditioning**
iv. **Endothelial integrity and Anti-inflammatory pathways**
v. **Exercise-induced protection**

**i) Antioxidant defense mechanisms:**
The body's antioxidant (both enzymatic and nonenzymatic) system drives effectively through a sequential complex, interconnected, and supportive network of mechanisms [27]. These mechanisms demonstrate several antioxidants as cardioprotective. Important antioxidants include superoxide dismutase (SOD), glutathione peroxidase (GPx), catalase, peroxiredoxin (Prx), and glutathione.

- SOD contributes significantly to the transformation of superoxide anions into hydrogen peroxide [28, 29] and is in charge of preventing peroxynitrite generation [30].
- Catalase helps in neutralization of negative charge by turning hydrogen peroxide into water; it is mainly found in the liver and kidneys.
- GPx has a similar effect to catalase, converting hydrogen peroxide into water, and is found in cytoplasmic, mitochondrial, and nuclear compartments.
- Glutathione serves many antioxidant roles as a cofactor for GPx, a metal chelator, and a vitamin C and E regenerator. It may also act as a peroxide by interacting with hydroxyl radicals [31].
- Prx will reduce peroxides from various molecules [32], like hydrogen peroxide and peroxynitrite, and exists in six distinguishable isoforms.

**ii) Mitochondrial protection and energy balance:**
Mitochondria are central to cardiomyocyte survival. To achieve mitochondrial stabilization and ultimately safeguard against cell death via connexin-43, low levels of reactive oxygen species (ROS) signaling and p66HC are essential. Connexin-43 is involved in mitochondrial respiration, adenosine triphosphate (ATP) generation, and mitochondrial potassium influx. Mild oxidative stress stimulates protective responses that precondition cardiac tissue against later, severe insults. p66SHC catalyzes electron transfer between oxygen and cytochrome c, which results in ROS production. Blockade of all these substances may lead to loss of cardioprotection [33].

**iii) Ischemic conditioning and cellular preconditioning:**
Ischemic conditioning and cellular preconditioning are powerful mechanisms by which the body protects cardiac tissue from the effects of ischemia and reperfusion [34]. Triggers, mediators, and effectors are the three categories of factors that are released during ischemic preconditioning. Bradykinin, adenosine, and endorphins are the stimulating factors released during brief episodes of ischemia. In the first phase, all these factors attach to their respective receptors (guanine protein-coupled receptors [GPCRs]),

which causes message transduction through extracellular signal-regulated kinase ½ (ERK ½), protein kinase, Akt, and phosphatidylinositol 3-kinase (PI3-K). These leads to obstruction of the 1-methyl-4-phenyl-1,2,3,6-tetrahydropyri dine (mPTP) opening. Its opening results in cell membrane rupture, mitochondrial enlargement, and the cessation of ATP synthesis.

Several processes, including the activation of cytoprotective proteins like heat shock proteins and antioxidant enzymes like SOD and heme oxygenase-1, are involved in the second window of protection [35]. These proteins provide sustained resistance to oxidative and inflammatory injury during subsequent ischemic events.

**iv) Endothelial integrity and Anti-inflammatory pathways:**
Endothelial integrity and anti-inflammatory pathways are interlinked through barrier regulation, immune modulation, and inhibition of oxidative and metabolic stress. Endothelial integrity depends on cell–cell junctions composed primarily of vascular endothelial cadherin (VE-cadherin) complexes, which link to the actin cytoskeleton to maintain tight adhesion and barrier function. Disruption of these junctions increases vascular permeability, leading to edema and inflammation. Remodeling of actin filaments ensures a balance between stability and responsiveness to stimuli [36].

Inflammation drives vascular pathology by impairing endothelial function and promoting plaque formation. Anti-inflammatory pathways stabilize VE-cadherin junctions, maintain nitric oxide bioavailability, and minimize leukocyte adhesion. In parallel, intact endothelial barriers prevent excessive immune cell infiltration and cytokine diffusion into the vessel wall, preserving vascular tone and reducing atherogenic stimuli [37].

**v) Exercise-induced protection:**
Exercise is a practical and effective nonpharmacological intervention that enhances intrinsic cardiac defense mechanisms, reduces ischemic injury, improves recovery, and lowers cardiovascular disease (CVD) risk. Exercise-induced cardioprotection arises from mitochondrial resilience, antioxidant enhancement, favorable signaling adaptations, and systemic risk modification, collectively fortifying the heart against ischemic and reperfusion injury [38].

### 7.3.2 ROLE OF HERBAL DRUGS IN CARDIOPROTECTION

The available synthetic agents are potent, rapid, and effective in acute and chronic cardiovascular care, but require careful dose adjustment and monitoring due to risks of bleeding and drug interactions.

Herbal plants offer several advantages over commercially used anticoagulant, antiplatelet, and fibrinolytic agents, primarily due to their multifactorial mechanisms, lower toxicity, and accessibility. However, while they hold promise for cardiovascular health, standardization and clinical validation remain ongoing challenges. The main CVDs, like stroke, coronary artery disease, and peripheral artery disease, are operated by several factors, such as chronic inflammation, oxidative stress, and coagulation abnormalities. Many herbal agents produce cardiovascular protection by targeting these two important central pathways.

1. Inflammation and atherosclerosis
2. Coagulation and thrombosis

**1. Inflammation and atherosclerosis:**
Inflammation is an important factor in the evolution and increased risk of atherosclerosis. Plaque is developed in three phases:

- Endothelial dysfunction
- Foam cell formation and plaque growth
- Plaque instability

*Endothelial dysfunction:*
Endothelial dysfunction is a main and intense early event in the progression of CVDs, especially atherosclerosis, hypertension, and thrombosis. This mainly refers to an imbalance in the general functions of the endothelial cells. In pathological states, endothelial cells will lose their function due to several risk factors, such as oxidized low-density lipoprotein (LDL), hyperglycemia, smoking, hypertension, and systemic inflammation [39].

*Foam cell formation and plaque growth:*
These processes indicate an important factor where lipid accumulation, immune response, and inflammation progress to form atherosclerotic plaques. These plaques can cause obstruction to blood flow or their rupture can lead to heart attacks and strokes. Foam cells are lipid-loaded macrophages [40].

The process of foam cell formation and plaque development is indicated in Figure 7.4.

*Plaque instability:*
Persistent inflammation activates enzymes such as matrix metalloproteinases (MMPs), which degrade the fibrous cap of plaques. A weakened cap increases the risk of rupture and subsequent thrombosis.

Most herbal plants target the above-mentioned steps in plaque formation and exert their cardioprotective functions. The preferred targets of herbal agents are cytokines, LDL, nitrous oxide synthase (NOS), and nuclear factor kappa B (NF-κB) [41].

**2. Coagulation and thrombosis:**
A detailed discussion on coagulation and thrombosis is mentioned in Section 2 (hemostasis). Some herbs interfere with coagulation by inhibiting various blood-coagulating factors (e.g., Xa, IIa, and Va), which play a major role in extrinsic and intrinsic pathways of coagulation. Certain herbals directly degrade fibrin or activating plasminogen to breakdown the formed clots. Examples include *Panax ginseng, Glycyrrhiza glabra, Terminalia arjuna,* etc.

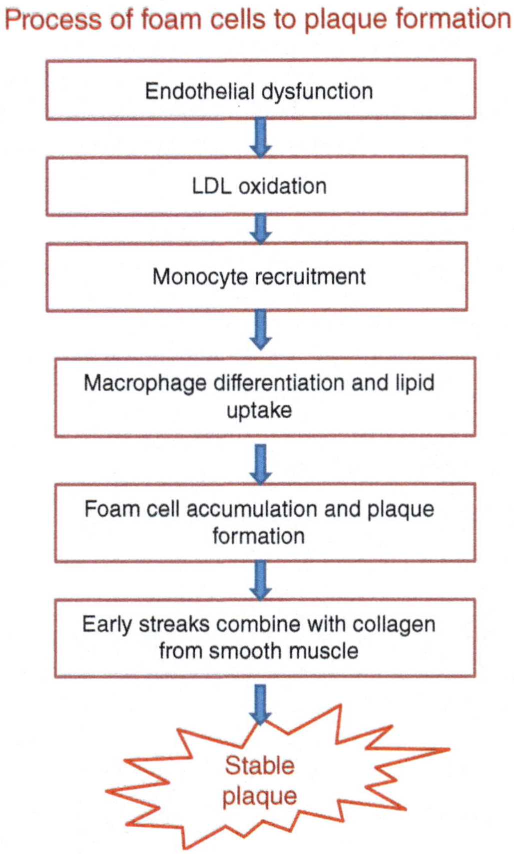


**FIGURE 7.4** Plaque formation.

## 7.4 PLANT BIOACTIVE COMPOUNDS

Because of their valuable medicinal properties, plants have been used extensively for therapeutic or preventive purposes from ancient times [42, 43]. Research on bioactive compounds that are extracted from plant species is currently gaining popularity because of their potential for use in particular therapeutic applications and activities. The type, amount, and chemical makeup of plant extracts greatly influence their activity and possible uses [44]. Plant-derived natural compounds are divided into primary and secondary metabolites. The key bioactive compounds with anticoagulant, immunostimulatory, toxicological, therapeutic, and preventive properties are secondary metabolites [45]. Terpenoids, phenolic compounds, and alkaloids are the three main groups that make up the basic classification of bioactive compounds. Others include lipids, saponins, essential oils, carbohydrates, ketones, and others bioactives. Phenolic substances, primarily flavonoids and polyphenols, are strong antioxidants with anti-inflammatory, antiplatelet, and anticoagulant properties are secondary metabolites, which are abundant in plants and their extracts [20, 46, 47]. Polyphenols, flavonoids, and plant extracts rich in polyphenols and flavonoids may be very helpful in preventing and treating thromboembolic complications due to their described properties.

### 7.4.1 HERBAL ANTICOAGULANTS

Herbs are used in cardiovascular care frequently work through the mechanisms that may impact both the clotting system (coagulation) and the body's inflammatory responses. These pathways are deeply interconnected, and targeting them broadly can help to reduce major cardiovascular risks such as atherosclerosis, heart attacks, and strokes. A separate discussion for coagulation and inflammation of herbal drugs with their specific targets is given below.

**Anticoagulation mechanisms:**
As discussed in the previous section (2.2), the natural coagulation process, especially primary hemostasis, involves clotting factors that play an important role in coagulation process, and these are the main targets for herbal anticoagulants. Herbal anticoagulants work by targeting various stages of the blood-clotting process. Their natural compounds can help prevent thrombus (clot) formation and promote healthier blood rate, reducing the risk of cardiovascular effects like myocardial infarction and strokes. The important targets for most of the herbal anticoagulants are factors Xa, Va, and IIa. Some plants also target direct fibrinogen levels and endogenous anticoagulants. Here are the some important mechanisms of the respective plant products. The following are the major mechanisms:

i. **Inhibition of thrombin (Factor IIa)**
ii. **Inhibition of factor Xa**
iii. **Reduction of fibrinogen levels**
iv. **Enhancement of endogenous anticoagulants**
v. **Calcium chelation**

**i) Inhibition of thrombin (Factor IIa)**:
Factor IIa (thrombin) is the main enzyme of the clotting cascade, playing a dual role as both a procoagulant and an anticoagulant. Its initial role is modification of soluble fibrinogen into insoluble clot to seal damaged vessels. Secondly, it activates other clotting factors (V, VIII, and XI) to amplify the process. Thrombin also stimulates platelets to promote clotting. Because of its lead role in coagulation, most of the drugs choose it as a target for its anticoagulation activity. The herbals that target this thrombin are *Allium sativum* and *Curcuma longa*.

*A. sativum (garlic):*
Garlic is a powerhouse herb for cardiovascular health, known for its anticoagulant properties. The main phytochemicals responsible for the activity are allicin and ajoene. These phytochemicals directly attach to thrombin and inhibit its function, which leads to prolongation of prothrombin time (PT) and partial thromboplastin time [48].

*C. longa (turmeric):*
Turmeric, with its active compound curcumin, is familiar for its anti-inflammatory and anticoagulant activity. Curcumin helps to reduce the formation of clots by preventing platelets from sticking together. This leads to low levels of fibrin formation and provides anti-inflammatory synergy with endothelial protection [49].

**ii) Inhibition of Factor Xa:**
Factor Xa act as central point where the intrinsic and extrinsic pathways converge to form a blood clot. Its main role is to convert prothrombin to thrombin, which acts as an enzyme in the conversion of fibrinogen to fibrin clot. Due to its central role, Xa is a major target for herbal anticoagulant agents. The herbals that act on Xa are *Ginkgo biloba* and *C. longa*.

*G. biloba:*
It is a popular herbal supplement known for improving blood flow and oxygen delivery throughout the body. Terpenoids such as "ginkgolide" are the main phytochemicals responsible for its anticoagulant activity. It has anticoagulant effects, which help to prevent the formation of clots by inhibiting platelet aggregation. *Ginkgo* also protects blood vessels from damage, making it an important addition to any cardiovascular health regimen [50].

**iii) Reduction of fibrinogen levels:**
When a blood vessel is damaged, fibrinogen is activated by thrombin. Fibrinogen is mainly produced by some pro-inflammatory mediators (interleukin 6 [IL-6], tumor necrosis factor-alpha [TNF-$\alpha$]). Fibrinogen serves as a precursor to fibrin. Fibrinogen releases fibrino peptides and creates fibrin monomers. These fibrin monomers spontaneously polymerize to form a net-like structure over the wound, strengthening the temporary platelet plug (i.e., soluble clot). Some herbals directly target this fibrinogen to reduce the coagulation process. Examples include *Zingiber officinale* and *Crataegus oxyacantha*.

*Z. officinale* (ginger):
Some researchers found that chronic consumption of ginger extracts has been shown to reduce plasma fibrinogen concentration, lower blood viscosity, and improve microcirculation. The phytochemical "gingerol" produces this effect by targeting the mediators (IL-6, TNF-$\alpha$) needed for the synthesis of fibrinogen. This mechanism is responsible for its anticoagulation activity [51].

*C. oxyacantha* (hawthorn):
*C. oxyacantha* (hawthorn) is a well-established cardiotonic herb belonging to the Rosaceae family. Flavonoid-rich phytochemicals are responsible for its anticoagulant activity, including hyperoside, vitexin, quercetin, rutin, and oligomeric proanthocyanidins. Experimental research suggests that hawthorn extracts can downregulate hepatic synthesis of fibrinogen, likely through inhibition of IL-6– and TNF-$\alpha$–mediated inflammatory signaling. This reduces plasma fibrinogen levels, a critical substance of blood viscosity and cardiovascular risk [52].

**iv) Enhancement of endogenous anticoagulants:**
The human body maintains hemostatic balance through intrinsic anticoagulant mechanisms that oppose excessive thrombin generation and clot formation. Key physiological anticoagulants include AT-III, protein S, cofactor II, protein C, heparin, and tissue factor pathway inhibitor (TFPI). Several herbal medicines have demonstrated the ability to enhance the synthesis, activation, or functional efficiency of these endogenous anticoagulants. Such activity represents a natural and physiologically harmonious approach to thromboprotection without the excessive bleeding risks often associated with synthetic anticoagulants. Some herbal plants which are involved in the enhancement of endogenous anticoagulants are *C. longa, Z. officinale, G. biloba, C. sinensis, P. ginseng, Salvia miltiorrhiza*, and *G. glabra*.

*P. ginseng:*
*P. ginseng* belongs to the family Araliaceae, widely known as "Asian ginseng." It is one of the most extensively studied adaptogenic herbs. It is popular for its immunomodulatory and neuroprotective activities. *P. ginseng* also exhibits potent antithrombotic, antiplatelet, and anticoagulant effects mediated through both direct inhibition of coagulation enzymes and enhancement of endogenous anticoagulant systems [53]. Protopanaxatriol-type ginsenosides are the important phytochemicals that enhance the synthesis and activity of AT-III, a key serine protease inhibitor that neutralizes thrombin and Factor Xa. Elevated levels of AT-III increases PT and thromboplastin time it leads to its anticoagulant enhancement [54].

*G. glabra:*
*G. glabra* L., belonging to the family Fabaceae, popularly known as licorice, is a traditional medicinal herb extensively used in Ayurvedic, Unani, and Chinese medicine. It is well known for its anti-inflammatory, hepatoprotective, and antiviral activities. Along with these effects, it also exhibits significant anticoagulant, antiplatelet, and fibrinolytic effects. The anticoagulant action of *G. glabra* is primarily attributed to its triterpenoid saponins (glycyrrhizin and glycyrrhetinic acid) and flavonoids (liquiritigenin, isoliquiritigenin, glabridin, liquiritin), which modulate multiple components of the hemostatic cascade and enhance endogenous anticoagulant defenses. Glycyrrhizin and 18$\beta$-glycyrrhetinic acid increase AT-III expression in hepatocytes via Nrf2-mediated antioxidant signaling, improving the inhibition of thrombin (Factor IIa) and Factor Xa [55, 56].

**v) Calcium chelation:**
Intracellular calcium ($Ca^{2+}$) is a regulatory element in platelet activation, aggregation, and coagulation. Excessive cytosolic $Ca^{2+}$ also facilitates activation of coagulation enzymes (e.g., Factor X, prothrombinase complex) and fibrin formation. Therefore, chelating or reducing bioavailable $Ca^{2+}$ can suppress coagulation and thrombus formation. The plants with this calcium chelation activity are *Vitis vinifera, T. arjuna, A. sativum, etc.*

*V. vinifera: (Grape seed):*
*V. vinifera L.* (Vitaceae) is cultivated worldwide, and its seeds, skins, and leaves are rich in polyphenols, particularly catechin, epicatechin, and their gallates (collectively called proanthocyanidins), as well as resveratrol, and quercetin, and kaempferol. Proanthocyanidins and resveratrol bind divalent calcium ions ($Ca^{2+}$) through their multiple hydroxyl groups, forming stable complexes. Chelation limits cytosolic $Ca^{2+}$ rise

in platelets, thereby inhibiting activation of protein kinase C, phospholipase C (PLC), and GPIIb/IIIa receptor exposure. This may result in decreased fibrinogen binding, platelet aggregation, and $TXA_2$ synthesis [57, 58].

*T. arjuna:*

*T. arjuna*, known as Arjuna, is an important cardiotonic in Ayurvedic medicine. It contains phytochemicals such as triterpenoid saponins, including arjunolic acid, arjungenin, and arjunic acid, and flavonoids like quercetin and kaempferol. Arjunolic acid possesses multiple hydroxyl and carboxyl groups capable of chelating divalent cations like $Ca^{2+}$. This chelation reduces cytosolic $Ca^{2+}$ availability in platelets and smooth muscle cells, which will lead to its anticoagulant activity [59].

Apart from the above popular herbal plants other plants also can show powerful anticoagulant activity with unknown mechanisms such as *Erigeron canadensis* L., *Fragaria vesca, and Echinacea purpurea, Thymus atlanticus, Thymus zygis, Fumaria officinalis* with proven activity. Several emerging herbal plant-derived bioactive compounds from recent researches are found, but these are not approved clinically. Examples include *S. miltiorrhiza*, quercetin, and luteolin. Some plants are under study only *in vitro* studies. Examples include *Jatropha gossypiifolia, Terminalia bellirica, Origanum vulgare,* and *Astragalus arbusculinus*. Table 7.1 presents some herbal anticoagulants along with their mechanisms and effects.

## 7.4.2 HERBAL ANTIPLATELETS

Antiplatelets are the pharmacologically active compounds that prevent the aggregation of the platelets, thereby preventing thrombus formation. Platelets are enucleate, tiny cells of blood responsible for blood clot formation during vascular injury; this process is called hemostasis. However, excessive activation of platelets results in abnormal blood clots within the blood vessels, contributing to various life-threatening CVDs associated with heart attack (myocardial infarction), ischemic stroke, etc. Hence, antiplatelet agents play a crucial role in thrombotic disorders by acting through different mechanisms and maintaining a physiological balance between normal hemostasis and thromboembolic diseases. Figure 7.5 outlines the platelet plug formation.

**Antiplatelet mechanisms:**

i. **Inhibition of arachidonic acid (A.A) pathway**
ii. **Inhibition of ADP-mediated platelet activation:**
iii. **Protection of nitric oxide and endothelial cell integrity**
iv. **Inhibition of intracellular calcium mobilization**

**Table 7.1** Herbal anticoagulants.

| Plant name | Major phytochemicals | Mechanism | Effect |
|---|---|---|---|
| *Allium sativum* | Allicin, ajoene | Factor IIa inhibition | Prolongation of PTT and PT |
| *Curcuma longa* | Curcumin | | |
| *Ginkgo biloba* | Ginkgolide B | Factor Xa inhibition | Prevention of clot formation |
| *Zingiber officinal* | Gingerol | Direct fibrinogen inhibition | Decreased fibrinogen synthesis |
| *Crataegus oxyacantha* | Hyperoside, vitexin | | |
| *Panax ginseng* | Berberine | Enhancement of endogenous anticoagulants | Prolongation of PTT and PT |
| *Glycyrrhiza glabra* | Glycyrrhizin | | |
| *Vitis vinifera* | Resveratrol | $Ca^{2+}$ chelation | Decreased fibrinogen binding |
| *Terminalia arjuna* | Arjunolic acid | | |

**General mechanisms of platelet plug formation:**

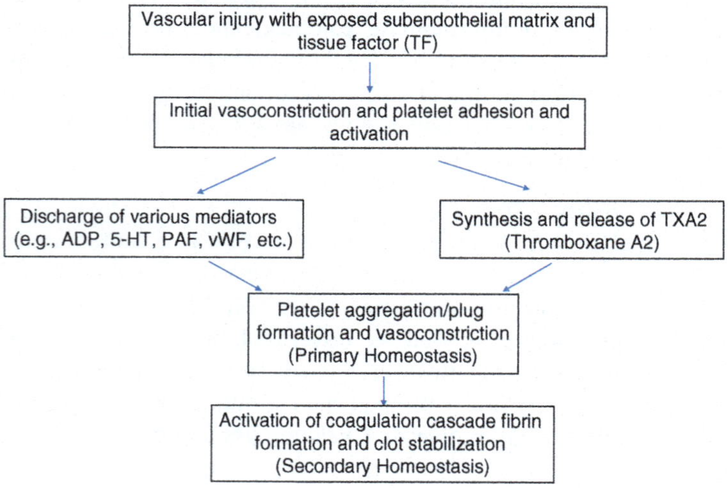


**FIGURE 7.5** Platelet aggregation.

**i) Inhibition of arachidonic acid pathway:**
Arachidonic acid plays an important role in platelet activation. Membrane phospholipids releases A.A on the stimulation of phospholipases $A_2$, which converts cyclooxygenase-1 (COX-1) into prostaglandin $G_2$ and $H_2$, thereby subsequently causes the release of $TXA_2$ by $TXA_2$ synthase which is a potent vasoconstrictor and inhibits platelet aggregation [60].

Examples: Curcumin, allicin *(A. sativum)*, apigenin (*Chamomilla recutita*), and hydroxytyrosol (*Olea europaea*) suppress COX-1 and downregulate $TXA_2$.

*O. europaea*:
*O. europaea* L., well known as olive tree, belongs to the family Oleaceae. Flavonoids like oleuropein and hydroxytyrosol are the most significant principal bioactives that possess cardioprotective and blood-thinning properties. The mechanism of phytoconstituents such as hydroxytyrosol and oleuropein, in particular hydroxytyrosol, suppress the thromboxane $B_2$ ($TXB_2$) synthesis [61] by downregulating COX-1 and lipoxygenase pathways, thereby preventing aggregation of platelets induced by ADP, A.A, and collagen. Additionally, these polyphenols also reduce the expression of platelet surface glycol proteins such as GPIIb/IIIa and P-selectin, which are crucial for platelet adhesion and aggregation.

**ii) Inhibition of ADP-mediated platelet activation:**
ADP acts as a physiological platelet activator by binding to $P2Y_{12}$ and $P2Y_1$ receptors. This interaction promotes intracellular calcium mobilization and activates glycoprotein IIb/IIIa, thereby facilitating fibrinogen cross-linking between platelets.

Examples: Ginkgolides (*G. biloba*) and (Z)-ligustilide (*Angelica sinensis*), (phenolic acids) *(Rosmarinus officinalis)* acts as platelet-activating factor (PAF) receptor antagonist, thereby reducing ADP-dependent aggregation.

*Angelica sinensis*:
Radix *A. sinensis* (Olivacea) Diels, commonly known as *Dang-gui,* is the dried root of *A. Sinensis* (Oliv.) Diels It consists of a complex mixture of bioactive constituents, including volatile oils (mainly phthalides such as (Z)-ligustilide and butylidenephthalide), ferulic acid, polysaccharides, coumarins, organic acids, and flavonoids. Among them (Z)-ligustilide is recognized as the principle bioactive pthalide, which exhibits potent antithrombotic and antiplatelet activity. (Z)-ligustilide exhibits antiplatelet and anti-thrombotic effects through multiple mechanisms, including inhibition of ADP-induced platelet aggregation, $TXA_2$ formation, modulation of prostacyclin ($PGI_2$) production, and amelioration of oxidative endothelial injury [62].

*R. officinalis* L.:
This aromatic shrub, popularly known as "rosemary," is a culinary and medicinal herb widely cultivated in Mediterranean regions. Rosemary consists of a wide range of rich components such as phenolic diterpenes (carnosic acid and carnosol) and phenolic acids (rosmarinic and caffeic acids) along with other volatile derivatives. These compounds demonstrate potent antiplatelet activity by inhibiting ADP-induced platelet aggregation. The polyphenols [63] also modulate intracellular calcium ions, thereby decreasing platelet reactivity.

*G. biloba* L.:
*G. biloba* belongs to the family Ginkgoaceae and has synonyms such as *Salisburia adiantifolia, Salisburia macrophylla,* and *Pterophylla salisburiensis.* It consists of ginkgolides (A, B, C), bilobalide, and flavonoid glycosides. Among them, particularly ginkgolide B, acts as a specific potent platelet-activating factor (receptor) antagonist, thereby preventing platelet aggregation and decreases $TXA_2$ [64] biosynthesis without affecting bleeding time. In addition, flavonoids also enhance nitric oxide (NO) release, providing endothelial protection leading to improved vascular tone, thereby reducing thrombotic risk.

**iii) Protection of nitric oxide and endothelial cell integrity:**
Elevating the synthesis of cyclic guanylyl monophosphate (cGMP) levels through the release of nitric oxide (NO) from endothelial cells activates guanylate cyclase in the platelets, thus decreasing the calcium ion concentration intracellularly and thereby preventing platelet adhesion and aggregation.

Examples: Flavonoids (*Vitis vinifera*), polyphenols (*O. europaea*), and curcumin increase NO bioavailability.

*Curcumin longa* L.:
Curcumin, a yellow polyphenolic pigment derived from the plant *Curcuma longa* L., commonly known as turmeric, belongs to the family Zingiberaceae traditionally. Curcumin, the main constituent of this plant, acts by inhibiting platelet aggregation by collagen, adrenaline, and A.A. It decreases the synthesis of thromboxane $B_2$ production but enhances 1,2-lipoxygenase (LOX) pathways. It also suppresses the platelet/endothelial cell adhesion molecule-1, netrin G1, delta-like-1, and plasma cell endoplasmic reticulum protein-1, which decrease platelet cell adhesion [65]. Curcumin also possesses anti-inflammatory and antioxidant properties, which protect endothelial cells and preserve nitric oxide (NO) synthesis and decreases platelet hyper activation [66]. These combined actions help to improve vascular hemostasis, making it a natural antithrombotic and cardiovascular protective agent.

*V. vinifera* (Vitaceae):
It is well known as "grape vine," which belongs to the family" Vitaceae" and is broadly cultivated worldwide. Due to the presence of its rich poly phenolic composition, it has gained considerable attention as an antiplatelet. The plant contains flavonoids [67], such as stilbenes, proanthocyanidins, and phenolic acids, which together contribute to antiplatelet and cardioprotective effects. By interfering with intracellular calcium ion signaling, it maintains the platelets in a resting state, inhibiting degranulation [68] and adhesion, thereby showing potent antiplatelet activity.

**iv) Inhibition of intracellular calcium mobilization:**
Calcium ions ($Ca^{+2}$) play a significant role in granule shape, secretion, and platelet activation. Blocking or modulating the intracellular $Ca^{+2}$ ions[3] from influx through membrane channels inhibits platelet aggregation.

**Table 7.2** Herbal antiplatelets.

| Plant source | Principal compounds | Target/pathway | Pharmacological effect |
|---|---|---|---|
| *Olea purpurea* | Oleuropein and hydroxytyrosol | Inhibition of arachidonic pathway | ↓ Platelet aggregation |
| *Angelica sinensis* | (Z)-ligustilide | Inhibition of ADP | ↓ Platelet aggregation |
| *Rosmarinus officinalis* | Caffeic acids | | |
| *Ginkgo biloba* | Ginkgolides B | | |
| *Curcuma longa* | Curcumin | Endothelial protection | ↓ ADP-induced aggregation |
| *Vitis vinifera* | Proanthocyanidins | | |
| *Chamomilla recutita* | Apigenin, quercetin, patuletin, luteolin | Inhibition of intracellular $Ca^{2+}$ | Fibrin degradation |

Examples: Apigenin (*Chamomilla*) and curcumin (*C. longa*) decreases intracellular $Ca^{+2}$ ions.

*Chamomilla recutita* L.:
*C. recutita* belongs to the family Asteraceae. Traditionally, it was used as an anti-inflammatory, spasmolytic, and antioxidant agent. The important constituents of this herbaceous plant are various phenolics and flavonoids, such as patuletin, apigenin, quercetin, luteolin and their glucoside derivatives. It was evidenced that mostly flavonoid derivatives (apigenin) shows anti platelet and antithrombotic activity by inhibiting platelet aggregation stimulated by collagen or ADP [69] through inhibition of COX-1 and reduces ($TXA_2$) synthesis preventing excessive platelet activation. The constituents of *Chamomilla* also raise endothelial nitric oxide (NO) and decrease intracellular calcium mobilization which lowers oxidative stress and enhances endothelial function. The plant decreases fibrin deposition and prolongs the bleeding time without altering the activated partial thromboplastin time (APTT) [70]. Table 7.2 presents herbal antiplatelet agents with their mechanisms and effects.

### 7.4.3 HERBAL THROMBOLYTICS

Fibrinolytic therapy is necessary to remove issues brought on by blood clots or thrombi and restore function to the afflicted area [71]. Blood vessel or venous thrombosis, PE, myocardial infarction, arterial thromboembolism, and acute ischemic stroke [72] are all treated with fibrinolytic substances.

The main side effect of thrombolytics is excessive bleeding, or hemorrhage, although they are generally safe and effective in treating thrombosis. According to recent epidemiological data, 11% of all ill patients who received thrombolytic medication experienced side effects like bleeding (hemorrhage) [73]. Hence, thrombolytic therapy remains a cornerstone in managing acute myocardial infarction, ischemic stroke, and PE. Traditional substances like urokinase, streptokinase, and recombinant tissue plasminogen activator (rtPA) effectively dissolve fibrin clots but carry significant risks of hemorrhage, short plasma half-life, and immunogenicity. The thrombolytic qualities of plant parts and their isolated forms of few plants have been the subject of numerous studies. Herbal thrombolytics offer an alternative with multi-target mechanisms, reduced side effects and better biocompatibility. Herbal thrombolytics augment process either by stimulating endogenous tPA, suppressing PAI-1, or directly exhibiting fibrinolytic protease activity [74]. Herbal agents with milder, multi-targeted effects may offer synergistic benefits but need careful standardization and clinical validation.

Examples: *S. miltiorrhiza* extracts elevate tPA levels, while nattokinase from fermented soybean (*Bacillus subtilis* var. *natto*) directly hydrolyzes fibrin.

**Herbal fibrinolytic agents mechanisms:**
In previous sections of this chapter, natural fibrinolysis under the section "hemostasis" and the enzymes responsible for fibrin (clot) breakdown have been discussed. The following are the some of the important fibrinolytic mechanisms of herbal plants.

i. **Direct fibrin degradation**
ii. **Plasminogen activation**
iii. **Suppression of PAI-1**
iv. **Antioxidant and endothelial-protective effects**

**i) Direct fibrin degradation:**
*B. subtilis:*
A serine protease produced during the fermentation of soybeans by *B. subtilis* directly cleaves cross-linked fibrin and also enhances endogenous fibrinolysis by converting prourokinase to urokinase. *In vitro* studies show nattokinase possesses stronger fibrin-degrading capacity than plasmin and improves blood rheology. It also directly promotes fibrinolysis by enhancing plasmin activity, increasing tPA activity, and reducing PAI-1[75]. Clinical trials indicate that oral nattokinase significantly reduces plasma fibrinogen and factor VII levels in hypercoagulable subjects. Due to its safety and oral bioavailability, nattokinase is among the most promising natural thrombolytic agents.

*Carica papaya*:
Papain, a cysteine protease from *C. papaya,* is widely used in industry and traditional medicine. Papain, with enzymatic activity, can directly cleave fibrin and fibrinogen chains and shows clot-dissolving potential. It may also act on plasminogen/plasmin pathways [76].

**ii) Suppression of PAI-1:**
PAI-1 plays a primary role in fibrinolysis by inhibiting it through inactivation of key enzymes, tissue plasminogen activator-1,

Table 7.3 Herbal thrombolytics.

| Plant name | Active phytochemical | Mechanism | Effect |
|---|---|---|---|
| *Bacillus subtilis* var. *natto* | Nattokinase | Direct fibrin hydrolysis; activation of urokinase | Reduces fibrinogen and factor VII in humans |
| *Carica papaya* | Papain | | |
| *Camellia sinensis* | Epigallocatechin, epicatechin gallate, epigallocatechin, and epicatechin | Enhancement of tissue plasminogen activator (tPA) and PAI-1 | Fibrin degradation |
| *Enhydra fluctuans* | Chlorogenic acid, caffeic acid | | |
| *Streblus asper* | Quercetin, kaempferol, catechin | Plasminogen activation | Fibrin degradation |
| *Salvia miltiorrhiza* | Salvianolic acid B | | |
| *Tinospora cordifolia* | Phenolics | t-PA inhibition | Endothelial protection |
| *Ocimum sanctum* | Carvacrol, ursolic acid, apigenin, rosmarinic acid, and eugenol | Inhibition of $TXA_2$ | |

and urokinase plasminogen activator. This leads to prevention of plasmin from plasminogen. Plasmin is the main enzyme that breaks down fibrin clots. An imbalance in the levels of PAI-1 can lead to pathological conditions such as "Thrombosis."

*Camellia sinensis:*
*C. sinensis* belongs to the family Theaceae. Green tea is the common name for *C. sinensis. C. sinensis* (green tea) contains several polyphenolic compounds, primarily catechins such as epigallocatechin gallate, epicatechin gallate, epigallocatechin, and epicatechin, which mainly enhance tPA activity and/or lower plasminogen levels. This shifts the balance toward plasmin formation, leading to fibrin degradation [77].

*Enhydra fluctuans* Lour.:
*Enhydra fluctuans* Lour. is a small herb that grows in tropical and subtropical areas and is a member of the Asteraceae family [78]. Certain phenolic acids and flavonoids in *E. fluctuans* may facilitate the conversion of plasminogen to plasmin, either by forming complexes that expose the activation site on plasminogen or stimulating endogenous plasminogen activators (t-PA).

**iii) Plasminogen activation:**
Plasminogen is the precursor to plasmin, an important enzyme in fibrinolysis. Once plasminogen is activated to plasmin, it breaks down the fibrin, which forms the structure of the clot.

*Streblus asper:*
*Streblus asper* is a plant that belongs to the family Moraceae. Certain bioactive compounds, such as quercetin, kaempferol, and catechin in *S. asper,* may promote the conversion of plasminogen into plasmin [79]. This mimics the action of streptokinase or tissue-type plasminogen activator (tPA).

*S. miltiorrhiza:*
*S. miltiorrhiza* Bunge, commonly called as Danshen (Chinese), red sage root, belongs to the family Lamiaceae. Salvianolic acid B (Sal B) upregulates tPA mRNA and protein expression, leading to direct enhancement of plasminogen activation [80].

**iv) Antioxidant and endothelial protective effects:**
*Tinospora cordifolia:*
The herbaceous vine *T. cordifolia* (Menispermaceae) is native to the tropical regions of Sri Lanka, Myanmar, and India. Phenolics are the key phytochemicals, and they mainly act by reducing oxidative stress, preserving endothelial function, and potentially supporting tPA release or lowering PAI-1. Thus, it may indirectly enhance the endogenous fibrinolytic system [81].

*Ocimum sanctum:*
*O. sanctum* is rich in carvacrol, ursolic acid, apigenin, rosmarinic acid, and eugenol, which are substances that are known for strong ROS-scavenging and anti-inflammatory properties. The effect is believed to be due to enzyme-like proteolytic activity and polyphenol-induced activation of the plasminogen–plasmin system, facilitating fibrin breakdown. *O. sanctum* also inhibits platelet aggregation and reduces $TXA_2$ synthesis, preventing excessive fibrin formation [82]. Table 7.3 presents herbal fibronolytics with their mechanisms and effects.

## 7.5 CONCLUSION

The decline in cardiovascular health is a progressive cause of pathological states and fatality worldwide, responsible for pathological conditions like heart failure, heart attacks, and high blood pressure. Pharmacological treatments, including anticoagulants, thrombolytics, and antiplatelet agents are effective; however, they often carry risks of side effects and long-term complications. Many medicinal plants possess bioactive compounds that exhibit cardioprotective functions like curcumin, ginsenosides, allicin, gingerols, ginkgolides, and nattokinase with strong anticoagulant, antiplatelet, and thrombolytic properties. Through multiple mechanisms, ranging from platelet inhibition to fibrin dissolution, they provide complete vascular protection.

## REFERENCES


1. Raskob, G.E., Angchaisuksiri, P., Blanco, A.N. et al. (2014). Thrombosis: a major contributor to global disease burden. In: *Seminars in Thrombosis and Hemostasis*, vol. 40 (ed. E.J. Favaloro), 724–735. Thieme Medical Publishers.
2. Wolberg, A.S., Rosendaal, F.R., Weitz, J.I. et al. (2015). Venous thrombosis. *Nat. Rev. Dis. Primers* 1 (1): 1–7.
3. Ay, C., Beyer-Westendorf, J., and Pabinger, I. (2019). Treatment of cancer-associated venous thromboembolism in the age of direct oral anticoagulants. *Ann. Oncol.* 30 (6): 897–907.
4. Seca, A.M. and Pinto, D.C. (2018). Plant secondary metabolites as anticancer agents: successes in clinical trials and therapeutic application. *Int. J. Mol. Sci.* 19 (1): 263.
5. Hrachovinová I. Diagnostic strategies in disorders of hemostasis. *VnitrLek* 2018; 64: 537–544. https://doi.org/10.36290/vnl.2018.076.
6. Sadek, M. and Kabnick, L.S. (2021). Endothermal heat induced thrombosis. *Phlebologie* 50 (04): 258–262.
7. Sun, J.C. and Joffe, H. (2007). *The Most Common Inpatient Problems in Internal Medicine: Ward Survival*. Elsevier Health Sciences.
8. Chapin, J.C. and Hajjar, K.A. (2015). Fibrinolysis and the control of blood coagulation. *Blood Rev.* 29 (1): 17–24.
9. Burnett, A.E., Mahan, C.E., Vazquez, S.R. et al. (2016). Guidance for the practical management of the direct oral anticoagulants (DOACs) in VTE treatment. *J. Thromb. Thrombolysis* 41 (1): 206–232.
10. Song, A.B., Rosovsky, R.P., Connors, J.M. et al. (2019). Direct oral anticoagulants for treatment and prevention of venous thromboembolism in cancer patients. *Vasc. Health Risk Manag.* 15: 175–186.
11. Berndt, M.C., Metharom, P., and Andrews, R.K. (2014). Primary haemostasis: newer insights. *Haemophilia* 20: 15–22.
12. Mahaut-Smith, M.P. (2012). The unique contribution of ion channels to platelet and megakaryocyte function. *J. Thromb. Haemost.* 10 (9): 1722–1732.
13. Clemetson, K.J. (2012). Platelets and primary haemostasis. *Thromb. Res.* 129 (3): 220–224.
14. Stalker, T.J., Newman, D.K., Ma, P. et al. (2012). Platelet signaling. *Handb. Exp. Pharmacol.* 210: 59–85.
15. Andrews, R.K. and Berndt, M.C. (2004). Platelet physiology and thrombosis. *Thromb. Res.* 114 (5–6): 447–453.
16. Barkhan, P., Silver, M.J., Da Costa, P.B. et al. (1958). Phosphatidyl serine and blood coagulation. *Nature* 182 (4641): 1031.
17. Hou, Y., Carrim, N., Wang, Y. et al. (2015). Platelets in hemostasis and thrombosis: novel mechanisms of fibrinogen-independent platelet aggregation and fibronectin-mediated protein wave of hemostasis. *J. Biomed. Res.* 29 (6): 437.
18. Lisman, T., Weeterings, C., and de Groot, P.G. (2005). Platelet aggregation: involvement of thrombin and fibrinogen. *Front. Biosci.* 10 (1–3): 2504–2517.
19. Ramström, S., Rånby, M., and Lindahl, T.L. (2002). The role of platelets in blood coagulation—effects of platelet agonists and GPIIb/IIIa inhibitors studied by free oscillation rheometry. *Thromb. Res.* 105 (2): 165–172.
20. Lopez, J.J., El Haouari, M., and Jardin, I. (2019). Flavonoids and platelet-derived thrombotic disorders. *Curr. Med. Chem.* 26 (39): 7035–7047.
21. Smith, S.A., Travers, R.J., and Morrissey, J.H. (2015). How it all starts: initiation of the clotting cascade. *Crit. Rev. Biochem. Mol. Biol.* 50 (4): 326–336.
22. Tankersley, D.L. and Finlayson, J.S. (1984). Kinetics of activation and autoactivation of human factor XII. *Biochemistry* 23 (2): 273–279.
23. Morrissey, J.H. and Broze, G.J. Jr. (2013). Tissue factor and the initiation and regulation (TFPI) of coagulation. In: *Hemostasis and Thrombosis: Basic Principles and Clinical Practice*, 6e (ed. V.J. Marder, W.C. Aird, J.S. Bennett, et al.), 163–178. Philadelphia, PA: Lippincott Williams & Wilkins.
24. Norris, L.A. (2003). Blood coagulation. *Best Pract. Res. Clin. Obstet. Gynaecol.* 17 (3): 369–383.
25. Rang, H.P., Dale, M.M., Ritter, J.M. et al. (2011). *Rang & Dale's Pharmacology*. Elsevier Health Sciences.
26. Kumar, S., Joseph, L., George, M., and Sharma, A. (2011). A review on anticoagulant/antithrombotic activity of natural plants used in traditional medicine. *Int. J. Pharm. Sci. Rev. Res.* 8 (1): 70–74.
27. Baharuddin, B. (2024). Antioxidant protection mechanisms in the cardiovascular system. *Asian J. Med. Health* 22 (6): 140–146.
28. Batool, R., Umer, M.J., Hussain, B. et al. (2022). Molecular mechanisms of superoxide dismutase (SODs)-mediated defense in controlling oxidative stress in plants. In: *Antioxidant Defense in Plants: Molecular Basis of Regulation* (ed. M. Hasanuzzaman, K. Nahar, and M. Fujita), 157–179. Singapore: Springer Nature.
29. Gao, W., He, J., Chen, L. et al. (2023). Deciphering the catalytic mechanism of superoxide dismutase activity of carbon dot nanozyme. *Nat. Commun.* 14 (1): 160.
30. Andrés, C.M., Pérez de la Lastra, J.M., Juan, C.A. et al. (2022). Chemistry of hydrogen peroxide formation and elimination in mammalian cells, and its role in various pathologies. *Stress* 2 (3): 256–274.
31. Kalyanaraman, B. (2013). Teaching the basics of redox biology to medical and graduate students: oxidants, antioxidants and disease mechanisms. *Redox Biol.* 1 (1): 244–257.
32. Sies, H. and Jones, D.P. (2020). Reactive oxygen species (ROS) as pleiotropic physiological signaling agents. *Nat. Rev. Mol. Cell Biol.* 21 (7): 363–383.
33. Cabrera-Fuentes, H.A., Aragones, J., Bernhagen, J. et al. (2016). From basic mechanisms to clinical applications in heart protection, new players in cardiovascular diseases and cardiac theragnostics: meeting report from the third international symposium on "New frontiers in cardiovascular research". *Basic Res. Cardiol.* 111 (6): 69.
34. Tomai, F., Crea, F., Chiariello, L. et al. (1999). Ischemic preconditioning in humans: models, mediators, and clinical relevance. *Circulation* 100 (5): 559–563.
35. Downey, J.M. and Cohen, M.V. (1996). Mechanisms of preconditioning: correlates and epiphenomena. In: *Ischemia: Preconditioning and Adaptation* (ed. M.S. Marber and D.M. Yellon), 21–34. Oxford: BIOS Scientific Publishers Limited.
36. Duong, C.N. and Vestweber, D. (2020). Mechanisms ensuring endothelial junction integrity beyond VE-cadherin. *Front. Physiol.* 11: 519.
37. Mensah, G.A., Arnold, N., Prabhu, S.D. et al. (2025). Inflammation and cardiovascular disease: 2025 ACC scientific statement: a report of the American College of Cardiology. *J. Am. Coll. Cardiol.* 87: 1–13.
38. Quindry, J.C. and Michalak, R.E. (2025). Exercise-induced cardioprotection: from endogenous to exogenous mechanisms. *Sports Med. Health Sci.* 7: 366–374.
39. Lerman, A. and Zeiher, A.M. (2005). Endothelial function: cardiac events. *Circulation* 111 (3): 363–368.
40. Moore, K.J., Sheedy, F.J., and Fisher, E.A. (2013). Macrophages in atherosclerosis: a dynamic balance. *Nat. Rev. Immunol.* 13 (10): 709–721.
41. Kaur, N., Chugh, V., and Gupta, A.K. (2011). Anti-atherosclerotic potential of plants: a review. *J. Pharm. Bioallied Sci.* 3 (1): 13–19.
42. Nyakudya, T.T., Tshabalala, T., Dangarembizi, R. et al. (2020). The potential therapeutic value of medicinal plants in the management of metabolic disorders. *Molecules* 25 (11): 2669.

43. Gholipour, S., Sewell, R.D., Lorigooini, Z. et al. (2018). Medicinal plants and atherosclerosis: a review on molecular aspects. *Curr. Pharm. Des.* 24 (26): 3123–3131.
44. Segneanu, A.E., Velciov, S.M., Olariu, S. et al. (2017). Bioactive molecules profile from natural compounds. In: *Amino acid—New Insights and Roles in Plant and Animal* (ed. T. Tanaka and A. Sakurai), 209–228. InTechOpen.
45. Thirumurugan, D., Cholarajan, A., Raja, S.S. et al. (2018). An introductory chapter: secondary metabolites. In: *Secondary Metabolites-Sources and Applications*, vol. 1 (ed. H.E.I.-D.M. Saleh and R.F. Aglan), 13. InTechOpen.
46. Marimoutou, M., Le Sage, F., Smadja, J. et al. (2015). Antioxidant polyphenol-rich extracts from the medicinal plants *Antirhea borbonica*, *Doratoxylon apetalum* and *Gouania mauritiana* protect 3T3-L1 preadipocytes against $H_2O_2$, TNFα and LPS inflammatory mediators by regulating the expression of superoxide dismutase and NF-κB genes. *J. Inflamm.* 12 (1): 10.
47. Bijak, M., Saluk, J., Szelenberger, R. et al. (2016). Popular naturally occurring antioxidants as potential anticoagulant drugs. *Chem. Biol. Interact.* 257: 35–45.
48. Srivastava, R., Singh, S., and Singh, R. (2017). Anticoagulant activity of garlic (*Allium sativum*) extract. *J. Ethnopharmacol.* 205: 65–74.
49. Gupta, S.C., Patchva, S., and Aggarwal, B.B. (2013). Therapeutic roles of curcumin: lessons learned from clinical trials. *AAPS J.* 15 (1): 195–218.
50. Volken, T. (2025). Natural blood thinners: herbs and foods for optimal circulation. *Herb Health* .
51. Verma, S.K., Singh, R., Singh, R.K. et al. (2011). Effect of *Zingiber officinale* on blood coagulation system – an experimental study. *Thromb. Res.* 127 (6): 565–571.
52. Zhang, Z., Wang, Y., Hu, X. et al. (2017). Hawthorn flavonoid extract modulates plasma fibrinogen and hemostatic parameters in hyperlipidemic rats. *J. Ethnopharmacol.* 207: 118–126.
53. Kim, J.H., Park, S.H., Kang, K.S. et al. (2019). Ginsenoside Rb1 prolongs coagulation times and enhances endogenous anticoagulants in rats. *J. Ethnopharmacol.* 235: 210–218.
54. Yun, T.K., Choi, S.Y., and Lee, J.H. (2021). Ginseng and blood coagulation: modulation of antithrombin and fibrinolytic pathways. *Front. Pharmacol.* 12: 658907.
55. Kao, T.C., Wu, C.H., and Yen, G.C. (2014). Bioactivity and potential health benefits of licorice. *J. Agric. Food Chem.* 62 (3): 542–553.
56. Yu, S.M. and Kim, S.J. (2014). The molecular mechanism of liquiritigenin-mediated vascular relaxation and endothelial protection. *J. Pharmacol. Exp. Ther.* 350 (2): 340–348.
57. Bagchi, D., Garg, A., Krohn, R.L. et al. (2018). Protective effects of grape seed proanthocyanidins on platelet function and calcium homeostasis. *Phytother. Res.* 32 (9): 1652–1661.
58. Li, W., Wu, J., Jiang, X. et al. (2019). Antithrombotic and anticoagulant effects of grape seed extract through fibrinogen inhibition and fibrinolysis. *Phytomedicine* 61: 152848.
59. Dwivedi, S. and Pandey, R. (2019). Arjunolic acid attenuates calcium-mediated platelet aggregation and thrombosis. *Indian J. Exp. Biol.* 57: 407–413.
60. Patrono, C. and Rocca, B. (2010). The future of antiplatelet therapy in cardiovascular disease. *Annu. Rev. Med.* 61 (1): 49–61.
61. Petroni, A., Blasevich, M., Salami, M. et al. (1995). Inhibition of platelet aggregation and eicosanoid production by phenolic components of olive oil. *Thromb. Res.* 78 (2): 151–160.
62. Shen, X., Wu, Y., Chen, P. et al. (2024). Anti-platelet aggregation activities of different grades of *Angelica sinensis* and their therapeutic mechanisms in rats with blood deficiency: insights from metabolomics and lipidomics analyses. *Front. Pharmacol.* 14: 1230861.
63. Andrade, J.M., Faustino, C., Garcia, C. et al. (2018). *Rosmarinus officinalis* L.: an update review of its phytochemistry and biological activity. *Future Sci. OA* 4 (4): FSO283.
64. Zhang, M., Sun, J., Chen, B. et al. (2018). Ginkgolide B inhibits platelet and monocyte adhesion in TNFα-treated HUVECs under laminar shear stress. *BMC Complement. Altern. Med.* 18 (1): 220.
65. Maheswaraiah, A., Jaganmohan Rao, L., and Naidu, K.A. (2015). Anti-platelet activity of water dispersible curcuminoids in rat platelets. *Phytother. Res.* 29 (3): 450–458.
66. Hussain, Y., Abdullah, K.F., Alsharif, K.F. et al. (2022). Regulatory effects of curcumin on platelets: an update and future directions. *Biomedicine* 10 (12): 3180.
67. Ciumărnean, L., Milaciu, M.V., Runcan, O. et al. (2020). The effects of flavonoids in cardiovascular diseases. *Molecules* 25 (18): 4320.
68. Balykina, A., Naida, L., Kirkgöz, K. et al. (2024). Antiplatelet effects of flavonoid aglycones are mediated by activation of cyclic nucleotide-dependent protein kinases. *Int. J. Mol. Sci.* 25 (9): 4864.
69. McKay, D.L. and Blumberg, J.B. (2006). A review of the bioactivity and potential health benefits of chamomile tea (*Matricaria recutita* L.). *Phytother. Res.* 20 (7): 519–530.
70. Bijak, M., Saluk, J., Tsirigotis-Maniecka, M. et al. (2013). The influence of conjugates isolated from *Matricaria chamomilla* L. on platelets activity and cytotoxicity. *Int. J. Biol. Macromol.* 61: 218–229.
71. Perler, B. (2005). Thrombolytic therapies: the current state of affairs. *J. Endovasc. Ther.* 12 (2): 224–232.
72. Tripathi, K.D. (2018). *Essentials of Medical Pharmacology*, 8e. New Delhi: Jaypee Brothers Medical Publishers.
73. Einarson, T.R. and Mikhailidis, D.P. (2009). Benefit-risk assessment of fibrinolytic therapy in acute myocardial infarction. *Drug Saf.* 32 (5): 391–410.
74. Prajapati, R., Kalariya, M., Parmar, S., and Sheth, N. (2011). Herbal remedies for thrombosis: a review. *Pharmacogn. Rev.* 5 (9): 30–37.
75. Weng, Y., Yao, J., Sparks, S., and Wang, K.Y. (2017). Nattokinase: an oral antithrombotic agent for the prevention of cardiovascular disease. *Int. J. Mol. Sci.* 18 (3): 523.
76. Fathima, S.N. and Begum, R. (2010). Papain: a protease with potential thrombolytic activity. *J. Enzyme Inhib. Med. Chem.* 25 (6): 861–867.
77. Nagao, T., Hase, Y., and Tokimitsu, I. (2007). Catechin-rich tea and its effect on blood coagulation and fibrinolysis. *Clin. Hemorheol. Microcirc.* 37 (1): 27–35.
78. Ali, R.M.D. (2013). Preliminary phytochemical screening and *in vitro* thrombolytic potential of the methanolic extract of *Enhydra fluctuans* Lour (Leaves). *Int. J. Pharmamedix India* 1 (2): 270–280.
79. Rahman, M.A., Islam, M.S., Biswas, M. et al. (2014). Evaluation of thrombolytic and membrane stabilizing activities of methanolic extracts of four medicinal plants. *Bangladesh J. Pharmacol.* 9: 310–314.
80. Liu, J., Shen, H.M., and Ong, C.N. (2013). Role of *Salvia miltiorrhiza* in the modulation of tissue plasminogen activator and plasminogen activator inhibitor-1 expression in human endothelial cells. *J. Ethnopharmacol.* 149 (1): 98–104.
81. Mishra, A., Kumar, S., and Pandey, A.K. (2013). Scientific validation of the medicinal efficacy of *Tinospora cordifolia*. *Sci. World J.* 2013 (1): 292934.
82. Mondal, S., Mirdha, B.R., and Mahapatra, S.C. (2009). The science behind sacredness of Tulsi (*Ocimum sanctum* Linn.). *Indian J. Physiol. Pharmacol.* 53 (4): 291–306.

CHAPTER 8

# Barriers and Breakthroughs in Herbal Drug Formulation and Delivery Systems

**Thummala Udaya Kumar**

*Department of Pharmaceutics, School of Pharmacy, Aditya University, Surampalem, Andhra Pradesh, India*

## 8.1 INTRODUCTION

Across centuries, various cultures have utilized herbal medicines as a cornerstone of traditional healthcare. Despite their extensive history and documented therapeutic benefits, the integration of herbal remedies into modern healthcare has been inconsistent. While many people worldwide rely on these products for primary care, their incorporation into mainstream medicine faces significant hurdles, primarily due to challenges in formulation, delivery, quality control, and evidence-based validation [1].

The worldwide herbal medicine market has been growing consistently, fueled by heightened consumer interest in natural treatments, a rising occurrence of chronic illnesses, and a tendency toward comprehensive healthcare options. Recent forecasts indicate that the herbal medicine market is anticipated to exceed USD 400 billion by 2030, driven by advancements in formulation and delivery methods [2]. Nonetheless, in spite of this expansion, significant obstacles persist that hinder herbal medications from attaining parity with traditional pharmaceuticals. Challenges like inadequate water solubility, reduced bioavailability, instability in processing and storage, fluctuations in phytoconstituent levels, and absence of standardized regulations hinder the reliable application of herbal remedies [3].

From a pharmacokinetic standpoint, many herbal bioactives experience inadequate oral absorption, quick metabolism, and significant first-pass effects [4]. Curcumin, a primary polyphenol sourced from *Curcuma longa*, shows an oral bioavailability of under 1%, primarily due to its hydrophobic characteristics and swift hepatic metabolism [5]. Comparable difficulties have been reported for resveratrol, quercetin, and silymarin, hindering their therapeutic effectiveness despite robust preclinical support [6]. Tackling these challenges necessitates contemporary formulation approaches that improve solubility, safeguard bioactives from degradation, and guarantee targeted delivery.

A significant hurdle exists in the uniformity of herbal remedies. In contrast to synthetic medications made up of singular, clearly defined active compounds, herbal remedies are intricate combinations that can include numerous or even hundreds of phytochemicals. The therapeutic effect frequently relies on synergistic interactions among these components, complicating the establishment of quality control standards. Environmental elements like soil quality, farming techniques, harvest timing, and storage environments also affect the phytochemical levels, leading to variability between batches [7]. In the absence of standardization, achieving consistent efficacy and safety in clinical practice remains challenging.

Moreover, there are issues concerning safety and toxicity. Despite the common notion that natural is safe, numerous herbal remedies have been linked to negative effects, especially when taken in large amounts or alongside standard medications. For example, kava (*Piper methysticum*) has been associated with liver toxicity, whereas aristolochic acids from *Aristolochia* species are acknowledged carcinogens [8].

These issues emphasize the need for strong pharmacovigilance systems to oversee the safety of herbal products. In spite of these obstacles, recent advancements in drug delivery technologies and pharmaceutical sciences are slowly changing the field of herbal medicine research. Nanotechnology, lipid-derived carriers, phytosomes, and innovative extraction methods are being investigated to address solubility, stability, and bioavailability challenges [9]. Artificial intelligence (AI) and computational resources are increasingly assisting in formulation design, predicting drug–herb interactions, and optimizing clinical trials [10]. This section examines the challenges and advancements in the formulation and delivery of herbal medications. The initial part outlines the obstacles thoroughly, emphasizing solubility problems, stability issues, lack of standardization, low bioavailability, and regulatory hurdles. The following sections address technological advances, such as nanotechnology-based carriers, phytosomes, ethosomes, and AI-enhanced methods. Ultimately, regulatory considerations and upcoming trends are discussed to offer a comprehensive outlook on the present condition and future possibilities of herbal medication formulation and delivery systems.

## 8.2 BARRIERS IN HERBAL DRUG FORMULATION AND DELIVERY

The development of herbal formulations faces numerous barriers, which can be broadly categorized into physicochemical, biological, technical, and regulatory challenges. Understanding

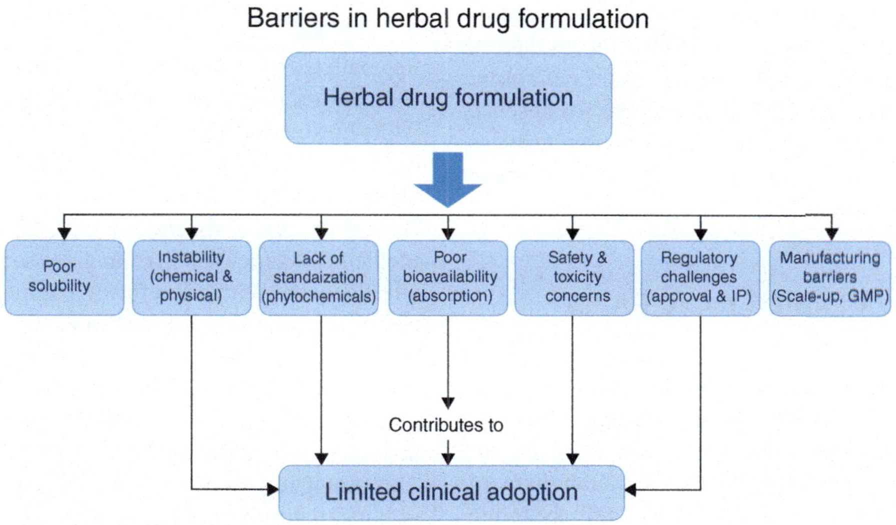


**FIGURE 8.1** Barriers in herbal drug formulation.

these barriers is crucial for developing effective solutions that ensure the therapeutic consistency of herbal medicines, as shown in Figure 8.1.

### 8.2.1 POOR SOLUBILITY AND DISSOLUTION

A prevalent problem with herbal bioactives is their low solubility in water, which affects both dissolution and absorption in the digestive system. About 40% of phytoconstituents are categorized within the Biopharmaceutics Classification System (BCS) as Class II or IV, noted for low solubility and/or permeability [11]. Examples include curcumin, quercetin, and resveratrol, each of which exhibits low solubility rates in biological fluids [12].

Limited solubility not only lowers oral absorption but also requires larger doses, potentially raising the risk of adverse effects. More sophisticated methods such as solid dispersions, cyclodextrin inclusion complexes, and lipid-based formulations have been explored but continue to encounter issues with scalability and reproducibility [13].

**Table 8.1** Key barriers in herbal drug formulation and delivery.

| Barrier type | Examples of herbal bioactives | Consequences |
|---|---|---|
| Poor solubility | Curcumin, Resveratrol | Low absorption, poor bioavailability |
| Instability | Catechins, Quercetin | Degradation during processing/storage |
| Lack of standardization | Ginseng, Ashwagandha | Batch variability inconsistent efficacy |
| Rapid metabolism | Silymarin, Piperine | Short half-life, reduced therapeutic effect |
| Toxicity | Kava, *Aristolochia* | Hepatotoxicity, carcinogenicity |

As shown in Table 8.1, multiple barriers collectively hinder the progress of herbal drug formulations. *Source:* [14]/MDPI/CC BY 4.0.

### 8.2.2 INSTABILITY OF HERBAL BIOACTIVES

Many herbal components are prone to instability due to environmental factors like heat, light, moisture, and oxygen. Catechins present in green tea, for instance, quickly oxidize in water-based solutions, greatly diminishing their shelf longevity [15]. Likewise, quercetin and anthocyanins are very responsive to alterations in pH and temperature [16].

Encapsulation techniques, like liposomes, nanoparticles, and polymeric matrices, are being investigated to safeguard unstable herbal bioactives from deterioration. Nonetheless, the production and stability evaluation of these sophisticated formulations on a large scale continue to be difficult [17].

### 8.2.3 LACK OF STANDARDIZATION AND QUALITY CONTROL

In contrast to synthetic drugs, which are generally single, well-defined chemical compounds, herbal medicines consist of intricate mixtures of phytochemicals. The therapeutic capacity of herbal products relies not just on the levels of single bioactive compounds but also on the cooperative interactions among various components [18]. This complexity renders it highly challenging to create consistent quality benchmarks.

For instance, ginseng (*Panax ginseng*) has numerous ginsenosides that differ according to the plant's age, growing area, and time of harvest [19]. Likewise, the active alkaloid levels in Ashwagandha vary based on soil quality and climate variations [20]. These differences lead to considerable inconsistency between batches, complicating the assurance of therapeutic reproducibility.

In recent years, methods for standardization, including chromatographic fingerprinting, spectroscopic profiling, and quantification of marker compounds, have been adopted [21].

Nevertheless, these approaches frequently do not encompass the entire pharmacological profile of the herbal formulation, especially when therapeutic effectiveness relies on synergistic interactions among phytochemicals. Additionally, the absence of unified global standards introduces further complexity, as regulatory bodies in various countries adhere to differing guidelines for herbal products [22].

### 8.2.4 POOR BIOAVAILABILITY AND RAPID METABOLISM

Even if herbal medications are sufficiently soluble and stable, their bioavailability can still be low because of quick metabolism and removal from the body. Numerous phytochemicals experience significant first-pass metabolism in the liver and intestines, which decreases their systemic availability [23].

For example, silymarin, sourced from *Silybum marianum*, exhibits hepatoprotective properties but has a brief half-life because of quick biliary excretion [24]. Bipstine, derived from *Piper nigrum* has low absorption and significant glucuronidation, which restricts its plasma levels [25]. In a similar manner, polyphenols such as quercetin and resveratrol are quickly converted into inactive conjugates, dampening their therapeutic efficacy [26].

Attempts to address these issues involve the combined use of bioenhancers like piperine, which hinders drug-metabolizing enzymes and enhances the bioavailability of substances such as curcumin [27]. However, the application of bioenhancers brings up safety issues, as enzyme inhibition may result in adverse herb–drug interactions [28].

### 8.2.5 SAFETY AND TOXICITY CONCERNS

While herbal remedies are often seen as safe because of their natural sources, numerous instances of negative reactions and toxicity have been documented. For example, kava (*Piper methysticum*) intake has been associated with hepatotoxicity, whereas nephrotoxicity and urothelial cancers have been linked to aristolochic acids derived from aristolochia species [29]. St. John's wort (*Hypericum perforatum*), a popular herbal remedy for depression, has been demonstrated to activate cytochrome $P_{450}$ enzymes, resulting in lower plasma levels of traditional medications like cyclosporine and warfarin [30].

A further issue is the contamination and adulteration of herbal products. Studies have indicated the existence of heavy metals, pesticides, microbial contaminants, and contamination with synthetic substances in herbal products [31]. These contaminants present considerable dangers to patients, particularly those who are taking herbal products in addition to their prescribed medications. In many areas, pharmacovigilance systems for herbal remedies are still poorly developed [32]. In the absence of systematic monitoring, establishing a dependable safety profile for numerous herbal medications is challenging.

### 8.2.6 REGULATORY CHALLENGES

Regulations for herbal medicines differ greatly among countries, with some Asian countries having more lenient systems, while Europe and North America impose stricter standards. For example, in India, herbal products can be sold under Ayurvedic, Siddha, or Unani classifications with comparatively minimal clinical trial data obligations [33]. Conversely, the European Medicines Agency (EMA) mandates comprehensive safety and effectiveness information for herbal medicinal products, especially for those that are not categorized as traditional medicines [34]. This absence of uniformity leads to confusion for producers and slows down worldwide market growth. Additionally, the regulatory routes for new herbal formulations, including nanoherbal medicines, are still inadequately outlined. This ambiguity hinders investment and delays the application of hopeful formulations in clinical settings [35].

### 8.2.7 TECHNICAL AND MANUFACTURING BARRIERS

The mass production of herbal formulations is frequently hindered by technical challenges. Extraction methods need to be meticulously refined to guarantee the consistency of phytochemical composition; however, traditional techniques like maceration and decoction frequently produce inconsistent outcomes [36]. Enhanced extraction techniques, such as supercritical fluid extraction (SFE), microwave-assisted extraction (MAE), and ultrasound-assisted extraction (UAE), provide greater efficiency but are costly and not broadly available [37].

Moreover, increasing the scale of herbal formulations based on nanotechnology presents difficulties related to cost, consistency, and quality management. Laboratory-scale encapsulation methods may not readily adapt to production on an industrial scale [38]. Additionally, stability testing, packaging, and shelf-life assessment for sophisticated herbal formulations are frequently insufficiently standardized, leading to inconsistencies in product effectiveness [39].

## 8.3 BREAKTHROUGHS IN HERBAL DRUG DELIVERY SYSTEMS

Despite significant hurdles in the formulation and delivery of herbal drugs, advancements in pharmaceutical technology have opened up possibilities to address these obstacles. Contemporary drug delivery systems (DDS) seek to improve solubility, stability, bioavailability, and therapeutic effectiveness of plant-derived compounds. Advancements in nanotechnology, lipid carriers, vesicular systems, polymer matrices, and computational methods have greatly enhanced the potential of herbal medicines. These advancements can be generally classified into carriers based on nanotechnology, vesicular systems, lipid formulations, polymer systems, innovative extraction methods, and AI-driven optimization approaches [40].

## 8.3.1 NANOTECHNOLOGY-BASED APPROACHES

Nanotechnology has transformed herbal drug delivery by allowing the creation of nanoscale carriers that safeguard bioactives, enhance solubility, and enable regulated release. Nanoparticles generally fall within the 1–100 nm size range and display distinctive physicochemical characteristics, including a larger surface area and improved permeability through biological membranes [41].

### 8.3.1.1 Polymeric Nanoparticles

Polymeric nanoparticles consist of biodegradable polymers like polylactic-co-glycolic acid (PLGA), chitosan, and polycaprolactone. These systems are extensively researched for enclosing hydrophobic plant-based compounds. Curcumin-loaded PLGA nanoparticles showed notably enhanced oral bioavailability and anticancer effectiveness in comparison to free curcumin [42]. In a similar manner, chitosan nanoparticles loaded with quercetin displayed improved stability and antioxidant properties [43].

Polymeric nanoparticles enable regulated release, decreased dosing intervals, and targeted delivery. Nevertheless, scalability and reproducibility continue to pose challenges in applying these formulations in clinical settings [44].

### 8.3.1.2 Solid Lipid Nanoparticles and Nanostructured Lipid Carriers

Solid lipid nanoparticles (SLNs) and nanostructured lipid carriers (NLCs) consist of biocompatible lipids that solidify at both room and body temperatures, offering structural integrity. These carriers merge the benefits of polymeric nanoparticles with improved safety profiles. Herbal ingredients like resveratrol, silymarin, and baicalein have been effectively developed into SLNs, demonstrating enhanced oral absorption and liver-protective effects [45].

NLCs combine solid and liquid lipids to address certain drawbacks of SLNs, like restricted drug-loading capacity. For instance, NLCs loaded with resveratrol showed greater stability and improved antioxidant activity in comparison to SLNs [46].

## 8.3.2 VESICULAR DRUG DELIVERY SYSTEM

Vesicular systems including liposomes, niosomes, phytosomes, and ethosomes, have gained prominence in enhancing the solubility and targeted delivery of herbal bioactives.

### 8.3.2.1 Liposomes

Liposomes are round vesicles made of phospholipid bilayers that can encapsulate drugs that are both hydrophilic and lipophilic. Their structural resemblance to cell membranes enables effective fusion and medication delivery. Herbal ingredients like ginseng saponins, curcumin, and glycyrrhizin have been effectively integrated into liposomal carriers [47].

Liposomes increase stability, lower toxicity, and boost therapeutic effectiveness. Nevertheless, factors like elevated production expenses and limited shelf life hinder their market use [48].

### 8.3.2.2 Niosomes

Niosomes are vesicles made from nonionic surfactants that provide benefits over liposomes regarding stability and affordability. Curcumin and quercetin in liposomal formulations have shown greater solubility, regulated release, and increased anticancer efficacy [49]. Niosomes are considered promising options for commercial herbal formulations due to their comparatively simple scale-up and chemical stability [50].

### 8.3.2.3 Phytosomes

Phytosomes signify an innovation specifically created for herbal bioactive compounds. These systems entail the complexation of phytochemicals with phospholipids, improving solubility, absorption, and bioavailability [51].

Silymarin planes, for example, showed around 4–7 times greater bioavailability than traditional silymarin extracts [52]. Curcumin and polyphenols from green tea have been effectively developed into phytosomes, resulting in improved therapeutic effects, as shown in Figure 8.2[53].

As shown in Table 8.2, diverse nanocarriers have been applied to overcome solubility, stability, and bioavailability barriers of herbal actives.

### 8.3.2.4 Ethosomes

Ethosomes are vesicular carriers made of phospholipids, ethanol, and water, intended to enhance delivery through the skin and across it. Herbal formulations incorporating *Curcuma longa*, and *Aloevera*, have demonstrated improved skin penetration and therapeutic benefits in topical uses [54]. In contrast to traditional liposomes, ethosomes, demonstrate increased deformability, facilitating greater penetration into the skin layers, as shown in Figure 8.3[55].

## 8.3.3 LIPID-BASED FORMULATIONS

Lipid-based systems have been investigated to enhance the solubility and absorption of lipophilic herbal substances. Self-emulsifying drug delivery systems (SEDDS) and micro emulsion rank among the most extensively researched. For instance, formulations of curcumin and resveratrol as SEDDS showed increased oral absorption because of better solubilization and lymphatic transport [56]. Likewise, quercetin microemulsions notably enhanced antioxidant and anti-inflammatory effects in preclinical research [57].

## 8.3.4 POLYMERIC AND HYDROGEL SYSTEMS

Hydrogels and polymeric matrices provide prolonged release and precise delivery of herbal bioactives. Hydrogel formulations of *Aloevera* and curcumin have demonstrated promise for applications in wound healing [58]. Likewise, hydrogels loaded

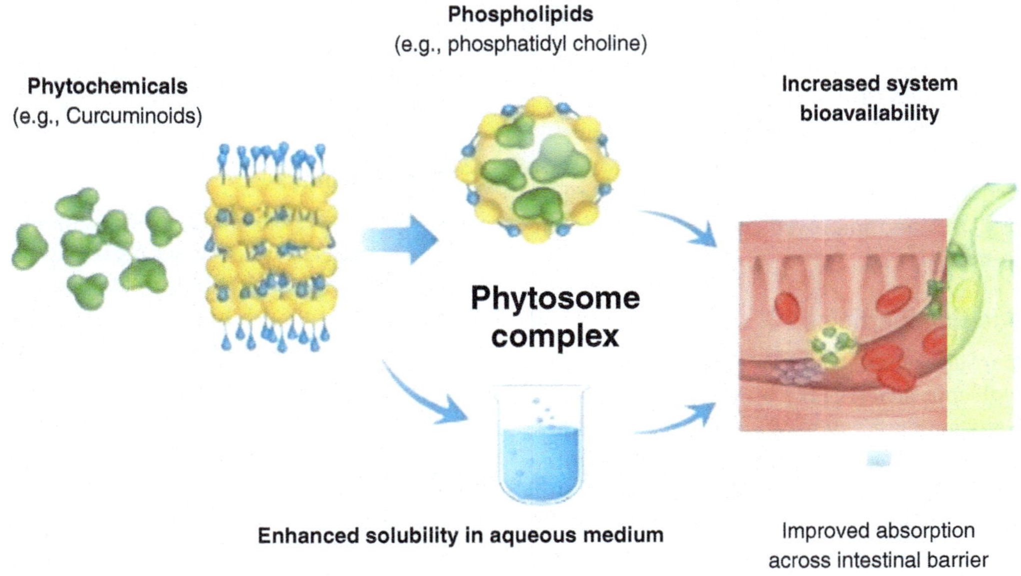


FIGURE 8.2 Phytosome preparation.

Table 8.2 Novel nanocarriers and herbal applications.

| Carrier | Herbal active | Outcome |
|---|---|---|
| Polymeric nanoparticles | Curcumin | Increased oral bioavailability, anticancer effect |
| SLNs | Silymarin | Increased hepatoprotective activity |
| NLNs | Resveratrol | Increased stability, antioxidant effect |
| Liposomes | Ginseng | Increased absorption and bioactivity |
| Niosomes | Quercetin | Increased solubility, anticancer efficacy |
| Phytosomes | Silymarin | Increased bioavailability |

with quercetin have been studied for delivering anticancer drugs, showing extended release and lower toxicity [59].

Polymeric systems enable the tailoring of release profiles and can be designed for particular administration routes, such as oral, topical, and parenteral.

## 8.4 ADVANCES IN EXTRACTION AND PROCESSING TECHNIQUES

Breakthroughs in extraction technologies have also contributed to improving the quality and reproducibility of herbal formulations

SFE: Provides high-purity extracts of thermolabile compounds without solvent residues [60].

MAE: Enhances extraction efficiency and reduces processing time [61].

UAE: Improves yield of bioactive compounds with minimal solvent use [62]. These techniques reduce degradation of phytoconstituents and ensure reproducible phytochemical profiles, addressing one of the major barriers in herbal medicine standardization.

## 8.5 ARTIFICIAL INTELLIGENCE AND COMPUTATIONAL APPROACHES

The use of AI and computational modeling is growing in herbal drug research. Algorithms in machine learning assist in forecasting interactions between herbs and drugs, enhancing formulation parameters, and simulating pharmacokinetics [63].

AI-based molecular docking research has revealed possible synergistic effects of curcumin and resveratrol in cancer treatment applications [64]. Models are also being created to predict solubility and permeability profiles of intricate herbal combinations [65].

## 8.6 REGULATORY FRAMEWORK FOR HERBAL DRUG FORMULATION AND DELIVERY SYSTEMS

The oversight of herbal medication formulations and distribution methods is among the most intricate and contested elements of contemporary pharmaceutical policy. In contrast to synthetic medications, which typically comprise single, well-defined molecules, herbal products are frequently multicomponent mixtures obtained from various plant sources. This complexity creates difficulties in quality control, standardization, safety evaluation, and efficacy confirmation [66]. Simultaneously, there is a rising worldwide demand for herbal remedies, fueled by patients' inclination toward natural treatments and the increasing market for nutraceuticals and phytopharmaceuticals [67].

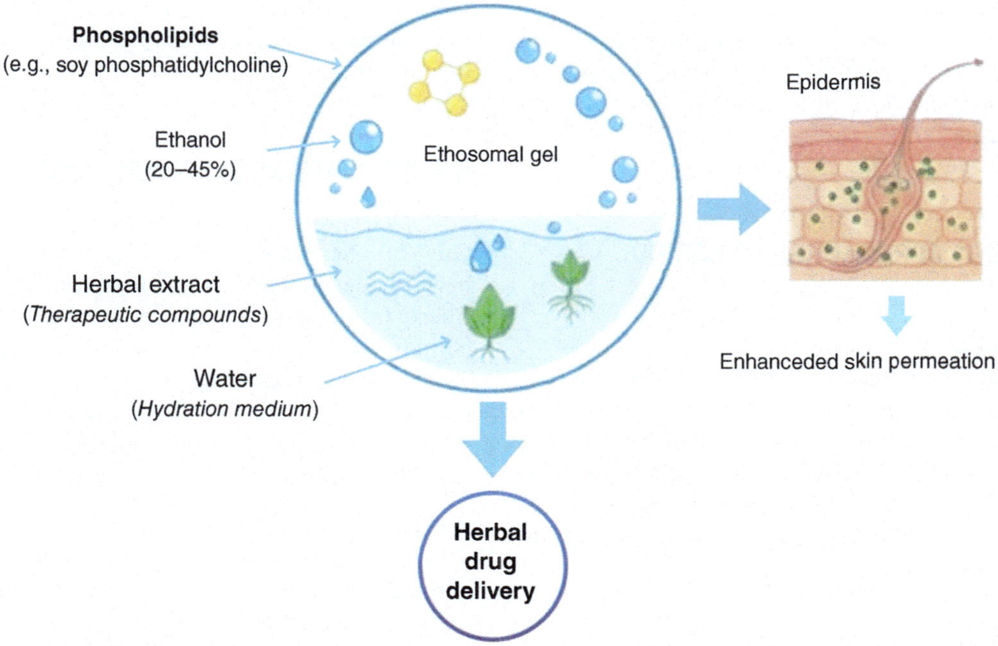


**FIGURE 8.3** Ethosomal gel preparation.

Proper oversight of herbal products necessitates a careful equilibrium. Regulations need to protect public health by guaranteeing the safety and effectiveness of products; however, they should also acknowledge the cultural and historical significance of traditional medicines that have been safely utilized for centuries. This shared responsibility sets apart the regulation of herbal medications from that of traditional pharmaceuticals [68].

## 8.7 PILLARS OF HERBAL DRUG REGULATION

Across different regions, regulatory frameworks, though diverse, are built upon four conceptual pillars:

1. Safety: Prevention of toxicity from herbal constituents, adulterants, or contaminants is essential. For example, reports of hepatotoxicity linked to certain plant alkaloids have highlighted the risks of inadequate toxicological screening [69].
2. Efficacy: Establishing therapeutic benefits supported by either traditional usage data or modern clinical trials is essential. Many regulatory bodies allow evidence from long-standing traditional use in place of randomized controlled trials, although this remains controversial [70].
3. Quality: Ensuring reproducibility through standardization of raw materials, marker compounds, and manufacturing processes is essential. Herbal extracts often vary depending on geographical origin, harvesting season, and extraction method [71].
4. Pharmacovigilance: Post-marketing surveillance for adverse reactions is essential but often underdeveloped in herbal regulation. Consumer self-reporting remains inconsistent, and many adverse events go unrecorded [72].

Together, these pillars provide a framework for evaluating herbal medicines while recognizing their unique nature compared to synthetic drugs.

Unique Challenges in Herbal Drug Regulation

1. Complexity of herbal formulations
   Herbal products are inherently complex, often containing dozens or even hundreds of phytochemicals. Interactions between these constituents may contribute to therapeutic effects but also complicate reproducibility and safety testing [73].
2. Standardization difficulties
   Unlike synthetic drugs, which can be precisely synthesized, the concentration of active compounds in herbal extracts can vary depending on cultivation practices, environmental conditions, and postharvest processing [74]. This variability often leads to inconsistent clinical outcomes.
3. Adulteration and contamination
   Herbal products are vulnerable to contamination with heavy metals, pesticides, and microorganisms. Additionally, intentional adulteration with synthetic drugs has been reported, undermining consumer trust [75].
4. Lack of global harmonization
   Regulatory frameworks differ widely across regions, creating barriers to international trade and limiting the global availability of certain herbal products [76].

5. Limited clinical evidence
While centuries of traditional use provide a foundation for safety, the lack of rigorous clinical trials for many formulations restricts their acceptance within evidence-based medicine [77].

## 8.8 REGULATORY APPROACHES TO HERBAL MEDICINES

*Traditional use pathway*
A frequent regulatory method is to allow the endorsement of herbal remedies grounded in recorded traditional application. In this framework, a product might receive approval if it has been utilized for many years without significant safety issues. This method recognizes the cultural significance of herbal remedies and lessens the demands of performing expensive clinical trials, as shown in Figure 8.4 [78].

*Evidence-based pathway*
Conversely, the evidence-based route demands clinical data similar to that of synthetic drugs. Products undergo preclinical toxicology research and sequential clinical trials to determine effectiveness [79]. This model improves scientific validity but could be less attainable for smaller producers or conventional practitioners.

*Overlap with nutraceuticals and functional foods*
An intricate aspect of herbal regulation is the intersection with categories like nutraceuticals, dietary supplements, and functional foods. Numerous herbal products are promoted as health supplements, allowing them to avoid more rigorous pharmaceutical regulations [80]. Nonetheless, this merging of categories heightens the chances of consumer misunderstanding and weakens the effectiveness of safety regulations.

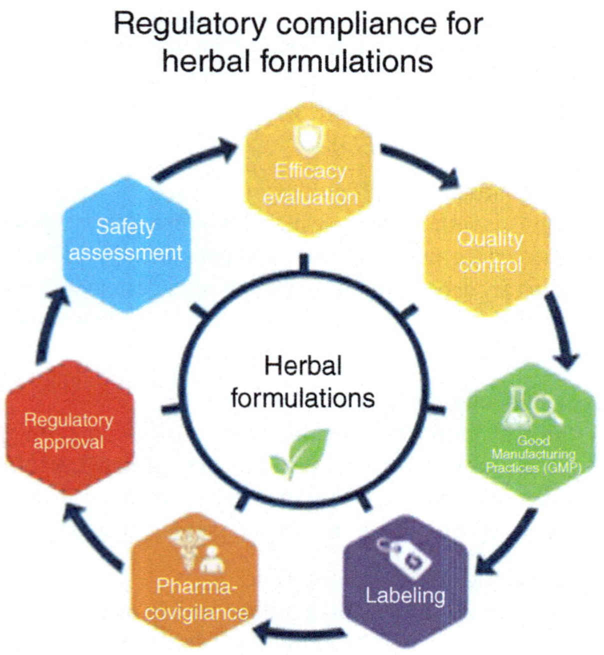


**FIGURE 8.4** Regulatory compliance for herbal formulations.

## 8.9 INNOVATIONS IN HERBAL DRUG REGULATION

*Phytopharmaceuticals Frameworks*
One of the most notable regulatory innovations has been the development of phytopharmaceuticals categories. These frameworks recognize plant-derived formulations containing defined active constituents and subject them to modern drug evaluation processes, including preclinical and clinical studies [81]. This represents an attempt to integrate traditional herbal wisdom with contemporary scientific validation

*Advanced analytical techniques*
Recent years have seen significant advances in the use of chromatographic and spectroscopic fingerprinting to standardize herbal extracts. Techniques such as high-performance liquid chromatography (HPLC), liquid chromatography–tandem mass spectrometry (LC–MS/MS), and nuclear magnetic resonance (NMR) are increasingly applied to identify and quantify phytochemical markers [82]. Regulatory guidelines now encourage manufacturers to adopt such methods to improve reproducibility.

*Artificial intelligence and machine learning*
AI is beginning to play a role in herbal drug regulation. Machine learning algorithms can analyze complex chemical fingerprints to predict batch consistency, detect adulteration, and even forecast herb–drug interactions [83]. This shift toward data-driven oversight is likely to revolutionize quality control in the coming decade.

*Blockchain in supply chain authentication*
Blockchain-based systems are being tested to ensure traceability of herbal raw materials, preventing counterfeiting and ensuring sustainability. This innovation allows regulators and consumers to track the journey of a product from farm to pharmacy [84].

*Challenges in regulating nanoformulations*
The advent of herbal nanomedicines such as curcumin nanoparticles and silymarın liposomes poses additional regulatory challenges. Conventional frameworks often lack clear guidelines for assessing nanocarriers in herbal products, leaving regulatory agencies to adopt a case-by-case approach [85].

## 8.10 BREAKTHROUGH CONCEPTS IN HERBAL REGULATION

*Global pharmacovigilance networks*
One emerging concept is the establishment of international pharmacovigilance systems for herbal medicines. Such networks would allow cross-border sharing of safety data, reducing delays in detecting and responding to adverse effects [86].

*Sustainability and Ethical Regulation*
The growing demand for certain herbal drugs has led to over-harvesting and ecological concerns. Regulatory frameworks are beginning to integrate sustainability guidelines, such as requirements for Good Agricultural and Collection Practices (GACP) [87].

*Adaptive Clinical Trial Models*
Traditional randomized controlled trials may not always be feasible for multi-constituent herbal formulations. Innovative models such as adaptive trials, pragmatic trials, and real-world evidence studies are being explored to better evaluate herbal drug efficacy without losing methodological rigor [88].

*Integration of Traditional Knowledge*
Regulatory frameworks are increasingly considering traditional knowledge databases to safeguard against biopiracy and to guide research priorities. This integration ensures that intellectual property rights are respected and that communities benefit from the commercialization of their knowledge [89].

## 8.11 FUTURE OUTLOOK

Looking ahead, the regulation of herbal drugs must evolve to meet the needs of an expanding global market while maintaining consumer protection. Several trends are anticipated:

1. Dedicated guidelines for herbal nanomedicines – Clear standards for evaluating bioavailability, safety, and stability of herbal nanoformulations
2. Personalized herbal medicine– Leveraging genomics and metabolomics to tailor herbal therapies to individual patients [90]
3. Digital pharmacopeias– Expansion of global digital databases containing standardized monographs, safety profiles, and clinical evidence
4. Cross-regional harmonization –Development of international standards to facilitate trade and enhance consumer confidence
5. Holistic safety models– Integration of traditional safety records with modern toxicology and pharmacogenomics

## 8.12 CONCLUSION

The oversight of herbal medicine formulation and distribution systems exists at an essential crossroads of tradition and modernity. In contrast to synthetic drugs, which are assessed on single, well-defined molecules, herbal remedies constitute a broad and diverse group, including raw plants, standardized extracts, phytopharmaceuticals, and innovative nanoformulations. This variety highlights the urgent requirement for strong but flexible regulatory systems. A key takeaway from years of herbal usage is that while long-standing traditional wisdom should be honored, it cannot be the only foundation for worldwide acceptance. Historical evidence supports safety, but in the absence of thorough toxicological testing, current pharmacovigilance, and consistent manufacturing standards, numerous herbal products continue to face examination. Consequently, regulatory frameworks need to advance into a dual-level model – one that appreciates ethnomedicine while also mandating evidence from preclinical and clinical trials for novel claims or new delivery methods. A significant obstacle remains the issue of standardization. Variations in phytochemical makeup among different plant batches compromise reproducibility, consequently diminishing clinical results and eroding regulatory confidence. New tools, like chromatographic fingerprinting, spectroscopic profiling, and AI algorithms, present chances to surpass this obstacle. Incorporating these innovations into regulatory standards can enhance consistency in oversight of herbal drugs while preserving the natural diversity of botanicals. Another domain requiring regulatory attention is safety and pharmacovigilance. Herbal medications are frequently viewed as "safe due to being natural", yet numerous case reports and toxicological studies show that this belief can be deceptive. A well-organized and clear post-marketing surveillance system, ideally linked across areas, is crucial. The idea of a worldwide pharmacovigilance system for herbal products signifies a potential advancement, enabling collective knowledge and quicker identification of adverse reactions.

The emergence of herbal nanomedicines, like phytosomes, nanoparticles, and liposomes, introduces a fresh aspect to the regulatory discussion. Although these technologies improve bioavailability and therapeutic effectiveness, they introduce new safety and stability issues that current herbal regulations frequently do not cover. The lack of clear nanotechnology guidelines for botanicals leads to uncertainty among researchers, manufacturers, and regulators. Filling this gap will be essential for advancement in the future. Anticipating the future, herbal drug regulation is closely linked to wider trends in digitalization, personalization, and sustainability. The emergence of digital pharmacopeias and blockchain-supported supply chains could ultimately address enduring challenges related to authenticity and traceability. The integration of genomics and metabolomics may advance personalized herbal medicine, providing customized solutions that combine traditional knowledge with precise scientific methods. Simultaneously, the ecological impact of high volume herbal demand cannot be overlooked. Regulatory frameworks need to incorporate sustainable farming practices and responsible sourcing to ensure that worldwide herbal supply chains are robust and environmentally sustainable.

In the end, the outcome is evident: the effective regulation of herbal medication formulation and delivery systems relies on equilibrium. Regulation should be stringent enough to ensure quality, safety, and effectiveness while remaining adaptable to accommodate diversity, cultural heritage, and innovation. By achieving this equilibrium, herbal remedies can transition from their historical origins into recognized, globally esteemed treatments. The regulatory pathway is more than just a legal obligation; it serves as a connection between the traditional and the contemporary, the experiential and the scientific, the regional and the international. If constructed with vision, this bridge will enable herbal medicines to play a significant role in addressing the health issues of the 21st century, while preserving the authenticity of traditional knowledge for upcoming generations.

## REFERENCES


1. Ekor, M. The growing use of herbal medicines: issues relating to adverse reactions and challenges in monitoring safety. *Front. Pharmacol.* 2021; 12: 611722. https://doi.org/10.3389/fphar.2021.611722.
2. Market Research Future (2023). Herbal medicine market research report 2023–2030. MRFR reports.https://www.marketresearchfuture.com/reports/herbal-medicine-market-2023 (accessed 20 August 2025).
3. Parasuraman, S., Thing, G.S., Dhanaraj, S.A. Polyherbal formulation: concept of Ayurveda. *Pharmacogn. Rev.* 2020; 14 (27): 80–89. https://doi.org/10.4103/phrev.phrev_8_20.
4. Liu, Y., Li, H., Wang, X. Pharmacokinetics and bioavailability challenges of herbal medicines. *Drug Metab. Rev.* 2021; 53(2): 199–215. https://doi.org/10.1080/03602532.2021.1879864.
5. Hewlings, S.J., Kalman, D.S. Curcumin: a review of its effects on human health. *Foods* 2020; 9(10): 1214. https://doi.org/10.3390/foods9101214.
6. Salehi, B., Mishra, A.P., Nigam, M., et al. Resveratrol: a double-edged sword in health benefits. *Biomedicine* 2021; 9(9): 1046. https://doi.org/10.3390/biomedicines9091046.
7. Kunle, O.F., Egharevba, H.O., Ahmadu, P.O. Standardization of herbal medicines: a review. *Int. J. Biodivers. Conserv.* 2022; 14(3): 128–138. https://doi.org/10.5897/IJBC2020.1404.
8. Xu, J., Zhao, W., Pan, J., et al. Impact of environmental factors on active constituents in medicinal plants. *Front. Plant Sci.* 2021; 12: 630735. https://doi.org/10.3389/fpls.2021.630735.
9. Teschke, R., Xuan, T.D., Lebot, V. Herbal hepatotoxicity: review and criteria for causality assessment. *World J. Hepatol.* 2020; 12(7): 389–398. https://doi.org/10.4254/wjh.v12.i7.389.
10. Alam, F., Shafique, Z., Khalil, A., et al. Nanotechnology-based drug delivery systems for herbal medicines: a review. *J. Drug Deliv. Sci. Technol.* 2021; 61: 102158. https://doi.org/10.1016/j.jddst.2020.102158.
11. Benet, L.Z. The role of BCS in herbal drug classification. *Eur. J. Pharm. Sci.* 2020; 153: 105495. https://doi.org/10.1016/j.ejps.2020.105495.
12. Gupta, S.C., Sung, B., Kim, J.H., et al. Multitargeting by curcumin: How molecular advances can help improve cancer therapy. *Cancer* 2020; 12(7): 1959. https://doi.org/10.3390/cancers12071959.
13. Patel, A.R., Velikov, K.P. Advances in solubility enhancement of poorly soluble phytochemicals. *Adv. Drug Deliv. Rev.* 2021; 177: 113915. https://doi.org/10.1016/j.addr.2021.113915.
14. Yuan, H., Ma, Q., Ye, L., Piao, G. The traditional medicine and modern medicine from natural products. *Molecules* 2020; 21(5): 559. https://doi.org/10.3390/molecules21050559.
15. Ahmad, M., Ashraf, M.A., Ghaffar, A. Stability issues of catechins in herbal formulations. *J. Food Sci. Technol.* 2020; 57(2): 447–455. https://doi.org/10.1007/s13197-019-04092-7.
16. Dias, M.I., Sousa, M.J., Alves, R.C., Ferreira, I.C. Exploring plant polyphenols: characterization, bioavailability, and stability. *Compr. Rev. Food Sci. Food Saf.* 2020; 19(1): 3323–3342. https://doi.org/10.1111/1541-4337.12647.
17. Chen, H., Li, X., Sun, J. Lipid nanoparticles for the stabilization of unstable herbal actives. *Pharmaceutics* 2021; 13 (12): 2022. https://doi.org/10.3390/pharmaceutics13122022.
18. Kong, J.M., Chia, L.S., Goh, N.K., et al. Standardization of complex herbal mixtures: challenges and solutions. *Planta Med.* 2020; 86 (12): 856–865. https://doi.org/10.1055/a-1165-0423.
19. Lee, M.S., Yang, E.J., Kim, J.I., Ernst, E. Ginseng for cognition: systematic review and meta-analysis. *J. Alzheimer's Dis.* 2020; 77(2): 1157–1167. https://doi.org/10.3233/JAD-200536.
20. Mirjalili, M.H., Moyano, E., Bonfill, M., et al. Phytochemical variability in *Withania somnifera*. *Phytochem. Rev.* 2021; 20(3): 713–727. https://doi.org/10.1007/s11101-020-09714-2.
21. Li, X., Chen, J., Zhang, L. Analytical advances in herbal standardization. *J. Pharm. Biomed. Anal.* 2022; 209: 114494. https://doi.org/10.1016/j.jpba.2021.114494.
22. EMA (2021). Guideline on quality of herbal medicinal products. https://www.ema.europa.eu/en/documents/scientific-guideline/herbal-medicinal-products-guideline-quality_en.pdf (accessed 29 August 2025).
23. Zhao, X., Wang, Y., Sun, W. First-pass metabolism and pharmacokinetics of herbal drugs. *Curr. Drug Metab.* 2020; 21(9): 654–664. https://doi.org/10.2174/1389200221666200914101452.
24. Bijak, M., Saluk, J. Hepatoprotective potential of silymarin nanoformulations. *Nutrients* 2020; 12(7): 2067. https://doi.org/10.3390/nu12072067.
25. Srinivasan, K. Black pepper and piperine: bioavailability enhancement and health benefits. *Crit. Rev. Food Sci. Nutr.* 2021; 61 (15): 2533–2557. https://doi.org/10.1080/10408398.2020.1774468.
26. Fang, J.Bioavailability of dietary polyphenols and strategies to improve delivery. *Nutrients* 2020; 12(6): 1719. https://doi.org/10.3390/nu12061719.
27. Shoba, G., Joy, D., Joseph, T., et al. Influence of piperine on the pharmacokinetics of curcumin in animals and human volunteers. *Planta Med.* 2021; 87(3): 186–193. https://doi.org/10.1055/a-1294-4696.
28. Posadzki, P., Watson, L., Ernst, E. Adverse effects and drug-herb interactions: an overview of systematic reviews. *Drugs* 2020; 80(7): 679–713. https://doi.org/10.1007/s40265-020-01325-7.
29. Stickel, F., Shouval, D. Hepatotoxicity of herbal and dietary supplements: an update. *Arch. Toxicol.* 2021; 95(2): 749–758. https://doi.org/10.1007/s00204-020-02934-9.
30. Borrelli, F., Izzo, A.A. Herb-drug interactions with St. John's wort (*Hypericum perforatum*): evaluation of clinical evidence. *Expert Opin. Drug Saf.* 2020; 19(3): 297–310. https://doi.org/10.1080/14740338.2020.1718752.
31. Ernst, E.Adulteration of traditional herbal medicines with synthetic drugs: a systematic review. *Br. J. Clin. Pharmacol.* 2020; 86(6): 1377–1386. https://doi.org/10.1111/bcp.14251.
32. Pal, D., Mitra, A.K. Pharmacovigilance for herbal medicines: current state and future directions. *J. Clin. Pharm. Ther.* 2021; 46(3): 688–697. https://doi.org/10.1111/jcpt.13323.
33. Gogtay, N.J., Bhatt, H.A., Dalvi, S.S., Kshirsagar, N.A. Regulatory requirements for herbal medicines in India. *J. Assoc. Physicians India* 2020; 68(5): 72–76. PMID: 32501236.
34. European Medicines Agency (2021). Guideline on the assessment of herbal medicinal products. https://www.ema.europa.eu/ (accessed 17 September 2025.)
35. Sharma, R., Martins, N., Chaudhary, A. Regulatory perspectives on herbal nanomedicines: opportunities and challenges. *Biomed. Pharmacother.* 2021; 141: 111900. https://doi.org/10.1016/j.biopha.2021.111900.

36. Azwanida, N.N. A review on extraction methods for medicinal plants: maceration, percolation and soxhlet. *Pharmacogn. Rev.* 2020; 14 (27): 7–15. https://doi.org/10.4103/phrev.phrev_7_19.
37. Chemat, F., Rombaut, N., Meullemiestre, A., et al. Alternative extraction processes for natural products: towards green and sustainable techniques. *Ultrason. Sonochem.* 2020; 63: 104953. https://doi.org/10.1016/j.ultsonch.2019.104953.
38. Danaei, M., Dehghankhold, M., Ataei, S., et al. Impact of particle size and polydispersity index on the clinical applications of lipidic nanocarrier systems. *Int. J. Pharm.* 2020; 576: 118982. https://doi.org/10.1016/j.ijpharm.2020.118982.
39. Katiyar, D., Singh, V., Ali, J., Baboota, S. Quality control considerations for herbal nanomedicines. *Drug Dev. Ind. Pharm.* 2020; 46(5): 745–754. https://doi.org/10.1080/03639045.2020.1752628.
40. Prasad, S., Gupta, S.C., Tyagi, A.K. Modern drug delivery systems for herbal formulations: recent advances and future prospects. *Drug Discov. Today* 2021; 26 (12): 2707–2715. https://doi.org/10.1016/j.drudis.2021.05.019.
41. Khan, I., Gothwal, A., Sharma, A.K. Nanotechnology-enabled delivery of phytochemicals for improved therapeutic outcomes. *Curr. Pharm. Des.* 2020; 26 (25): 2970–2985. https://doi.org/10.2174/1381612826666200611145342.
42. Yallapu, M.M., Jaggi, M., Chauhan, S.C. Curcumin nanoformulations for cancer therapy and imaging. *Drug Discov. Today* 2020; 25(4): 473–474. https://doi.org/10.1016/j.drudis.2020.01.001.
43. Alam, M.N., Almoyad, M., Huq, F. Development and application of quercetin-based nanoparticles. *Front. Pharmacol.* 2021; 12: 628898. https://doi.org/10.3389/fphar.2021.628898.
44. Delaney, J.T., Smith, J., Johnson, T.Scaling-up issues for herbal nanoparticle drug products: a translational perspective. *Nanomedicine* 2021; 16 (11): 889–901. https://doi.org/10.2217/nnm-2021-0014.
45. Naseri, N., Valizadeh, H., Zakeri-Milani, P. Solid lipid nanoparticles and nanostructured lipid carriers for herbal drug delivery. *Adv. Pharm. Bull.* 2020; 10(3): 437–443. https://doi.org/10.34172/apb.2020.053.
46. Ganesan, P., Narayanasamy, D. Lipid nanoparticles for resveratrol delivery: formulation, characterization and in vitro evaluation. *J. Food Sci. Technol.* 2021; 58(1): 825–833. https://doi.org/10.1007/s13197-020-04565-5.
47. Fang, Y., Li, L., Meng, L. Liposomal delivery systems for botanical therapeutics. *Int. J. Nanomed.* 2020; 15: 9917–9932. https://doi.org/10.2147/IJN.S285397.
48. Akbarzadeh, A., Rezaei-Sadabady, R., Davaran, S., et al. Liposomes in medicine and pharmacy: current applications and future perspectives. *J. Liposome Res.* 2020; 30(4): 336–348. https://doi.org/10.1080/08982104.2020.1749754.
49. Moghassemi, S., Hadjizadeh, A. Niosomes as effective nanocarriers: recent advances in design and applications. *J. Control. Release* 2021; 335: 103–116. https://doi.org/10.1016/j.jconrel.2021.05.016.
50. Touitou, E., Dayan, N., Bergelson, L., Godin, B., Eliaz, M. Ethosomes – novel vesicular carriers for enhanced delivery. *J. Control. Release* 2020; 327: 326–336. https://doi.org/10.1016/j.jconrel.2020.07.018.
51. Kumar, R., Singh, B., Bakshi, M. Ethosomal systems for dermal and transdermal delivery of herbal bioactives. *Curr. Drug Deliv.* 2021; 18(6): 777–788. https://doi.org/10.2174/1567201818666210212153551.
52. Bombardelli, E.Phytosome: a new patented delivery system for herbal molecules. *Fitoterapia* 2020; 141: 104485. https://doi.org/10.1016/j.fitote.2019.104485.
53. Riva, A., Ronchi, M., Petrangolini, G., Bosisio, S., Allegrini, P. Improved bioavailability of silybin by phytosome complexation. *Fitoterapia* 2020; 145: 104634. https://doi.org/10.1016/j.fitote.2020.104634.
54. Cuomo, J., Appendino, G., Dern, A.S., et al. Meriva®: a curcumin delivery system. *Phytomedicine* 2021; 90: 153554. https://doi.org/10.1016/j.phymed.2021.153554.
55. Di Pierro, F., Bressan, A., Riva, A. Clinical efficacy of curcumin phytosome (Meriva®) in osteoarthritis. *Panminerva Med.* 2020; 62(1): 7–13. https://doi.org/10.23736/S0031-0808.20.03845-2.
56. Kidd, P.M. Bioavailability and activity of phytosome complexes from botanical extracts. *Altern. Med. Rev.* 2020; 25(1): 58–66. PMID: 32525632.
57. Upadhyay, S., Dixit, M. Nanophytomedicine: advances in phytosome research. *J. Drug Deliv. Sci. Technol.* 2021; 63: 102443. https://doi.org/10.1016/j.jddst.2021.102443.
58. Jain, S., Jain, A.K., Pohekar, M. Advances in phytophospholipid complexes for herbal drug delivery. *Curr. Pharm. Des.* 2021; 27 (28): 2989–3000. https://doi.org/10.2174/1381612827666210519124731.
59. Ashrafizadeh, M., Ahmadi, Z., Farkhondeh, T., Samarghandian, S. Nanotechnology-based strategies for enhanced curcumin delivery. *Int. J. Nanomed.* 2020; 15: 7929–7950. https://doi.org/10.2147/IJN.S278210.
60. Singh, P., Garg, A., Aggarwal, A. Microwave-assisted extraction of phytoconstituents: greener perspectives. *Ind. Crop. Prod.* 2020; 145: 112103. https://doi.org/10.1016/j.indcrop.2019.112103.
61. Azmir, J., Zaidul, I.S.M., Rahman, M.M., et al. Techniques for extraction of bioactive compounds from plant materials: a review. *J. Food Eng.* 2020; 278: 109937. https://doi.org/10.1016/j.jfoodeng.2020.109937
62. Mandal, S.C., Mandal, V., and Das, A.K. (2020). *Essentials of Botanical Extraction*. Amsterdam: Elsevier.
63. Verma, N., Shukla, S. Impact of supercritical fluid extraction on bioactive retention in herbal medicines. *J. Supercrit. Fluids* 2020; 165: 104986. https://doi.org/10.1016/j.supflu.2020.104986.
64. Chemat, F., Abert-Vian, M., Fabiano-Tixier, A.S., et al. Green extraction of natural products: sustainable perspectives. *TrAC Trends Anal. Chem.* 2020; 118: 248–263. https://doi.org/10.1016/j.trac.2019.05.037.
65. Gaba, B., Khan, T., Haider, M.F. AI-driven prediction models for herbal pharmacokinetics. *Comput. Biol. Med.* 2022; 143: 105288. https://doi.org/10.1016/j.compbiomed.2022.105288.
66. Ekor, M. (2014). The growing use of herbal medicines: issues relating to adverse reactions and challenges in monitoring safety. *Front. Pharmacol.* 4: 177.
67. Robinson, M.M. and Zhang, X. (2011). *The World Medicines Situation 2011: Traditional Medicines: Global Situation, Issues and Challenges*. Geneva: World Health Organization.
68. Heinrich, M., Barnes, J., Prieto, J.M. et al. (2012). *Fundamentals of Pharmacognosy and Phytotherapy*, 2ee. Edinburgh: Elsevier.
69. Teschke, R., Larrey, D., Melchart, D. et al. (2013). Traditional herbal medicines and hepatotoxicity: a clinical and regulatory perspective. *Br. J. Clin. Pharmacol.* 75 (3): 630–636.
70. Vickers, A. and Zollman, C. (1999). ABC of complementary medicine: herbal medicine. *BMJ* 319 (7216): 1050–1053.
71. Calixto, J.B. (2019). The role of natural products in modern drug discovery. *An. Acad. Bras. Cienc.* 91 (Suppl 3): e20190105.
72. Kunle, O.F., Egharevba, H.O., and Ahmadu, P.O. (2012). Standardization of herbal medicines – a review. *Int. J. Biodivers. Conserv.* 4 (3): 101–112.
73. Bent, S. (2008). Herbal medicine in the United States: review of efficacy, safety, and regulation. *J. Gen. Intern. Med.* 23 (6): 854–859.
74. Barnes, J., Anderson, L.A., and Phillipson, J.D. (2007). *Herbal Medicines*, 3ee. London: Pharmaceutical Press.
75. Posadzki, P., Watson, L.K., and Ernst, E. (2013). Contamination and adulteration of herbal medicinal products (HMPs): an overview of systematic reviews. *Eur. J. Clin. Pharmacol.* 69 (3): 295–307.

76. Capasso, R., Izzo, A.A., Pinto, L. et al. (2000). Phytotherapy and quality of herbal medicines. *Fitoterapia* 71 (Suppl 1): S58–S65.
77. Tilburt, J.C. and Kaptchuk, T.J. (2008). Herbal medicine research and global health: an ethical analysis. *Bull. World Health Organ.* 86 (8): 594–599.
78. Williamson, E.M., Lorenc, A., Booker, A., and Robinson, N. (2013). The rise of traditional Chinese medicine and its incorporation into global healthcare. *Eur. J. Integr. Med.* 5 (2): 114–118.
79. Walji, R., Boon, H., Barnes, J. et al. (2010). Regulatory and legislative barriers to the incorporation of complementary medicine into primary care. *Integr. Healthc. Policy* 6 (3): 260–266.
80. Izzo, A.A. and Ernst, E. (2009). Interactions between herbal medicines and prescribed drugs. *Drugs* 69 (13): 1777–1798.
81. Patel, D.N., Low, W.L., Tan, L.L. et al. (2012). Adverse events associated with herbal medicines. *Clin. Pharmacol. Ther.* 92 (4): 478–484.
82. EMA (2022). Guideline on quality of herbal medicinal products/traditional herbal medicinal products. https://www.ema.europa.eu/en/documents/scientific-guideline/final-guideline-quality-herbal-medicinal-productstraditional-herbal-medicinal-products-revision-3_en.pdf. (accessed 16 October 2025).
83. Li, S., Han, Q., Qiao, C. et al. (2008). Chemical markers for the quality control of herbal medicines: an overview. *Chin. Med.* 3: 7.
84. Choi, D.W., Kim, J.H., Cho, S.Y. et al. (2011). Regulatory approach and status of herbal medicines in Korea. *J. Ethnopharmacol.* 137 (2): 587–595.
85. Mackey, T.K. and Nayyar, G. (2017). A review of existing and emerging digital technologies to combat the global trade in fake medicines. *Expert Opin. Drug Saf.* 16 (5): 587–602.
86. Bhattacharya, S. (2013). Phytosomes: emerging strategy in delivery of herbal drugs. *J. Drug Deliv. Ther.* 3 (3): 91–101.
87. Barnes, J. (2003). Quality, efficacy and safety of complementary medicines: fashions, facts and the future. Part II: efficacy and safety. *Br. J. Clin. Pharmacol.* 55 (4): 331–340.
88. WHO (2003). *Guidelines on Good Agricultural and Collection Practices (GACP) for Medicinal Plants*. Geneva: World Health Organization.
89. Fonnebo, V., Grimsgaard, S., Walach, H. et al. (2007). Researching complementary and alternative treatments – the gatekeepers are not at home. *BMC Med. Res. Methodol.* 7: 7.
90. Ginsburg, G.S. and Willard, H.F. (2009). Genomic and personalized medicine: foundations and applications. *Transl. Res.* 154 (6): 277–287.

# Targeted Delivery of Herbal Compounds for Cardiovascular Health Using Liposomes, Phytosomes, and Self Nano-Emulsified Drug Delivery Systems

CHAPTER 9

**Pathuri Raghuveer[1], Haya Khader Ahmed Yasin[2], Shakil Akthar[3], and Grandhi Srikar[4]**

[1] *School of Pharmaceutical Sciences, GITAM University, Hyderabad, Telangana, India*

[2] *Department of Pharmaceutical Sciences, College of Pharmacy and Health Sciences, Ajman University, Ajman, United Arab Emirates*

[3] *Department of Pharmacy, Central University of South Bihar, Gaya, Bihar, India*

[4] *Department of Pharmaceutical Sciences, Vignan's Foundation for Science, Technology and Research, Guntur, Andhra Pradesh, India*

## 9.1 INTRODUCTION

### 9.1.1 ROLE OF PHYTOCHEMICALS IN CARDIOVASCULAR DISEASE TREATMENT

As per the World Health Organization (WHO), each year, more than 17.9 million people suffer from life-threatening conditions due to cardiovascular diseases (CVDs) [1]. Oxidative stress, chronic inflammation, endothelial dysfunction, and metabolic abnormalities are some of the intricate etiologies of CVDs. These complications in etiology stress the importance of the investigation of new therapeutic alternatives. Among all phytochemicals, were emerged as prominent agents due to their pleiotropic bioactivities, advantages in safety profiles, and natural origin [2].

Phytochemicals are secondary metabolites from plants, categorized into classes including flavonoids, polyphenols, alkaloids, terpenoids, saponins, and lignans. These chemicals exert major protective effects on the heart and blood vessels by changing important metabolic processes. Phytochemicals have been shown to inhibit lipid peroxidation, decrease low-density lipoprotein (LDL) oxidation, enhance endothelial nitric oxide synthase (eNOS) activity, and suppress inflammatory mediators, including nuclear factor kappa B (NF-κB) and tumor necrosis factor-alpha (TNF-α) [3–5]. There has been a significant development in translating herbal medicines into clinically useful formulations. Many commercial products of phytochemicals are available for the treatment of CVDs. Some examples are ResVantage (resveratrol), Greenselect® Phytosome (green tea extract), and Meriva® (curcumin phytosome). Nonetheless, despite their potential, numerous phytochemicals have inadequate aqueous solubility, low permeability, and fast biotransformation, thereby limiting their therapeutic utility [6].

Researchers are increasingly working on nanotechnology-based delivery technologies to alleviate the problems with the conventional phytochemical formulations. Nanocarriers like, liposomes, phytosomes, nanoemulsions, polymeric micelles, dendrimers, and solid lipid nanoparticles (SLNs) have shown a lot of promise in making the phytochemicals more soluble, permeable, and stable to have improved pharmacokinetics [7, 8]. Not only can these nanocarriers improve pharmacokinetics, but they also lower systemic toxicity and allow for site-specific delivery. This makes them perfect for cardiovascular therapy, where precision targeting is important. Recent studies concentrate on optimizing these systems regarding size, surface charge, drug-loading efficiency, and biocompatibility to attain superior therapeutic results [9].

Even though integration of nanotechnology with the phytochemicals is attracting more attention by the researchers, still it is facing numerous challenges. A significant problem is lack of proper standardization of the phytochemicals, which actually constitute various active and inactive chemicals with varied compositions. This further makes it challenging in carrying out quality control and dose adjustment [10]. Besides, no proper regulatory guidelines have been developed for approving these nanocarrier-based formulations of phytochemicals [11]. Despite these challenges, research on therapeutic potential of the phytochemicals with nanocarriers is growing. To make safe and complete use of these systems in the treatment of CVDs, it will be important to encourage strategic investments in interdisciplinary research, improve regulatory policies, and build strong clinical evidence.

## 9.2 PHYTOCHEMICALS FOR CARDIOVASCULAR DISEASE THERAPY

Phytochemicals form the basis of many traditional and modern strategies for treating CVDs, as they are safe and effective. Among the various phytochemicals investigated, curcumin, resveratrol, and green tea catechins are notable for their significant cardioprotective effects, as evidenced by both preclinical and clinical research. However, because of their natural physicochemical limitations, they often need improved delivery systems to reach their full therapeutic potential. Table 9.1 summarizes the pharmacodynamics, physicochemical limitations, and explored drug delivery strategies.

## 9.3 PHYSICOCHEMICAL AND PHARMACOKINETIC CHALLENGES

Despite the widespread use of phytochemicals in CVD management, their full therapeutic potential is limited by critical pharmacokinetic and physicochemical barriers, like poor solubility, low permeability, instability under physiological conditions, and rapid systemic clearance. In order to assess their accurate clinical efficacy, addressing these limitations is necessary. In the current section, some of these pharmacokinetic limitations of phytochemical-derived agents, such as curcumin, resveratrol, EGCG, as well as other agents, which have established promising responses, such as berberine, quercetin, and baicalin that have been widely practiced for cardiovascular therapy, are summarized in Figure 9.1 and discussed in detail further.

### 9.3.1 POOR SOLUBILITY AND BIOAVAILABILITY

Starting with the most renowned compound, curcumin dissolves in water at a concentration of only nanomolar levels [29]. Other well-cited phytochemicals, resveratrol and EGCG, also exhibit poor solubility. This poor solubility causes them to have irregular systemic uptake due to the dissolution-limited oral bioavailability [21]. An alkaloid, berberine, utilized for lipid control, also exhibits a very minimal aqueous solubility (<1 mg/ml), resulting in its limited oral bioavailability (<5%) [30]. Similarly, quercetin, a flavonol prevalent in onions and apples, demonstrates minimal solubility in gastrointestinal (GI) fluids, thereby substantially restricting its absorption [31]. *Scutellaria baicalensis*-derived glycosylated flavone baicalin exhibits restricted intestinal permeability and necessitates microbial degradation for absorption, leading to heterogeneity in therapeutic effects [32]. Challenges associated with solubility and permeability result in the administration of higher doses leading to enhanced systemic toxicity or utilizing sophisticated dosage forms to enhance the bioavailability of these compounds.

### 9.3.2 RAPID METABOLISM AND SYSTEMIC ELIMINATION

The bioactivity of phytochemicals is often dramatically reduced due to phase I and phase II metabolic transformations. Rapid hepatic and intestinal metabolism are primarily responsible for converting curcumin into therapeutically less active compounds such as glucuronide and sulfate conjugates [15]. Resveratrol is also prone to extensive first-pass metabolism, leading to the formation of less bioactive

**Table 9.1** A comparative summary of the pharmacological mechanisms, limitations, and delivery strategies for the major phytochemicals.

| Phytochemical | Source | Mechanisms of cardiovascular protection | Key molecular targets | Limitations | Advanced delivery approaches |
|---|---|---|---|---|---|
| Curcumin [12–17] | *Curcuma longa* (turmeric) | Anti-inflammatory, antioxidant, anti-atherosclerotic, improves endothelial function | NF-κB, Nrf2, intercellular adhesion molecule 1 (ICAM-1), vascular cell adhesion molecule 1 (VCAM-1), eNOS | Poor solubility, rapid metabolism, low oral bioavailability | Liposomes, phytosomes, polymeric nanoparticles |
| Resveratrol [18–23] | Grapes, red wine, peanuts | Enhances vasodilation, inhibits inflammation, antioxidant, antiplatelet | Sirtuin 1 (SIRT1), AMP-activated protein kinase (AMPK), peroxisome proliferator-activated receptor gamma (PPARγ), eNOS, TNF-α | Extensive first-pass metabolism, short half-life | Liposomes, solid lipid nanoparticles, polymeric carriers |
| Green tea catechins (epigallocatechin-3-gallate [EGCG]) [24–28] | *Camellia sinensis* (green tea) | Reduces LDL oxidation, improves vascular reactivity, antioxidant, anti-inflammatory | NF-κB, phosphoinositide 3-kinase (PI3K/Akt), eNOS | Instability in GI tract, low permeability, rapid conjugation | Phytosomes, lipid-based nanoparticles, nanomicelles |

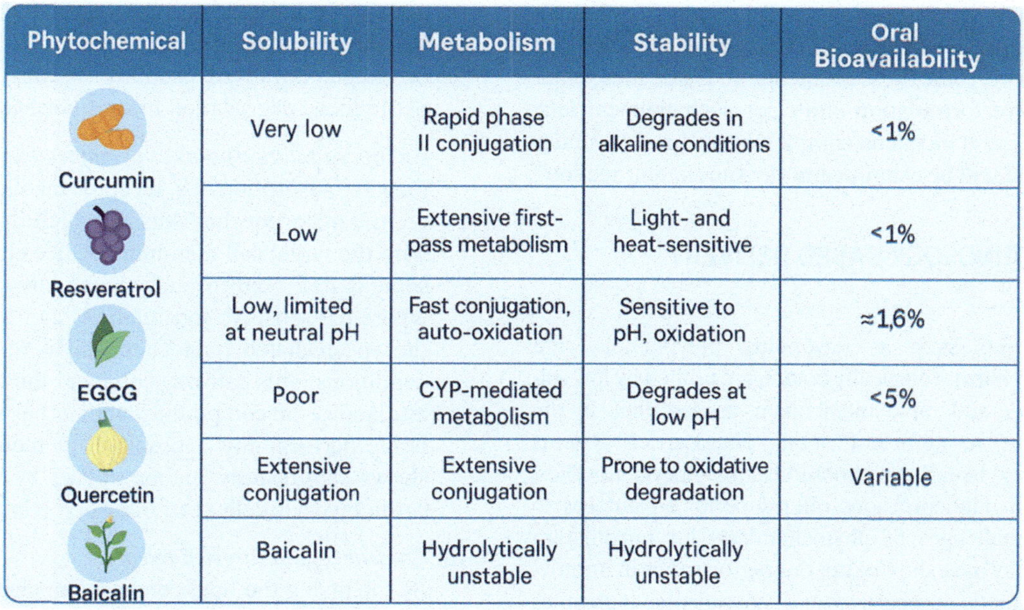


**FIGURE 9.1** Limitations of key phytochemicals relevant to cardiovascular therapy.

compounds [33]. A similar stability issue is also associated with EGCG, as it is unstable in the gastric environment. It will rapidly conjugate, resulting in reduced plasma half-life [27]. Multiple oxidized and demethylated metabolites of berberine were formed due to hepatic and gut metabolism. Some of these metabolites of berberine have little or no therapeutic activity [34]. 5′-diphospho-glucuronosyltransferases (UGTs) and sulfotransferases (SULTs) extensively metabolize quercetin resulting in variable plasma concentrations and wider interindividual differences in therapeutic action [35]. Baicalin utilizes gut metabolism for deglycosylation to baicalein, which is actively absorbed and bioactive in nature. Unfortunately, it also suffers from unpredictable bioavailability due to variations in gut microbiota [36]. Such metabolic vulnerabilities often necessitate multiple daily doses, leading to compliance issues in chronic CVD therapies.

### 9.3.3 INSTABILITY AND DEGRADATION

In addition to poor solubility and rapid metabolism, many phytochemicals are chemically unstable in physiological conditions, which limit their therapeutic efficacy. At alkaline pH and physiological temperature, curcumin degrades into ferulic acid and vanillin compounds, which lack the full biological effect of curcumin [37]. Upon UV exposure, resveratrol, which is a light-sensitive compound, undergoes isomerization from trans- to cis-resveratrol, reducing its pharmacological potency. The primary catechin in green tea, EGCG, is stable only in acidic environments and unstable in neutral and alkaline solutions; it also oxidizes in the presence of metal ions or heat [38]. Berberine shows instability under acidic gastric conditions and can hydrolyze before reaching systemic circulation [39]. Quercetin is prone to photodegradation and sensitive to light, temperature, and pH. This oxidative degradation decreases its shelf life and bioefficacy [40]. Similar to the above-discussed phytochemicals, baicalin also suffers instability in an aqueous environment and is predominantly susceptible to enzymatic degradation in the GI tract [41]. These stability issues are major challenges for formulation development, quality control, and scale-up of phytochemical formulation manufacturing.

### 9.3.4 CLINICAL CONSEQUENCES AND FORMULATION IMPLICATIONS

The combinational effect of poor solubility, extensive metabolism, instability at physiological pH, and rapid clearance results in decreased therapeutic efficacy. These limitations necessitate an enhanced dose or a more frequent dosing, which may enhance the risk of side effects, thereby decreasing patient adherence to the dosage regimen. Adherence to the dosage regimen is an important consideration in chronic diseases like atherosclerosis, hypertension, and heart failure. Additionally, inter-subject variability in the bioavailability of these compounds can be evident due to genetic polymorphisms in metabolizing enzymes and differences in gut microbiota composition, making dose standardization difficult [42]. Inconsistent pharmacokinetics also pose challenges in clinical trial design, endpoint validation, and regulatory approval processes.

For instance, whereas curcumin and resveratrol have shown major benefits in preclinical models, randomized controlled trials have not been able to reliably recreate these results, mostly because plasma concentrations in humans are not high enough [43]. In the same way, berberine has been found to work well for managing lipids, but its limited bioavailability means that it needs to be used with other drugs or improved delivery systems to reach therapeutic levels [44]. Table 9.1 shows the physicochemical and pharmacokinetic problems with important cardioprotective phytochemicals. It also shows how important it is to have sophisticated delivery mechanisms to overcome these problems. To tackle these challenges, innovative formulation strategies such nanocarriers, solid dispersions, and inclusion complexes are currently under development and will be examined in the subsequent section.

## 9.4 NANOTECHNOLOGY-BASED DELIVERY STRATEGIES

Herbal compounds such as flavonoids, polyphenols, and alkaloids, while pharmacologically potent, are limited by low solubility, instability, and rapid metabolism, as described in the previous sections in sufficient detail. Nanocarrier systems for drug delivery like SLNs, liposomes, polymeric micelles, phytosomes, and nanoemulsions offer superior advantages to overcome the challenges of phytochemicals for formulation development. They have shown superior performance in improving pharmacokinetic properties and therapeutic outcomes for compounds like curcumin, resveratrol, EGCG, berberine, and quercetin. Nanocarriers are colloidal systems with particle sizes ranging from 1 to 1000 nm, offering properties such as high surface-area-to-volume ratio, customizable surface charge, potential for active or passive targeting, and protection from enzymatic degradation. These carriers have been particularly effective in delivering phytochemicals to cardiovascular tissues by enhancing absorption, prolonging circulation time, and facilitating targeted release [45].

### 9.4.1 LIPOSOMES: COMPOSITION, MECHANISM, ADVANTAGES, AND ADVANCES

Liposomes are nanovesicles comprising one or more concentric phospholipid bilayers surrounding an aqueous core. Their amphiphilic structure allows for the encapsulation of both hydrophilic (in the core) and hydrophobic (within the lipid bilayer) phytochemicals. Liposomes are typically formulated using natural or synthetic phospholipids (e.g., phosphatidylcholine, phosphatidylethanolamine) and cholesterol to improve membrane stability [46].

#### 9.4.1.1 Applications in Drug Delivery

i. *Protection from enzymatic and acidic degradation:*
The active phytomolecules will be sequestered within the aqueous environment or in the bilayer of liposomes, thereby acting as a protective carrier, minimizing contact with gastric acid and metabolizing enzymes. For instance, encapsulation of EGCG in liposomes has demonstrated improved stability against oxidation and pH-induced degradation in simulated GI fluids [46–48].

ii. *Enhanced cellular uptake* via *endocytosis:*
Fusion, adsorption, or receptor-mediated endocytosis are the major mechanisms by which liposomes interact with the target cell membrane. Once engulfed, the liposome is trafficked through the endolysosomal pathway, where pH-sensitive formulations can trigger release of the encapsulated phytochemical in response to acidic conditions. This pathway enhances the intracellular bioavailability of compounds with otherwise poor membrane permeability. Liposomal quercetin, for example, shows significantly higher uptake by endothelial and cardiomyocyte cells than free quercetin [49].

iii. *Controlled and targeted release:*
By modifying the lipid composition, charge, and fluidity, liposomes can be engineered to provide sustained or stimulus-responsive release. Temperature-sensitive liposomes, for example, destabilize at hyperthermic conditions (~42°C), releasing the payload at inflamed cardiovascular tissues. Additionally, PEGylated or polymer-coated liposomes exhibit reduced clearance and prolonged systemic circulation, allowing the phytochemical to accumulate preferentially at pathological sites via the enhanced permeability and retention (EPR) effect [50].

#### 9.4.1.2 Phytochemicals Delivered via Liposomes

Beyond curcumin, resveratrol, and berberine, a wide array of phytochemicals has been successfully encapsulated in liposomal carriers for cardiovascular and metabolic disorders. Some of them are presented in Table 9.2.

These examples illustrate the adaptability of liposomal systems to encapsulate structurally diverse phytochemicals while enhancing their pharmacological performance.

#### 9.4.1.3 Technological Innovations in Liposomal Delivery

i. *Stealth liposomes (PEGylated liposomes):* These liposomes are surface-modified with polyethylene glycol (PEG), forming a hydrophilic shield that reduces recognition by the mononuclear phagocyte system (MPS). This prolongs the circulation half-life and

**Table 9.2** Key phytochemicals formulated into liposomes and their reported benefits in cardiovascular-related studies.

| Phytochemical | Therapeutic action | Liposomal benefits | Reference |
|---|---|---|---|
| Naringenin | Antioxidant, anti-atherogenic | ↑ Oral absorption, ↓ LDL oxidation | [51] |
| Luteolin | Anti-inflammatory, vasoprotective | ↑ Mitochondrial targeting, ↓ vascular damage | [52] |
| Apigenin | NO modulation, antihypertensive | ↑ Bioavailability, ↓ inflammatory cytokines | [53] |
| Kaempferol | Vasodilatory, antioxidant | ↑ Tissue retention, ↑ cardioprotection in I/R injury | [54] |
| Boswellic acids | Anti-inflammatory | ↓ Vascular inflammation, ↓ endothelial dysfunction | [55] |

facilitates passive accumulation in disease tissues via the EPR effect. For instance, PEGylated liposomal baicalin exhibits threefold higher plasma retention and superior neurological motor function in tumor-induced rat models [56].

ii. *Magnetic liposomes:* Super paramagnetic iron oxide nanoparticles (SPIONs) are incorporated into the lipid bilayer or core of liposomes to enable magnetic field-guided targeting. This enables us to control the drug release *in vivo* and promotes site-specific accumulation. Quercetin-loaded magnetic liposomes in a recent study were successfully directed to inflamed aortic plaques in mice, demonstrating reduced atherogenesis and localized anti-inflammatory action [57].

iii. *Multifunctional liposomes:* These engineered liposomes were designed to perform multiple tasks concurrently, such as co-delivery, stimuli responsiveness, and diagnostic purpose (imaging). For instance, a curcumin- and atorvastatin dual-loaded liposome exhibited synergistic anti-inflammatory and lipid-lowering effects in a rabbit model of hyperlipidemia [58]. These systems can also incorporate imaging agents (e.g., gadolinium for MRI), enabling real-time therapeutic monitoring.

iv. *Ligand-functionalized liposomes for site-specific targeting:* Conjugation of liposomes with ligands such as peptides (e.g., arginylglycylaspartic acid (RGD) for integrins on angiogenic vessels), antibodies (e.g., anti-VCAM-1 for atherosclerotic plaques), folic acid, hyaluronic acid, or aptamers can deliver the liposomes to the targeted sites like endothelial cells or cardiomyocytes. For example, folate-functionalized liposomal betulinic acid showed superior uptake by human hepatoblastoma cell line G2 (HepG2) cells compared with non-targeted liposomes [59].

These advances establish liposomes not only as passive delivery vehicles but also as intelligent, tunable systems that can adapt to complex cardiovascular pathophysiology. The specific applications of these advanced liposomes are illustrated in Figure 9.2.

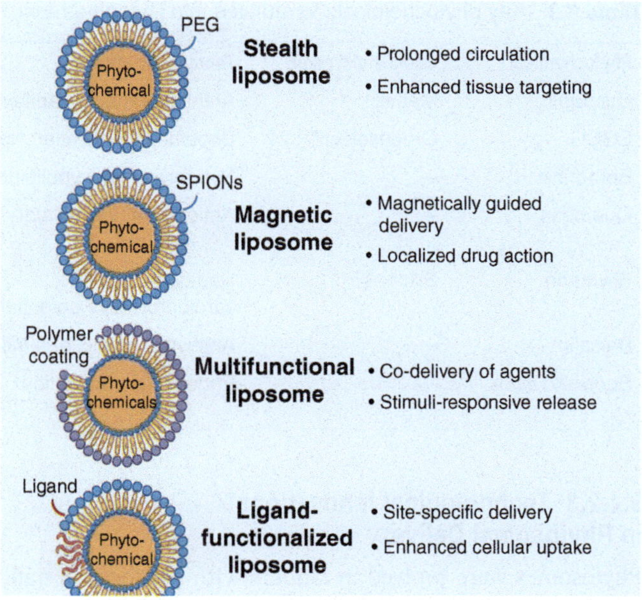


**FIGURE 9.2** Technologically modified liposomes for specific applications.

## 9.4.2 PHYTOSOMES: STRUCTURE, MECHANISM, ADVANTAGES, AND INNOVATIONS

Many herbal bioactive compounds are associated with poor solubility and low bioavailability limitations. To overcome these limitations, advanced phospholipid-based complexes, called phytosomes, were designed. In phytosomes, herbal bioactives were complexed with phospholipids, typically phosphatidylcholine, unlike liposomes, where bio-actives are entrapped in bilayer. This complexation makes phytosomes more lipid-compatible molecular entity that enhances absorption across biological membranes, improves systemic availability, and protects the active compounds from premature degradation – thus offering improved therapeutic benefits in CVDs [60].

### 9.4.2.1 Applications in Drug Delivery

i. *Enhanced lipophilicity and membrane permeability:* Hydrophilic phytochemicals, upon binding with phospholipids, will acquire a lipophilic nature that improves their passive diffusion across enterocyte membranes. For instance, quercetin–phospholipid complexes exhibit superior membrane affinity and increased systemic absorption [61].

ii. *Protection from enzymatic and pH-induced degradation:* As the compounds are complexed with phosphatidylcholine, phytosomes reduce exposure of phytochemicals to digestive enzymes (e.g., glucuronosyl transferases, sulfatases) and gastric acidity. Studies on sylibin-loaded phytosomes confirm their improved resistance to simulated GI environments [62].

iii. *Bypass of first-pass metabolism:* By nature, phytosomes are more lipophilic, which enables them for lymphatic absorption, thereby minimizing first-pass metabolism. This route has been exploited in berberine and EGCG-phytosome formulations to achieve greater plasma bioavailability [63].

iv. *Tissue-specific accumulation:* Phytosomes enhance biodistribution and tissue retention in cardiovascular targets such as myocardial, endothelial, and hepatic tissues. Baicalin and quercetin phytosomes have been shown to exhibit preferential accumulation in aortic tissue and cardiomyocytes, respectively.

### 9.4.2.2 Phytochemicals Delivered via Phytosomes

Numerous phytochemicals with cardiovascular benefits have been effectively delivered using phytosome technology. Table 9.3 summarizes the list of phytochemicals developed as phytosomes.

**Table 9.3** Key phytochemicals formulated into liposomes and their reported benefits in cardiovascular-related studies.

| Phytochemical | Commercial name | Therapeutic effects | Phytosomal advantages | Reference |
|---|---|---|---|---|
| Curcumin | Meriva® | Anti-inflammatory, antioxidant | ↑ Bioavailability, ↓ CRP and TNF-α | [64] |
| EGCG | Greenselect® | Endothelial protection, lipid-lowering | ↑ Antioxidant capacity, ↓ SBP and LDL | [65] |
| Berberine | — | Hypoglycemic, hypolipidemic | ↓ Triglycerides, ↑ oral tolerance | [66] |
| Quercetin | — | Antioxidant, vasodilatory | ↑ Plasma levels, ↑ NO production, ↓ oxidative markers | [67] |
| Silymarin | Siliphos® | Hepatoprotective, cardioprotective potential | ↓ Serum cholesterol, ↓ lipid peroxidation | [68] |
| Baicalin | — | Antihypertrophic, anti-inflammatory | ↑ Oral absorption, ↓ MAPK/NF-κB activation | [69] |
| Boswellic acids | — | Endothelial modulation | ↓ VCAM-1/ICAM-1, ↓ ROS, improved vascular relaxation | [70] |

#### 9.4.2.3 Technological Innovations in Phytosomal Delivery

Phytosomes were evolved in tandem with advances in nanotechnology and drug delivery systems, from simple lipid complexes to highly engineered, multifunctional systems tailored for precision therapeutics. Phytosomal technological innovations mainly focused on stability enhancement, targeted delivery, and pharmacokinetic control to address the limitations of conventional phytochemical formulations in cardiovascular applications.

i. *Solid-state phytosomes:* Traditional liposomes were in a liquid state, often suffer from instability, stability challenges during storage and formulation versatility. These necessities convert them into a solid state phytosomes by incorporating techniques like spray drying, freeze-drying, or lyophilization. This conversion may enhance their physicochemical stability, shelf life, and compatibility with solid dosage forms such as tablets, capsules, or powders.

ii. *PEGylated phytosomes:* PEG surface modification of phytosomes results in "stealth" phytosomes that evade opsonization by MPS, prolonging systemic circulation time. Steric stability enhancement and reduced aggregation were observed with PEGylated phytosomes. This is particularly beneficial in targeting vascular inflammation and ischemic cardiac tissue, where prolonged retention improves therapeutic efficacy. In a comparative study, PEGylated quercetin phytosomes exhibited significantly higher endothelial uptake and nitric oxide (NO) release compared to non-PEGylated variants [71].

iii. *Co-phytosomes (dual-drug complexes):* Co-phytosomes incorporate two or more phytochemicals or a phytochemical–pharmaceutical drug combination within the same lipid matrix, enabling synergistic therapeutic effects. These systems optimize pharmacodynamics while reducing pill burden and improving patient compliance.

iv. *Ligand-conjugated phytosomes:* Functionalizing the surface of phytosomes with targeting ligands (e.g., folic acid, galactose, peptides, or antibodies) facilitates receptor-mediated endocytosis by diseased tissues. This active targeting enables site-specific accumulation of the phytosome at inflamed endothelium, atherosclerotic plaques, or cardiac myocytes.

v. *Hydrogel-embedded phytosomes:* Integration of phytosomes into biocompatible hydrogels allows sustained, localized release and improved bioadhesion, especially in topical or transdermal cardiovascular applications (e.g., postsurgical cardiac dressings, ischemic limb therapy).

vi. *Effervescent and buccal phytosomes:* Innovative oral formats such as effervescent granules and buccal films are being developed to avoid GI degradation and enhance mucosal absorption. Buccal phytosomes bypass hepatic first-pass metabolism, offering rapid systemic onset.

vii. *Smart phytosomes – stimuli-responsive systems:* Smart phytosomes are engineered to release their payload in response to environmental stimuli such as pH, temperature, or redox gradients commonly found in inflamed or ischemic cardiovascular tissues. These smart systems improve drug localization and reduce off-target effects.

viii. *Phytosome–nanoparticle hybrids:* Combining phytosomes with inorganic or polymeric nanoparticles (e.g., gold, silica, or PLGA) can improve structural rigidity, loading capacity, and imaging capabilities. These hybrid phytosomes offer dual functionality for therapy and diagnostics (theranostics).

These technological advances have significantly broadened the potential of phytosomes, from simple delivery vehicles to multifunctional, responsive, and targeted nanosystems. They offer powerful solutions to current challenges in herbal cardiovascular therapy, especially in terms of site-specific action, reduced systemic toxicity, and enhanced clinical translation.

### 9.4.3 OTHER NANODELIVERY SYSTEMS: NANOEMULSIONS, POLYMERIC MICELLES, AND NANOPARTICLES

Although liposomes and phytosomes are the most clinically translated systems for herbal drug delivery, several other nanocarrier platforms have shown considerable potential in improving the solubility, stability, and therapeutic performance of phytochemicals for CVDs. These include nanoemulsions,

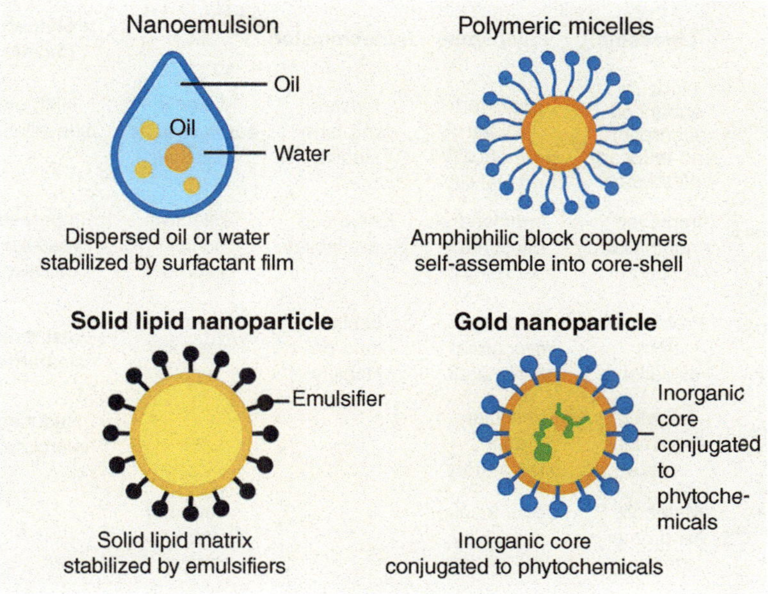


**FIGURE 9.3** Illustration of nanocarrier systems other than liposomes and phytosomes.

polymeric micelles, SLNs, nanostructured lipid carriers (NLCs), and inorganic/organic nanoparticles, which are illustrated in Figure 9.3.

#### 9.4.3.1 Nanoemulsions

Nanoemulsions are kinetically stable, thermodynamically unstable colloidal dispersions consisting of two immiscible liquids (typically oil and water) stabilized by surfactants, with droplet sizes ranging between 20 and 200 nm. They are advantageous in delivering lipophilic phytochemicals like terpenoids, flavonoids, and alkaloids due to their high interfacial surface area and low viscosity.

#### 9.4.3.2 Polymeric Micelles

Polymeric micelles are nanosized (10–100 nm) self-assembled structures formed from amphiphilic block copolymers, where the hydrophobic core solubilizes poorly water-soluble drugs and the hydrophilic shell enhances aqueous dispersibility and circulation time. Phytochemical-loaded micelles offer enhanced protection against degradation and controlled release. Curcumin-loaded polymeric micelles using Pluronics and Gelucires significantly improve oral bioavailability [72].

#### 9.4.3.3 Solid Lipid Nanoparticles and Nanostructured Lipid Carriers

SLNs consist of a solid lipid matrix stabilized by emulsifiers, offering high physical stability, controlled release, and protection against oxidative degradation. NLCs are an advanced form incorporating a blend of solid and liquid lipids, which increases drug-loading capacity and prevents expulsion during storage. SLNs encapsulating baicalin demonstrated enhanced oral bioavailability [73]. Rani et al. [74] demonstrated enhanced therapeutic efficacy of hesperidin via NLCs.

#### 9.4.3.4 Inorganic and Organic Nanoparticles

Inorganic nanoparticles from metals like gold (Au), silver (Ag), and silica have been developed and studied for their protective action against oxidation and inflammation and also for their targetability. On the other hand, organic NPs, especially those from biodegradable polymers like PLGA provide, controlled and targeted delivery in addition to their high stability. However, these NPs suffer some challenges like scalability owing to their complex manufacturing process, cytotoxicity of the carriers, and ambiguous regulatory approval process. Each type of system has its own advantage in improving the therapeutic efficiency of the herbal compounds. Their relative advantages for the loaded phytochemicals from different nanocarrier systems are presented in Figure 9.4.

## 9.5 LIMITATIONS OF NANO-BASED DELIVERY SYSTEMS

Nanocarrier systems provide solutions to the challenges of conventional delivery systems of phytochemicals for CVDs like low solubility, poor permeability, less stability, and lack of targetability. However, these systems also suffer several challenges at another level, like scalability and regulatory issues, such that their progression into mainstream drug delivery systems is still hampered.

### 9.5.1 TECHNICAL AND PRACTICAL LIMITATIONS

Here are some limitations regarding the design and development of formulation and quality control testing procedures:

- *Poor entrapment efficiency:* Herbal compounds with extreme hydrophilicity and lipophilicity often hinder their loading into nanocarriers.

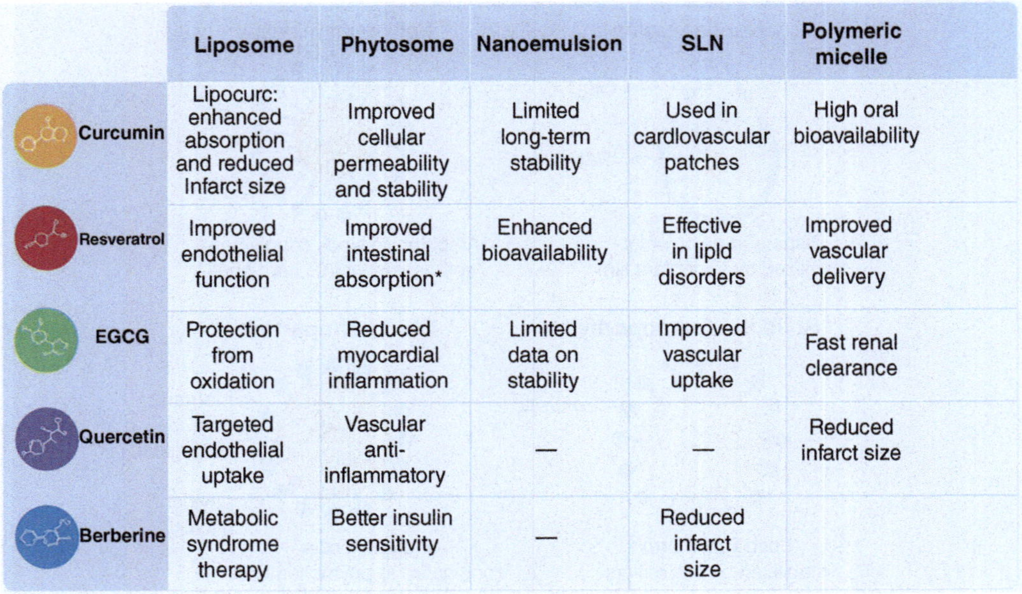

| | Liposome | Phytosome | Nanoemulsion | SLN | Polymeric micelle |
|---|---|---|---|---|---|
| Curcumin | Lipocurc: enhanced absorption and reduced Infarct size | Improved cellular permeability and stability | Limited long-term stability | Used in cardlovascular patches | High oral bioavailability |
| Resveratrol | Improved endothelial function | Improved intestinal absorption* | Enhanced bioavailability | Effective in lipld disorders | Improved vascular delivery |
| EGCG | Protection from oxidation | Reduced myocardial inflammation | Limited data on stability | Improved vascular uptake | Fast renal clearance |
| Quercetin | Targeted endothelial uptake | Vascular anti-inflammatory | — | — | Reduced infarct size |
| Berberine | Metabolic syndrome therapy | Better insulin sensitivity | — | Reduced infarct size | |

**FIGURE 9.4** Comparison of various nanocarrier systems for their advantages toward loaded herbal compounds used in the treatment of CVDs.

- *Inter-batch variability:* Manufacturing processes of these systems still suffer lack of robustness. Small variations in processing conditions, like source of raw lipidic materials, temperature, and homogenization pressure, exhibit a significant change in critical quality attributes (CQAs), like size, drug loading, zeta potential, and release kinetics. This will cause serious issues in pilot plant scale-up studies from lab to large-scale production for marketing [75].
- *Instability:* Systems like liposomes, phytosomes and nanoemulsions are sensitive to physical and chemical stability issues, like aggregation, leakage, oxidation, and hydrolysis. These issues shorten their shelf life and make them unsuitable for commercialization.
- *Short circulatory half-life:* Due to their lipophilic surface, these systems tend to be opsonized, followed by phagocytosis. This make them clear from the blood circulation, which is a concern for CVDs that require sustained plasma drug levels for long time.

### 9.5.2 STABILITY AND SCALABILITY CONCERNS

The evolution of nanocarrier-based phytochemicals from lab scale to commercialization level requires intense resources due to:

- *Exorbitant manufacturing technologies:* Production cost at a large scale level are very high with techniques like thin film hydration and high-pressure homogenization, as they require strict control over the processing conditions; otherwise, they may lead to batch-to-batch variability in CQAs [76].
- *Intricate storage conditions:* These products necessitate packing under inert atmospheres and low temperatures, and protection from light during their storage.

## 9.6 REGULATORY CHALLENGES

Even though these nanocarrier systems improve therapeutic efficiency of the phytochemicals, their regulatory approval process is still complicated. The lack of harmonization between pharmaceutical and nutraceutical products, together with heterogeneity in global guidelines, hinders the development and market authorization of these products [46].

### 9.6.1 CURRENT REGULATORY FRAMEWORK FOR PHYTOCHEMICALS

Based on the intended use, phytochemicals are covered under different regulatory guidelines in different countries. In India, these products come under AYUSH system, but it lacks confined guidelines. In United States, herbal compounds for nutritional compounds come under Dietary Supplement Health and Education Act (DSHEA), whereas those intended for therapeutic use come under New Drug Application (NDA) for their approval. In Europe, the Committee on Herbal Medicinal Products (HMPC) under the European Medicines Agency (EMA) provides guidelines for the phytochemicals. In case of the Meriva, it is marketed as a pharmaceutical product in some regions and as nutraceutical product in other regions [77].

### 9.6.2 CHALLENGES SPECIFIC TO NANO-BASED FORMULATIONS

Nanocarrier systems produce a new level of difficulty to regulatory evaluation:

- *Particle size-dependent performance:* Most of the performance indicators of these systems, like solubility, bioavailability, and biodistribution, depend on size. Regulatory agencies mandate full characterization of size-related properties, which is not necessary for the conventional products [78].

- *Reproducibility:* Particle size and uniform drug loading are critical for predicting pharmacokinetic and therapeutic outcomes. These systems pose challenges in maintaining consistency and reproducibility across batches during large-scale manufacturing. This causes difficulty in clearing regulator obligations [79].
- *Stability issues:* Nanocarriers made up of lipids and oils are highly prone for oxidation, leakage, and aggregation. Hence, detailed study data on physical and chemical stability is necessary for regulatory submissions [77].
- *Toxicological profiling:* Systemic toxicity, immunogenicity, and accumulation are concerns owing to the nano size and high surface area of these systems. Hence, regulatory bodies expect detailed toxicological profiling, which is actually unavailable for herbal compounds [80].

### 9.6.3 STRATEGIES TO OVERCOME REGULATORY BARRIERS

Several strategies have to be adopted by the nano-based herbal products developers to direct the developing regulatory ground:

- *Prior regulatory assignment:* Taking advice from the regulatory agencies prior to Investigational New Drug Application (IND) or NDA submissions on required data to be submitted will reduce delay in approvals [79].
- *Quality-by-design (QbD):* Regulatory compliance will be improved by adopting QbD principles in formulation design and development.
- *Strong preclinical study data:* Detailed pharmacokinetic and toxicological studies shall be carried out even the intended use is nutraceutical, so as to enhance regulatory acceptance.
- *Standardization and harmonization efforts:* Collective efforts among industry, academia, and regulatory agencies to develop guidelines for nano-based phytochemical products are important. ICH Q12 provides some fundamental initiatives for harmonization.

In conclusion, while nano-based herbal delivery systems hold immense therapeutic potential, their regulatory future depends on a proactive, evidence-based, and harmonized approach that balances innovation with public health safety.

## 9.7 FUTURE PERSPECTIVES AND RESEARCH DIRECTIONS

Even though significant improvements are reported in liposomal and phytosomal systems, still critical technological, translational, and regulatory gaps are unanswered. In this section, emerging trends and formulation strategies toward future clinical translation are discussed.

### 9.7.1 EMERGING INNOVATIONS IN NANO-FORMULATION TECHNOLOGY

New improvements in pharmaceutical materials and technology encouraged the creation of responsive and intelligent carriers, including:

- *Stimuli-responsive nanocarriers:* These systems respond to endogenous cues (e.g., pH, enzymes, redox state) or external stimuli (e.g., light, ultrasound, magnetic field) to trigger site-specific drug release. In a recent study, Zang et al. [81] developed phytosomes for baicalein delivery in infected tissues that are more acidic, so as to improve therapeutic efficacy.
- *Biomimetic nanocarriers:* Leveraging natural membranes or vesicles, such as exosomes, cell membrane-coated liposomes, and hybrid lipid–polymer systems avoid immune response to these systems. For example, Song et al., [82] developed liposomes coated with platelet membrane for targeted delivery to atherosclerotic lesions and found 5.91-fold improvement in accumulation in the target tissue.
- *Co-loaded Systems:* Phytochemicals can be combinedly loaded with other synthetic or herbal drugs to achieve additive or synergistic effects. Incorporation into liposomes or phytosomes can provide a multi-targeted approach. Sesarman et al., [83] developed such liposomes loaded with curcumin and doxorubicin, which were found to be produced additive effects.
- *Artificial intelligence (AI)-aided formulation:* Optimization of the nanocarrier formulation by predicting critical quality attributes, like drug-loading efficiency, drug release rate, and stability via AI and machine learning is increasing [84].

### 9.7.2 CLINICAL TRIALS AND FUTURE DEVELOPMENTS

Despite widespread success in preclinical studies on these systems, their progress into clinical practice is still limited. There are few products with development into controlled and randomized large-scale clinical trials: curcumin phytosome (Meriva) and silybin phytosome (Siliphos) exhibited enhanced bioavailability in phase I and II trials; berberine-loaded liposomes exhibited improved glycemic and lipid profiles in a small clinical trial performed in type 2 diabetes patients. Further clinical trials shall be necessary for establishing clear pharmacokinetics and long-term outcomes in cardiovascular endpoints.

## 9.8 CONCLUSION

Several highly effective herbal compounds, like curcumin and others as described above, face constraints in clinical use due to their poor physicochemical stability. The amalgamation of phytochemical delivery through phytosomes and liposomes has grown rapidly to address potential challenges of the phytochemicals, especially those used for

CVDs. Phytosomes, an upgraded system of liposomes for loading phytochemicals, can enhance drug loading, solubility, permeability, bioavailability, and stability. Besides, technological modifications such as PEGylation, impulse delivery, and multifunction loading have further improved therapeutic efficiency, pharmacokinetics, and pharmacodynamics of these herbal compounds.

Ultimately, liposomes and phytosomes are first-choice systems for phytochemical delivery. Nevertheless, these systems also face some limitations. Large-scale manufacturing, batch-to-batch variation, long-term stability, and complicated regulatory approval path limit their therapeutic benefits. A multifaceted approach with an amalgamation of pharmaceutics, pharmacology, quality control, and regulatory affairs is necessary to overcome these limitations. Collaboration among academic institutes, industries, and regulatory agencies is highly needed for their clinical application and to make them successful in commercial front. Proper development and application of these systems can redefine therapeutic approaches in the treatment and management of CVDs.

## REFERENCES


1. World Health Organization (2025). Cardiovascular diseases (CVDs). https://www.who.int/news-room/fact-sheets/detail/cardiovascular-diseases-(cvds) (accessed 06 May 2026)
2. Iqbal I, Wilairatana P, Saqib F, Nasir B, Wahid M, Latif MF, Iqbal A, Naz R, Mubarak MS. Plant polyphenols and their potential benefits on cardiovascular health: a review. *Molecules* 2023; 28 (17): 6403. https://doi.org/10.3390/molecules28176403.
3. Panche AN, Diwan AD, Chandra SR. Flavonoids: an overview. *J. Nutr. Sci.* 2016; 5: e47. https://doi.org/10.1017/jns.2016.41.Erratum.
4. Kumar S, Pandey AK. Chemistry and biological activities of flavonoids: an overview. *Sci. World J.* 2013; 2013: 162750. https://doi.org/10.1155/2013/162750.
5. Santangelo, C., Varì, R., Scazzocchio, B. et al. (2007). Polyphenols, intracellular signalling and inflammation. *Ann. Ist. Super. Sanita* 43 (4): 394–405. PMID: 18209273.
6. Manach C, Williamson G, Morand C, Scalbert A, Rémésy C. Bioavailability and bioefficacy of polyphenols in humans. I. Review of 97 bioavailability studies. *Am. J. Clin. Nutr.* 2005; 81 (1 Suppl): 230S–242S. https://doi.org/10.1093/ajcn/81.1.230S.
7. Bozzuto G, Molinari A. Liposomes as nanomedical devices. *Int. J. Nanomedicine* 2015; 10: 975–999. https://doi.org/10.2147/IJN.S68861.
8. Kathole KS, Hatwar PR, Bakal RL, Karule VG, Nano technology-based drug delivery systems and herbal medicine. *J. Drug Deliv. Ther.* 2025; 15(3): 133–141 https://doi.org/10.22270/jddt.v15i3.7017
9. Ahmad R, Srivastava S, Ghosh S, Khare SK. Phytochemical delivery through nanocarriers: a review. *Colloids Surf. B Biointerfaces* 2021; 197: 111389. https://doi.org/10.1016/j.colsurfb.2020.111389.
10. Kunnumakkara AB, Bordoloi D, Harsha C, Banik K, Gupta SC, Aggarwal BB. Curcumin mediates anticancer effects by modulating multiple cell signaling pathways. *Clin. Sci. (Lond.)* 2017; 131 (15): 1781–1799. https://doi.org/10.1042/CS20160935.
11. Tiwari G, Tiwari R, Sriwastawa B, Bhati L, Pandey S, Pandey P, Bannerjee SK. Drug delivery systems: an updated review. *Int. J. Pharm. Investig.* 2012; 2(1): 2–11. https://doi.org/10.4103/2230-973X.96920.
12. Hewlings SJ, Kalman DS. Curcumin: a review of its effects on human health. *Foods* 2017; 6(10): 92. https://doi.org/10.3390/foods6100092.
13. Gupta SC, Patchva S, Aggarwal BB. Therapeutic roles of curcumin: lessons learned from clinical trials. *AAPS J.* 2013; 15(1): 195–218. https://doi.org/10.1208/s12248-012-9432-8.
14. Yadav R, Mishra S, Chaturvedi R, Pandey A. Therapeutic potential of curcumin in cardiovascular disease: targeting atherosclerosis pathophysiology. *Biomed. Pharmacother.* 2025; 190: 118412. https://doi.org/10.1016/j.biopha.2025.118412.
15. Prasad S, Gupta SC, Tyagi AK, Aggarwal BB. Curcumin, a component of golden spice: from bedside to bench and back. *Biotechnol. Adv.* 2014; 32(6): 1053–1064. https://doi.org/10.1016/j.biotechadv.2014.04.004.
16. Bisht S, Mizuma M, Feldmann G, Ottenhof NA, Hong SM, Pramanik D, Chenna V, Karikari C, Sharma R, Goggins MG, Rudek MA, Ravi R, Maitra A, Maitra A. Systemic administration of polymeric nanoparticle-encapsulated curcumin (Nano Curc) blocks tumor growth and metastases in preclinical models of pancreatic cancer. *Mol. Cancer Ther.* 2010; 9(8): 2255–2264. https://doi.org/10.1158/1535-7163.MCT-10-0172.
17. Maiti K, Mukherjee K, Gantait A, Saha BP, Mukherjee PK. Curcumin-phospholipid complex: preparation, therapeutic evaluation and pharmacokinetic study in rats. *Int. J. Pharm.* 2007; 330 (1–2): 155–163. https://doi.org/10.1016/j.ijpharm.2006.09.025.
18. Baur JA, Sinclair DA. Therapeutic potential of resveratrol: the *in vivo* evidence. *Nat. Rev. Drug Discov.* 2006; 5(6): 493–506. https://doi.org/10.1038/nrd2060.
19. Li YR, Li S, Lin CC. Effect of resveratrol and pterostilbene on aging and longevity. *Biofactors* 2018; 44(1): 69–82. https://doi.org/10.1002/biof.1400.
20. Gal R, Deres L, Toth K, Halmosi R, Habon T. The effect of resveratrol on the cardiovascular system from molecular mechanisms to clinical results. *Int. J. Mol. Sci.* 2021; 22 (18): 10152. https://doi.org/10.3390/ijms221810152.
21. Walle T. Bioavailability of resveratrol. *Ann. N. Y. Acad. Sci.* 2011; 1215: 9–15. https://doi.org/10.1111/j.1749-6632.2010.05842.x.
22. Neves AR, Lucio M, Lima JL, Reis S. Resveratrol in medicinal chemistry: a critical review of its pharmacokinetics, drug-delivery, and membrane interactions. *Curr. Med. Chem.* 2012; 19 (11): 1663–1681. https://doi.org/10.2174/092986712799945085.
23. Neves AR, Lúcio M, Martins S, Lima JL, Reis S. Novel resveratrol nanodelivery systems based on lipid nanoparticles to enhance its oral bioavailability. *Int. J. Nanomedicine* 2013; 8: 177–187. https://doi.org/10.2147/IJN.S37840.
24. Suzuki T, Pervin M, Goto S, Isemura M, Nakamura Y. Beneficial effects of tea and the green tea catechin Epigallocatechin-3-gallate on obesity. *Molecules* 2016; 21 (10): 1305. https://doi.org/10.3390/molecules21101305.
25. Alvarez E, Campos-Toimil M, Justiniano-Basaran H, Lugnier C, Orallo F. Study of the mechanisms involved in the vasorelaxation induced by (−)-epigallocatechin-3-gallate in rat aorta. *Br. J. Pharmacol.* 2006; 147(3): 269–280. https://doi.org/10.1038/sj.bjp.0706507.
26. Kuriyama S, Shimazu T, Ohmori K, Kikuchi N, Nakaya N, Nishino Y, Tsubono Y, Tsuji I. Green tea consumption and mortality due to cardiovascular disease, cancer, and all causes in Japan: the Ohsaki study. *JAMA* 2006; 296 (10): 1255–1265. https://doi.org/10.1001/jama.296.10.1255.
27. Lambert JD, Sang S, Yang CS. Biotransformation of green tea polyphenols and the biological activities of those metabolites. *Mol. Pharm.* 2007; 4(6): 819–825. https://doi.org/10.1021/mp700075m.

28. Granja A, Frias I, Neves AR, Pinheiro M, Reis S. Therapeutic potential of epigallocatechin gallate nanodelivery systems. *Biomed. Res. Int.* 2017; 2017: 5813793. https://doi.org/10.1155/2017/5813793.
29. Anand P, Kunnumakkara AB, Newman RA, Aggarwal BB. Bioavailability of curcumin: problems and promises. *Mol. Pharm.* 2007; 4(6): 807–818. https://doi.org/10.1021/mp700113r.
30. Liu YT, Hao HP, Xie HG, Lai L, Wang Q, Liu CX, Wang GJ. Extensive intestinal first-pass elimination and predominant hepatic distribution of berberine explain its low plasma levels in rats. *Drug Metab. Dispos.* 2010; 38 (10): 1779–1784. https://doi.org/10.1124/dmd.110.033936.
31. Guo Y, Bruno RS. Endogenous and exogenous mediators of quercetin bioavailability. *J. Nutr. Biochem.* 2015; 26(3): 201–210. https://doi.org/10.1016/j.jnutbio.2014.10.008.
32. Li-Weber, M. (2009). New therapeutic aspects of flavones: the anticancer properties of Scutellaria and its main active constituents wogonin, baicalein and baicalin. *Cancer Treat. Rev.* 35 (1): 57–68.
33. Goldberg DM, Yan J, Soleas GJ. Absorption of three wine-related polyphenols in three different matrices by healthy subjects. *Clin. Biochem.* 2003; 36(1): 79–87. https://doi.org/10.1016/s0009-9120(02)00397-1.
34. Ai X, Yu P, Peng L, Luo L, Liu J, Li S, Lai X, Luan F, Meng X. Berberine: a review of its pharmacokinetics properties and therapeutic potentials in diverse vascular diseases. *Front. Pharmacol.* 2021; 12: 762654. https://doi.org/10.3389/fphar.2021.762654.
35. Graefe EU, Wittig J, Mueller S, Riethling AK, Uehleke B, Drewelow B, Pforte H, Jacobasch G, Derendorf H, Veit M. Pharmacokinetics and bioavailability of quercetin glycosides in humans. *J. Clin. Pharmacol.* 2001; 41(5): 492–499. https://doi.org/10.1177/00912700122010366.
36. Li P, Tian Y, Wang H, Ji Y, Zeng H, Zhang S, Gao X, Chen X. Effect of hepatic impairment on the pharmacokinetics of baicalin in rats: critical roles of gut microbiota and hepatic transporters. *Pharmaceutics* 2025; 17(7): 851. https://doi.org/10.3390/pharmaceutics17070851.
37. Tonnesen HH, Karlsen J. Studies on curcumin and curcuminoids. VI. Kinetics of curcumin degradation in aqueous solution. *Z. Lebensm. Unters. Forsch.* 1985; 180(5): 402–444. https://doi.org/10.1007/BF01027775.
38. Sang S, Lee MJ, Hou Z, Ho CT, Yang CS. Stability of tea polyphenol (−)-epigallocatechin-3-gallate and formation of dimers and epimers under common experimental conditions. *J. Agric. Food Chem.* 2005; 53 (24): 9478–9484. https://doi.org/10.1021/jf0519055.
39. Tan XS, Ma JY, Feng R, Ma C, Chen WJ, Sun YP, Fu J, Huang M, He CY, Shou JW, He WY, Wang Y, Jiang JD. Tissue distribution of berberine and its metabolites after oral administration in rats. *PLoS One* 2013; 8(10): e77969. https://doi.org/10.1371/journal.pone.0077969.
40. Boots AW, Haenen GR, Bast A. Health effects of quercetin: from antioxidant to nutraceutical. *Eur. J. Pharmacol.* 2008; 585 (2–3): 325–337. https://doi.org/10.1016/j.ejphar.2008.03.008.
41. Hu Z, Guan Y, Hu W, Xu Z, Ishfaq M. An overview of pharmacological activities of baicalin and its aglycone baicalein: new insights into molecular mechanisms and signaling pathways. *Iran. J. Basic Med. Sci.* 2022; 25(1): 14–26. https://doi.org/10.22038/IJBMS.2022.60380.13381.
42. Serra A, Macia A, Romero MP, Angles N, Morello J, Motilva MJ. Metabolic pathways of the colonic metabolism of procyanidins (monomers and dimers) and alkaloids. *Food Chem.* 2011; 126: 1127–1137. https://doi.org/10.1016/j.foodchem.2010.11.145.
43. Nelson KM, Dahlin JL, Bisson J, Graham J, Pauli GF, Walters MA. The essential medicinal chemistry of curcumin. *J. Med. Chem.* 2017; 60(5): 1620–1637. https://doi.org/10.1021/acs.jmedchem.6b00975.
44. Yin J, Xing H, Ye J. Efficacy of berberine in patients with type 2 diabetes mellitus. *Metabolism* 2008; 57(5): 712–717. https://doi.org/10.1016/j.metabol.2008.01.013.
45. Zhang L, Gu FX, Chan JM, Wang AZ, Langer RS, Farokhzad OC. Nanoparticles in medicine: therapeutic applications and developments. *Clin. Pharmacol. Ther.* 2008; 83(5): 761–769. https://doi.org/10.1038/sj.clpt.6100400.
46. Sercombe L, Veerati T, Moheimani F, Wu SY, Sood AK, Hua S. Advances and challenges of liposome assisted drug delivery. *Front. Pharmacol.* 2015; 6: 286. https://doi.org/10.3389/fphar.2015.00286.
47. Zarrabi A, Alipoor Amro Abadi M, Khorasani S, Mohammadabadi MR, Jamshidi A, Torkaman S, Taghavi E, Mozafari MR, Rasti B. Nanoliposomes and tocosomes as multifunctional nanocarriers for the encapsulation of nutraceutical and dietary molecules. *Molecules* 2020; 25(3): 638. https://doi.org/10.3390/molecules25030638.
48. Istenic K, Cerc Korosec R, Poklar Ulrih N. Encapsulation of (−)-epigallocatechin gallate into liposomes and into alginate or chitosan microparticles reinforced with liposomes. *J. Sci. Food Agric.* 2016; 96 (13): 4623–4632. https://doi.org/10.1002/jsfa.7691.
49. Goniotaki M, Hatziantoniou S, Dimas K, Wagner M, Demetzos C. Encapsulation of naturally occurring flavonoids into liposomes: physicochemical properties and biological activity against human cancer cell lines. *J. Pharm. Pharmacol.* 2004; 56 (10): 1217–1224. https://doi.org/10.1211/0022357044382.
50. Zhang YF, Wang JC, Bian DY, Zhang X, Zhang Q. Targeted delivery of RGD-modified liposomes encapsulating both combretastatin A-4 and doxorubicin for tumor therapy: *in vitro* and *in vivo* studies. *Eur. J. Pharm. Biopharm.* 2010; 74(3): 467–473. https://doi.org/10.1016/j.ejpb.2010.01.002.
51. Ji P, Yu T, Liu Y, Jiang J, Xu J, Zhao Y, Hao Y, Qiu Y, Zhao W, Wu C. Naringenin-loaded solid lipid nanoparticles: preparation, controlled delivery, cellular uptake, and pulmonary pharmacokinetics. *Drug Des. Devel. Ther.* 2016; 10: 911–925. https://doi.org/10.2147/DDDT.S97738.
52. Altamimi MA, Hussain A, AlRajhi M, Alshehri S, Imam SS, Qamar W. Luteolin-loaded elastic liposomes for transdermal delivery to control breast cancer: *in vitro* and *ex vivo* evaluations. *Pharmaceuticals (Basel)* 2021; 14 (11): 1143. https://doi.org/10.3390/ph14111143.
53. Shetti P, Jalalpure SS, Patil AS, Kaur K, Apigenin-loaded stealth liposomes: development and pharmacokinetic studies for enhanced plasma retention of drug in cancer therapy. *Top. Catal.* 2024; 67: 46–58.https://doi.org/10.1007/s11244-023-01818-3.
54. Fang Y, Liu Y, Cao K, Shen W, Wang L, Sun B, Zhang Y, Zhang Q, Xia H. Investigation of the anti-inflammatory and anti-oxidant activities of a novel kaempferol-liposome-loaded hydrogel for the treatment of acute eczema. *Gels* 2025; 11(2): 83. https://doi.org/10.3390/gels11020083
55. Mehta M, Dureja H, Garg M. Development and optimization of boswellic acid-loaded proniosomal gel. *Drug Deliv.* 2016; 23(8): 3072–3081. https://doi.org/10.3109/10717544.2016.1149744.
56. Yuan D, Xu W, Raza F, Zafar H, Guan S, Wang Z, Ullah KH, Shi H. Baicalein long-circulating liposomes improve histological and functional outcomes after traumatic brain injury. *Adv. Pharmacol. Pharm. Sci.* 2024; 2024: 2869332. https://doi.org/10.1155/adpp/2869332.
57. Poornima G, Gupta S, Dhayalan A, Lahiri BB, Philip J, Kannan S. Green synthesis of quercetin-loaded magneto-liposomes and their assessment of antioxidant efficacy, hyperthermia and MRI contrast features. *Mater. Chem. Phys.* 2024; 323: 129663. https://doi.org/10.1016/j.matchemphys.2024.129663.
58. Li X, Xiao H, Lin C, Sun W, Wu T, Wang J, Chen B, Chen X, Cheng D. Synergistic effects of liposomes encapsulating atorvastatin calcium

and curcumin and targeting dysfunctional endothelial cells in reducing atherosclerosis. *Int. J. Nanomedicine* 2019; 14: 649–665. https://doi.org/10.2147/IJN.S189819.

59. Guo B, Xu D, Liu X, Yi J. Enzymatic synthesis and *in vitro* evaluation of folate-functionalized liposomes. *Drug Des. Devel. Ther.* 2017; 11: 1839–1847. https://doi.org/10.2147/DDDT.S132841.
60. Lu M, Qiu Q, Luo X, Liu X, Sun J, Wang C, Lin X, Deng Y, Song Y. Phyto-phospholipid complexes (phytosomes): a novel strategy to improve the bioavailability of active constituents. *Asian J. Pharm. Sci.* 2019; 14(3): 265–274. https://doi.org/10.1016/j.ajps.2018.05.011.
61. Bombardelli, E., Curri, S.B., Loggia, R.D. et al. (1989). Complexes between phospholipids and vegetal derivatives of biological interest. *Fitoterapia* 60 (1): 1–9.
62. Yanyu X, Yunmei S, Zhipeng C, Qineng P. The preparation of silybin-phospholipid complex and the study on its pharmacokinetics in rats. *Int. J. Pharm.* 2006; 307(1): 77–82. https://doi.org/10.1016/j.ijpharm.2005.10.001.
63. Niu Z, Conejos-Sánchez I, Griffin BT, O'Driscoll CM, Alonso MJ. Lipid-based nanocarriers for oral peptide delivery. *Adv. Drug Deliv. Rev.* 2016; 106 (Pt B): 337–354. https://doi.org/10.1016/j.addr.2016.04.001.
64. Belcaro, G., Cesarone, M.R., Dugall, M. et al. (2010). Efficacy and safety of Meriva®, a curcumin-phosphatidylcholine complex, during extended administration in osteoarthritis patients. *Altern. Med. Rev.* 15 (4): 337–344. PMID: 21194249.
65. Belcaro G, Ledda A, Hu S, Cesarone MR, Feragalli B, Dugall M. Greenselect phytosome for borderline metabolic syndrome. *Evid. Based Complement. Alternat. Med.* 2013; 2013: 869061. https://doi.org/10.1155/2013/869061.
66. Solnier J, Zhang Y, Kuo YC, Du M, Roh K, Gahler R, Wood S, Chang C. Characterization and pharmacokinetic assessment of a new berberine formulation with enhanced absorption *in vitro* and in human volunteers. *Pharmaceutics* 2023; 15 (11): 2567. https://doi.org/10.3390/pharmaceutics15112567.
67. Riva A, Ronchi M, Petrangolini G, Bosisio S, Allegrini P. Improved oral absorption of quercetin from quercetin Phytosome®, a new delivery system based on food grade lecithin. *Eur. J. Drug Metab. Pharmacokinet.* 2019; 44(2): 169–177. https://doi.org/10.1007/s13318-018-0517-3.
68. Kidd, P. and Head, K. (2005). A review of the bioavailability and clinical efficacy of milk thistle phytosome: a silybin-phosphatidylcholine complex (Siliphos). *Altern. Med. Rev.* 10 (3): 193–203. PMID: 16164374.
69. Wang, W., Yang, R., Zhao, Z. et al. (2021). Baicalin phytosome inhibits myocardial hypertrophy via blocking MAPK and NF-κbsignaling pathways. *Cardiovasc. Toxicol.* 21 (3): 236–248.
70. Husch J, Bohnet J, Fricker G, Skarke C, Artaria C, Appendino G, Schubert-Zsilavecz M, Abdel-Tawab M. Enhanced absorption of boswellic acids by a lecithin delivery form (Phytosome®) of Boswellia extract. *Fitoterapia* 2013; 84: 89–98. https://doi.org/10.1016/j.fitote.2012.10.002.
71. Demirbolat GM, Erdogan O, Coskun GP, Cevik O. PEG4000 modified liposomes enhance the solubility of quercetin and improve the liposome functionality: *in vitro* characterization and the cellular efficacy. *Turk. J. Chem.* 2022; 46(4): 1011–1023. https://doi.org/10.55730/1300-0527.3411.
72. Patil S, Choudhary B, Rathore A, Roy K, Mahadik K. Enhanced oral bioavailability and anticancer activity of novel curcumin loaded mixed micelles in human lung cancer cells. *Phytomedicine* 2015; 22 (12): 1103–1111. https://doi.org/10.1016/j.phymed.2015.08.006.
73. Hao J, Wang F, Wang X, Zhang D, Bi Y, Gao Y, Zhao X, Zhang Q. Development and optimization of baicalin-loaded solid lipid nanoparticles prepared by coacervation method using central composite design. *Eur. J. Pharm. Sci.* 2012; 47(2): 497–505. https://doi.org/10.1016/j.ejps.2012.07.006.
74. Rani A, Kaur R, Aldahish A, Vasudevan R, Balaji P, Dora CP, Chandrasekaran B, Singh TG, Sharma R. Nanostructured lipid carriers (NLC)-based topical formulation of hesperidin for effective treatment of psoriasis. *Pharmaceutics* 2025; 17(4): 478. https://doi.org/10.3390/pharmaceutics17040478.
75. Basak S, Das TK. Liposome-based drug delivery systems: from laboratory research to industrial production—instruments and challenges. *ChemEngineering* 2025; 9(3): 56. https://doi.org/10.3390/chemengineering9030056.
76. Paliwal R, Babu RJ, Palakurthi S. Nanomedicine scale-up technologies: feasibilities and challenges. *AAPS Pharm. Sci. Tech.* 2014; 15(6): 1527–1534. https://doi.org/10.1208/s12249-014-0177-9.
77. EMA (2025). nanotechnology-based medicinal products for human use. EMA/20989/2025/Rev. 1 https://www.ema.europa.eu/en/documents/report/nanotechnology-based-medicinal-products-human-use-eu-horizon-scanning-report_en.pdf (accessed 06 May 2026)
78. Soares S, Sousa J, Pais A, Vitorino C. Nanomedicine: principles, properties, and regulatory issues. *Front. Chem.* 2018; 6: 360. https://doi.org/10.3389/fchem.2018.00360.
79. Muhlebach S. Regulatory challenges of nanomedicines and their follow-on versions: a generic or similar approach? *Adv. Drug Deliv. Rev.* 2018; 131: 122–131. https://doi.org/10.1016/j.addr.2018.06.024.
80. Kazi RNA, Hasani IW, Khafaga DSR, Kabba S, Farhan M, Aatif M, Muteeb G, Fahim YA. Nanomedicine: the effective role of nanomaterials in healthcare from diagnosis to therapy. *Pharmaceutics* 2025; 17(8): 987. https://doi.org/10.3390/pharmaceutics17080987.
81. Zang J, Zhang L, Guo R, Kong L, Yu Y, Li S, Liu M, Wang J, Zhang Z, Li X, Liu Y. Baicalein loaded liposome with hyaluronic acid and polyhexamethylene guanidine modification for anti methicillin-resistant *Staphylococcus aureus* infection. *Int. J. Biol. Macromol.* 2024; 276 (Pt 1): 133432. https://doi.org/10.1016/j.ijbiomac.2024.133432.
82. Song Y, Zhang N, Li Q, Chen J, Wang Q, Yang H, Tan H, Gao J, Dong Z, Pang Z, Huang Z, Qian J, Ge J. Biomimetic liposomes hybrid with platelet membranes for targeted therapy of atherosclerosis. *Chem. Eng. J.* 2021; 408: 127296. https://doi.org/10.1016/j.cej.2020.127296.
83. Sesarman A, Tefas L, Sylvester B, Licarete E, Rauca V, Luput L, Patras L, Porav S, Banciu M, Porfire A. Co-delivery of curcumin and doxorubicin in PEGylated liposomes favored the antineoplastic C26 murine colon carcinoma microenvironment. *Drug Deliv. Transl. Res.* 2019; 9(1): 260–272. https://doi.org/10.1007/s13346-018-00598-8.
84. Chou WC, Canchola A, Zhang F, Lin Z. Machine learning and artificial intelligence in nanomedicine. *Wiley Interdiscip. Rev. Nanomed. Nanobiotechnol.* 2025; 17(4): e70027. https://doi.org/10.1002/wnan.70027.

# Microneedles, Hydrogels, and Transdermal Patches for Cardiovascular Applications

CHAPTER 10

**Raghuveer Pathuri[1], S. M. Khamanga[2], M. V. N. L. Chaitanya[3], and Pavan Kumar Chintamaneni[1]**

[1] *Department of Pharmaceutics, GITAM School of Pharmacy, GITAM (Deemed to be) University, Hyderabad, Telangana, India*

[2] *Faculty of Pharmacy, Rhodes University, Makhanda, Eastern Cape, South Africa*

[3] *School of Pharmaceutical Sciences, Lovely Professional University, Phagwara, Punjab, India*

## 10.1 INTRODUCTION

Cardiovascular diseases (CVDs) are significant causes of death around the world, accounting for 17.9 million deaths annually. This accounts for 31% of deaths worldwide. Major CVDs include hypertension, coronary heart disease, arrhythmias, heart failure, and peripheral vascular disease. Further, comorbidities like diabetes and obesity, and lifestyle factors in the ageing population, increase the global burden of CVDs [1, 2]. Conventional treatment methods employ oral and parenteral administration of drugs such as beta-blockers, statins, antiplatelet agents, and angiotensin-converting enzyme (ACE) inhibitors offered fruitful results. However, long-term usage of these drugs can lead to several side effects, including electrolyte imbalance, metabolic disturbances, renal impairment, and tolerance. Moreover, CVD therapy is often linked with polypharmacy, with the possibility of drug–drug interactions. Due to rising awareness of these chronic side effects, therapeutic shift is now towards herbal drugs/bioactives, which are perceived to have less side effects and are safe for long-term usage.

Herbal drugs such as curcumin, garlic, guggulsterone, and resveratrol have achieved significant attention in CVD therapy due to their antioxidant, antihyperlipidemic, anti-inflammatory, and cardiotonic properties. These herbal drugs/bioactives help in reducing cholesterol, prevent oxidative damage of heart, and also improve endothelial function with less or no side effects, making them safe for chronic therapy. However, most of these herbal drugs, when administered orally, often endure poor bioavailability, instability, short half-life, and first-pass metabolism. Chromic parenteral administration is not patient-compliant [3, 4]. Hence, there is a growing need for advanced transdermal delivery systems such as microneedles, hydrogels, and transdermal patches to enhance therapeutic outcomes and improve patient compliance [5–7].

This book chapter aims to give an overview of microneedles, hydrogels, and transdermal patches in CVD therapy, with a focus on herbal drugs and formulation approaches for these advanced drug delivery systems. It also includes a comparative analysis of these three drug delivery systems, with a discussion on their regulatory and safety concerns. Furthermore, emerging trends like smart wearables, artificial intelligence (AI)-integrated devices, and future prospects of CVDs management were included.

## 10.2 PHYTOMEDICINE IN CVD THERAPY

Phytomedicine has emerged as a promising therapeutic approach in the management of CVDs. Extensive literature is available on plant-based bioactives in Ayurveda and traditional Chinese medicine for use in chronic CVD therapy. These herbal drugs/bioactives make a pharmacological repertoire of compounds showing antioxidant, antithrombotic, anti-inflammatory, and cardioprotective effects. Further, these herbal drugs/bioactives also help in improving endothelial function, reducing low-density lipoprotein (LDL) cholesterol, and preventing myocardial damage. In addition to the safety profile of these compounds, their multitargeted actions make them valuable, particularly in managing complex and chronic diseases such as CVDs [8].

### 10.2.1 KEY PHYTOCHEMICALS WITH CARDIOPROTECTIVE ACTION

Phytochemicals constitute a diverse group of plant secondary metabolites with several classes, such as flavonoids, polyphenols, alkaloids, saponins, and terpenoids. Extensive studies were available on their role in the prevention and management of CVDs.

- **Flavonoids** are polyphenolic compounds widely distributed in plants, fruits, and vegetables. Molecules such as quercetin, rutin, and kaempferol improve endothelial function, reduce low-density lipoprotein (LDL) oxidation, inhibit platelet aggregation, and improve microcirculation, aiding in the prevention of coronary artery disease and hypertension [9].
- **Alkaloids** are secondary metabolites with effective cardiovascular action. Berberine, an alkaloid from *Berberis aristata*, shows antihyperlipidemic, anti-arrhythmic, and vasodilatory properties. Berberine also improves insulin sensitivity, reduces LDL cholesterol, improves nitric oxide production, and activates AMP-activated protein kinase (AMPK), making it useful for treatment of metabolic syndrome-linked CVDs [10].
- **Terpenoids** are a large class of lipophilic compounds with cardiovascular significance. Compounds like arjunolic acid and guggulsterone are terpenoids with anti-inflammatory, hypolipidemic, and cardioprotective actions. These compounds help in lowering total cholesterol, prevent ischemia-induced myocardial injury, and improve myocardial function [11].
- **Polyphenols** are phytochemicals with antioxidant function, seen in grapes, berries, and tea. Resveratrol is a stilbene polyphenol that triggers the Sirtuin 1 (SIR T1) pathway and improves endothelial nitric oxide synthase. This produces antithrombotic, vasoprotective, and cardiotonic actions. Curcumin, another significant polyphenol from rhizomes of turmeric, inhibits NF-κB, Nrf2, AMPK, and TGF-beta signaling and various cytokines, preventing myocardial fibrosis and adverse remodeling of myocardial tissue [12].
- **Saponins** are glucosides with amphiphilic structure. Ginsenosides (from *Panax ginseng*) and dioscin from *Dioscorea* show antioxidant, antihyperlipidemic, and cardioprotective properties. These compounds lower triglycerides, stabilize cardiac membranes, and protect against oxidative damage of the myocardium. These compounds also improve cardiac contractility and enhance vascular tone [13].

### 10.2.2 CHALLENGES IN THE DELIVERY OF HERBAL DRUGS

Many herbal bioactives demonstrate poor aqueous solubility, chemical instability, and first-pass metabolism. Further, these molecules have high molecular weights, reducing their oral absorption and bioavailability (Table 10.1). These compounds also have low half-life, compelling frequent dosing, which may lead to poor patient compliance [14, 15].

Hence, the clinical translation of these phytochemicals remains limited due to these multiple delivery-related challenges. This calls for advanced drug delivery methods that can overcome the limitations and improve the therapeutic outcomes of these herbal bioactives without compromising patient compliance.

**Table 10.1** Herbal drugs in CVD therapy and their drug delivery limitations.

| Herbal bioactive | Source plant | Chemical class | Cardiovascular application | Limitations in drug delivery |
|---|---|---|---|---|
| Curcumin | *Curcuma longa* | Polyphenol | Anti-inflammatory, antithrombotic, reduces LDL cholesterol | Extremely poor water solubility, rapid clearance from systemic circulation, and low absorption |
| Resveratrol | *Vitis vinifera* | Polyphenol | Antioxidant, cardioprotective, anti-atherosclerotic | Poor aqueous solubility, rapid metabolism, and very low oral bioavailability |
| Quercetin | Green tea, onion, fruits | Flavonoid | Antioxidant, vasodilator, antihypertensive | Low solubility, GI instability, and extensive first-pass metabolism |
| Berberine | *Berberis aristata* | Isoquinoline alkaloid | Hypoglycemic, lipid-lowering, cardioprotective | Low permeability (P-gp efflux), low oral bioavailability (<1%), and poor solubility |
| Guggulsterone | *Commiphora mukul* | Steroidal terpenoid | Antihyperlipidemic, anti-inflammatory | Poor water solubility, rapid metabolism, and low systemic bioavailability |
| Boswellic acids | *Boswellia serrata* | Pentacyclic triterpenoid | Anti-inflammatory, antihypertensive | Poor solubility, limited bioavailability, poor pharmacokinetic profile |
| Ginsenosides | *Panax ginseng* | Saponin | Improves cardiac function | High-molecular weight, low permeability, and P-gp efflux |
| EGCG (epigallocatechin gallate) | Green tea | Polyphenol | Antioxidant, antihypertensive | Poor solubility in the GI tract, low solubility, rapid degradation |
| Diosgenin | *Dioscorea* spp. | Steroidal saponin | Cholesterol-lowering, anti-atherosclerotic | Poor solubility, limited GI absorption |

### 10.2.3 RATIONALE FOR TRANSDERMAL DRUG DELIVERY APPROACHES

Transdermal drug delivery has gained substantial attention in recent days as an alternative to oral administration, mainly in cases of drugs or herbal bioactives with low aqueous solubility, low oral bioavailability, extensive first-pass metabolism, and short half-life. Transdermal systems facilitate direct administration into systemic circulation through skin, bypassing first-pass metabolism and preventing gastrointestinal degradation, resulting in increased bioavailability and improved therapeutic efficiency. A further key advantage of transdermal drug delivery is controlled and sustained drug delivery, thereby maintaining steady-state plasma concentrations. This prevents fluctuations, which otherwise can cause adverse cardiovascular events, particularly in chronic disorders such as angina, hypertension, and dyslipidemia, where continuous therapeutic concentrations in plasma are essential. Furthermore, transdermal systems reduce dosing frequency, improving patient compliance, a critical factor in the chronic treatment of CVDs. The noninvasive or minimally invasive, painless transdermal drug delivery systems (TDDS) make them more patient-compliant. Collectively, transdermal drug delivery addresses significant limits of conventional drug delivery routes with improved therapeutic benefits for both synthetic and herbal drugs [16].

## 10.3 FUNDAMENTALS OF TRANSDERMAL DRUG DELIVERY SYSTEMS

The transdermal pathway has emerged as a noteworthy noninvasive alternative to conventional oral and parenteral delivery routes, specifically in the treatment of chronic diseases like CVDs. The shift of focus toward TDDS is mainly due to advances in formulation science and renewed focus on patient-centric drug delivery systems. A comprehensive understanding of skin structure, mechanism of permeation through skin, physicochemical properties for drugs/drug delivery systems required for transdermal permeation, and pharmacokinetic considerations, including its depot action, is essential [17].

### 10.3.1 ANATOMY AND PHYSIOLOGY OF SKIN IN RELATION TO DRUG TRANSPORT

Human skin is a complex, multilayered organ made up of epidermis, dermis, and hypodermis. The outermost layer is the epidermis, known for its barrier function, with the stratum corneum as the outermost sublayer. This layer is made of dead, keratinized cells, embedded in a layer of lipid-rich matrix, often referred to as the "brick and mortar model." Beneath this lies viable epidermis, which is metabolically active; however, it lacks blood vessels. Then lies the dermis, the bottom-most layer supplied with blood vessels, lymphatic vessels, sensory nerves, and connective tissue (Figure 10.1).

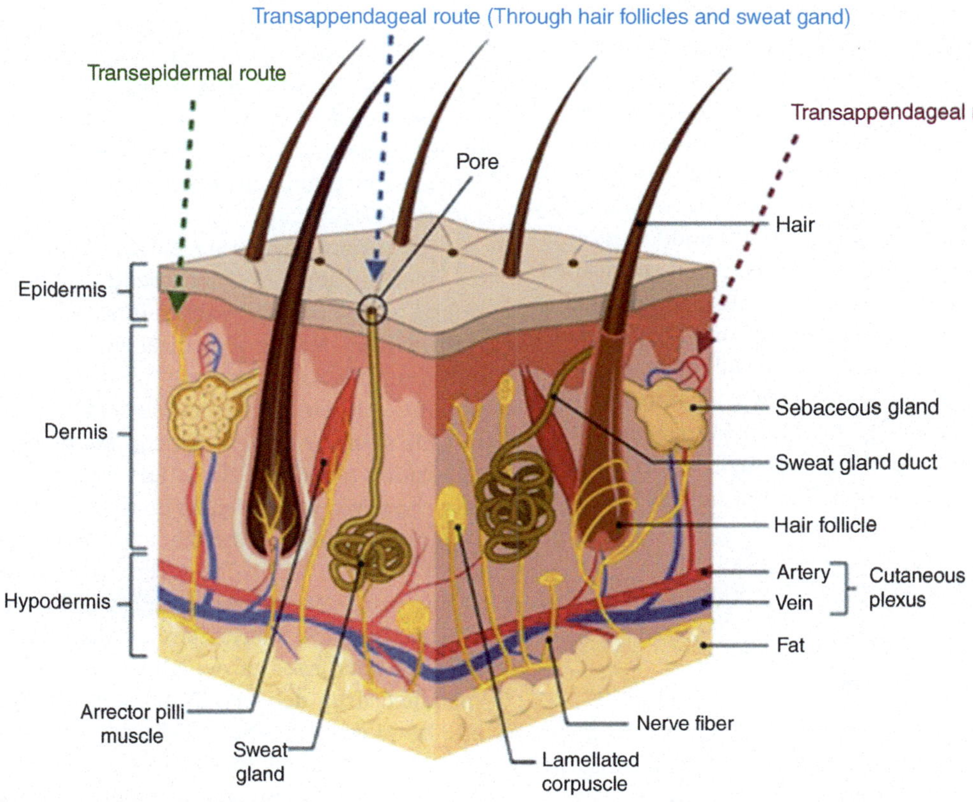


**FIGURE 10.1** Structure of skin and pathways for drug transport. *Source:* Yu et al. [18] / Frontiers Media SA / CC BY 4.0.

This tissue facilitates systemic absorption of drugs once they cross the stratum corneum. Subcutaneous tissue, also called hypodermis, is a tissue that mainly acts as fat storage and helps in thermal insulation. The skin also contains sweat glands, sebaceous glands, and hair follicles, which can offer an alternative route for drug administration. The rate and extent of drug delivery via skin are influenced by this microarchitecture and the barrier function of skin [19].

Drug molecules cross the skin via three principal pathways, namely the transcellular route, intercellular route, and appendageal routes. The transcellular route is the direct transport of drugs through corneocytes and is favored by lipophilic, low-molecular-weight compounds. The intercellular route is the diffusion of drugs between corneocytes, through lipid domains of the stratum corneum, suitable for lipophilic drugs. Finally, the appendageal route is the transport of drugs via skin appendages such as hair follicles and sweat glands, accounting for less than 0.1% of total skin area, making this route suited for hydrophilic drugs, larger molecules, and nanoparticles [20].

### 10.3.2 BARRIER FUNCTION OF THE STRATUM CORNEUM

The stratum corneum acts as the principal barrier for the delivery of drugs via skin due to its structural complexity. The corneocytes and the lipid matrix structure limit the passive diffusion of many pharmaceutical agents, particularly those that are hydrophilic, ionised, and have high molecular weight. As per Lipinski's Rule of Five, drugs ideal for passive transdermal drug delivery should have a molecular weight below 500 Da, a log P value between 1 and 4, hydrogen bond donors less than five, and hydrogen bond acceptors less than 10. Passive permeation drugs generally follow Fick's first law of diffusion, where the rate of transport of the drug is directly proportional to the concentration gradient and is inversely related to barrier thickness. Only the molecules that satisfy the Lipinski rule of five, generally lipophilic and low molecular weight, can undergo successful transdermal permeation, e.g., nitroglycerine, clonidine. Passive diffusion alone will be insufficient for therapeutic molecules that are high molecular weight, hydrophilic, macromolecules, and phytochemicals with poor permeability [21]. These anatomical and physiological considerations highlight the barrier function of skin and highlight innovative strategies such as microneedles, hydrogels, and transdermal patches for transdermal drug delivery [22].

## 10.4 MICRONEEDLE SYSTEMS IN CARDIOVASCULAR THERAPY

Microneedles are advanced TDDS, designed to overcome the barrier property of skin, particularly the stratum corneum. Microneedles create microscopic pathways without causing pain or discomfort. These microscopic pathways or projections facilitate drug transport and facilitate direct access to the viable epidermis and dermal microcirculation. This approach enhances the bioavailability of a wide range of molecules, including herbal bioactives, which are limited by poor oral bioavailability, in the management of CVDs. Microneedles facilitate consistent long-term drug administration with improved therapeutic outcomes and patient compliance [23].

### 10.4.1 TYPES OF MICRONEEDLES AND MATERIALS USED IN FABRICATION

Microneedles are microscopic projections of a typical 150–1500 μm length, fabricated from metals, silicon, and biodegradable polymers. Microneedles are mainly classified into five types based on their structure and drug delivery mechanism. These include solid microneedles, coated microneedles, dissolving microneedles, hollow microneedles, and hydrogel-forming microneedles [24, 25].

Solid microneedles create micropores in the skin and aid in subsequent topical drug application. In contrast, coated microneedles have drug layers coated on their surface and release the drug upon insertion into the skin. Dissolving microneedles, on the other hand, have drugs mixed in their matrix made of biodegradable polymers like hyaluronic acid, polyvinyl alcohol (PVA), and polyvinylpyrrolidone (PVP). These dissolving microneedles aid in drug release upon complete dissolution of the needles in layers of skin. Hollow microneedles, often made of metals, act like miniature hypodermic needles and deliver macromolecules and liquid formulations directly to dermal layers for faster absorption. Hydrogel-forming microneedles are similar to dissolving microneedles, where the drug is dissolved in the polymer matrix; however, these dissolving microneedles swell upon contact with interstitial fluid, thereby forming a gel-like matrix for controlled and sustained delivery of drugs (Table 10.2, Figure 10.2) [24, 25].

A variety of pharmaceutical-grade materials are used in the fabrication of microneedles (Table 10.3) to ensure safety, biocompatibility, mechanical integrity, and efficient drug delivery. Metals of medical grade, such as stainless steel and titanium, are commonly used in microneedle fabrication due to their mechanical strength, enabling precise and reliable skin permeation. Silicon manufacture using microfabrication technique also offers high precision and uniformity; however, its brittleness limits its large-scale therapeutic applications. Biocompatible and biodegradable polymers like PVP, PVA, PLGA (Poly [lactic-co-glycolic acid]), hyaluronic acid, CMC (carboxymethyl cellulose), and chitosan, are used in the fabrication of dissolving and hydrogel-forming microneedles, which aid in safer, controlled, and sustained drug delivery. Water-soluble sugars like maltose are employed in the fabrication of rapidly dissolving microneedles, used in peptide and vaccine delivery. The material selection further depends on its compatibility with the bioactive to be delivered [24, 25].

**Table 10.2** Microneedles: types, materials, and mechanism.

| Microneedle type | Material to make | Drug delivery mechanism | Key features |
|---|---|---|---|
| Solid microneedles | Metals (stainless steel, titanium), silicon | Creates microchannels in skin, a drug applied topically for diffusion via preformed microchannels | Simple design and two-step process |
| Coated microneedles | Metals, silicon, biodegradable polymers | Drugs coated on the microneedle surface are dissolved on insertion | Rapid onset, suitable for drugs with small doses |
| Dissolving microneedles | Biodegradable polymers (PVP, PVA, HA) | The drug is mixed in a polymer matrix and gets released as microneedles, which dissolve entirely in the skin | Single use, excellent biocompatibility, ideal for biomolecules and phytomedicine |
| Hollow microneedles | Metals, polymers, silicon | Liquid formulations and macromolecules reach the dermal microcirculation directly | Delivery of drugs with higher doses, controlled infusion is possible |
| Hydrogel from microneedles | Cross-linked polymers | Needles swell upon insertion and create a controlled/sustained drug diffusion | Long action, excellent biocompatibility |

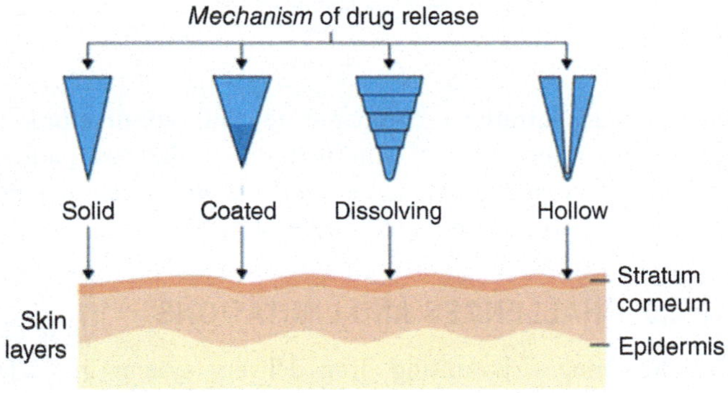


**FIGURE 10.2** Microneedle types and drug release mechanisms.

**Table 10.3** Materials used in microneedle fabrication and their herbal relevance.

| Material | Properties | Relevance to the delivery of herbal bioactives |
|---|---|---|
| Metals (SS steel, titanium) | High mechanical strength, rigid | Limited use, unsuitable for embedding herbal actives |
| Silicon | Brittle, precise microfabrication is possible | Not preferred, risk of breakage inside skin and no drug loading |
| Biodegradable polymers (PVS, PVP, HA, CMC) | Biocompatible, dissolvable, and swellable | Most suitable, excellent for herbal extracts and phytoconstituents |
| Sugars (maltose, trehalose) | Water soluble, generally regarded as safe (GRAS) | Suitable for fast-release herbal microneedles (antioxidant extracts) |
| Ceramics (calcium phosphates) | Rigid, bioactive | Brittle, low compatibility with herbal micromolecules |

### 10.4.2 MECHANISM OF ACTION OF MICRONEEDLES IN THE MANAGEMENT OF CVDs

Microneedles act by painlessly breaching the stratum corneum, the primary diffusion barrier of skin, thus creating a transient, aqueous microchannel that can access the dermal capillaries and thereby enable immediate systemic uptake. The localized disruption of skin layers significantly reduces the skin's resistance and enhances the flux, allowing the cardiovascular drugs to rapidly diffuse into the dermal microcirculation without much pain and tissue trauma. Depending on the design of microneedles, the drug release can be rapid, pulsatile, or sustained. In advanced systems, microneedles can even trigger drug release in response to physiological stimuli such as pH, enzyme activity, or oxidative stress, enabling smart and patient-centric cardiovascular therapy [26].

### 10.4.3 DELIVERY OF SYNTHETIC AND PHYTOCHEMICAL MOLECULES BY MICRONEEDLES

Researchers have extensively investigated the delivery of both synthetic and phytochemicals using microneedles. Among synthetic drugs, nicotine-loaded microneedles have been evaluated for smoking cessation, thereby reducing cardiovascular risk [27]. Similarly, Microneedle-based delivery of antihypertensive drugs like propranolol and atenolol has shown significant improvement of bioavailability compared to oral administration. In another study, hollow microneedles were used for the delivery of low-molecular-weight heparin and achieved adequate quantity for anticoagulant action [28–30].

Many herbal bioactives with established cardiovascular action have been successfully investigated via the microneedle platform, as given in Table 10.4. Curcumin, a potent anti-atherogenic and anti-inflammatory polyphenol, was evaluated using microneedle-assisted delivery via a nanocrystal formulation of curcumin. The study demonstrated a marked increase in *ex vivo* dermal penetration in porcine skin, compared to the

**Table 10.4** Herbal drugs investigated in microneedle-based delivery.

| Herbal bioactive | Cardiovascular relevance | Microneedle system type | Study model and key finding | Source |
|---|---|---|---|---|
| Curcumin | anti-inflammatory, anti-atherogenic, antioxidant | Microneedle-assisted delivery, curcumin nanocrystals vs. bulk curcumin | *Ex vivo* porcine skin, formulation showed a marked increase in dermal penetration vs. bulk, supports transdermal applicability | [31] |
| Resveratrol | Antihyperlipidemic, endothelial protection, cardiometabolic benefits | Dissolving microneedles | Dissolving microneedles improved transdermal absorption of resveratrol | [32] |
| Berberine | Antihyperlipidemic, | Chitosan microneedle arrays | Imaging-led delivery mapping, MALDI-MSI visualized berberine distribution throughout epidermal and dermal layers, confirming effective transdermal drug delivery. | [33] |
| Quercetin | Vasoprotective, antioxidant, endothelial modulator | Dissolving microneedle patches (Solid dispersion) | Microneedles enhanced drug loading and improved skin delivery of quercetin | [34] |
| Ginsenoside | Anti-ischemic, vasoprotective | Hydrogel-based microneedle with dissolving PVA/PVP tips | *In vivo* studies on mouse models showed prolonged drug release/ improved immunomodulatory effect, proangiogenic/antifibrotic effects. | [35] |

bulk of curcumin, confirming transdermal applicability [31]. Dissolving microneedles of resveratrol, known for its antioxidant and endotheilal protective effects, also showed significant improvement in transdermal bioavailability [32]. Similarly, berberine, known for its antihyperlipidemic and cardioprotective action, has been delivered via chitosan-based microneedles. These studies demonstrated deep permeation across epidermal and dermal layers [33]. Quercetin, a vasoprotective flavonoid with endothelial-modulating properties, has been loaded into dissolving polymeric microneedles and showed enhanced transdermal permeation in experimental models [34]. Ginsenoside RK3 from *Panax* spp. a saponin with anti-ischemic and vasoprotective action has been incorporated in a hydrogel microneedle with dissolving PVA/PVP tips and a hydrogel backing, demonstrating sustained drug delivery and immunomodulatory action [35]. These findings collectively support the strong potential of microneedle platforms in the delivery of herbal cardiovascular therapeutics.

### 10.4.4 ADVANTAGES OF MICRONEEDLE-BASED DELIVERY

Microneedle systems present several advantages for the delivery of cardiovascular drugs in comparison to oral and parenteral routes. As a minimally invasive, painless approach, microneedles potentially increase patient comfort and compliance, particularly in chronic CVD therapies. Microneedles, by precisely delivering drugs into the dermal circulation, dodging stratum corneum, prevent first-pass metabolism and increase bioavailability for both synthetic and herbal drugs with poor oral bioavailability. Additionally, their capacity to show rapid pharmacological action makes them appropriate for emergency interventions such as angina or hypertensive crisis. Furthermore, these microneedle systems allow dose sparing, as lower doses are sufficient to achieve therapeutic plasma concentrations compared to oral administration. Lastly, feasibility of self-administration enhances patient independence and convenience, limits their clinical dependency, and improves therapeutic effects [6, 36].

### 10.4.5 CHALLENGES AND LIMITATIONS

Despite being a promising drug delivery system in CVD, microneedles suffer from various technical, biopharmaceutical, and translational challenges. These challenges must be tackled for better clinical adoption. The major concern comes with the mechanical robustness of the microneedles, particularly those made of biodegradable polymers such as chitosan, PVA, and CMC, which may show an insufficient insertion force for thicker or highly elastic skins. To overcome this limitation, microneedles with a hybrid construction, fabricated using a combination of polymers, or nanomaterial reinforcements, or a composite gradient structure, have to be explored to enhance the mechanical strength and biocompatibility. Another major limitation of microneedles relates to the inherently low drug-loading capacity, especially for coated or dissolving microneedles, where the payload will be in a few milligrams, which may not be suitable for certain CVDs requiring greater systemic drug concentrations. Using hollow microneedles, multilayered architectures, and integrated patch-reservoir systems can enable increasing the payload [37].

Further, the instability of herbal bioactives, like resveratrol and curcumin, due to their sensitivity to heat, light, and oxidation, presents a significant challenge for the shelf life of the formulation and therapeutic efficiency. Advanced methodologies, including PEGylated hydrogel matrices, antioxidant coformulation, and nanoencapsulation, have been shown to enhance stability and controlled release. From the manufacturer's outlook, complex fabrication techniques like micromolding, photolithography, and high-resolution 3D printing can contribute to enhanced production costs and scalability issues. The implementation of emerging techniques like roll-to-roll fabrication, injection micromolding, and automated additive manufacturing can significantly reduce production time and costs. Further, usage of scalable polymer-based formulations, along with batch-level control automation, can allow Good Manufacturing Practice (GMP)-compliant, economic, and commercially scalable microneedle production [38]. Patient-centric challenges involve variability in skin physiology, movement limitations in older patients, microneedle adhesion, and overall usability. To enhance real-world applications, feedback insertion confirmation and a visual color-change indicator can improve user adherence and improve clinical outcomes.

### 10.4.6 FUTURE PROSPECTS OF MICRONEEDLES IN CVDs THERAPY

The potential of microneedle drug delivery systems in CVD drug delivery is driven by its merging with emerging personalized, multimodal, and smart therapeutic platforms. The combination of smart sensors in microneedles can enable real-time monitoring of cardiovascular biomarkers like blood pressure, nitric oxide levels, or enzymes of cardiac injury. Additionally, the addition of closed-loop feedback-controlled systems facilitates automatic dose adjustment as per the dynamic physiological status. Hybrid microneedle systems with integrated hydrogel matrices or transdermal patch reservoirs can achieve programmable extended-release kinetics, making once-a-week or once-a-month drug delivery systems, particularly advantageous in chronic cardiovascular conditions. In the modern era of pharmaceutical drug delivery, personalized medicine is gaining importance. Microneedles offer a potential platform for tailoring needle geometry, payload, release kinetics, and material used as per the patient's requirement. Collectively, advancements in drug delivery and precision medicine establish microneedles as next-generation, intelligent, and patient-centric CVD therapeutic systems. [39, 40]

## 10.5 HYDROGELS OF CARDIOVASCULAR DRUG DELIVERY

Hydrated, three-dimensional, viscoelastic polymeric networks characterize hydrogels. These systems have gained significant prominence as advanced drug delivery systems in cardiovascular drug delivery. The intrinsic biocompatibility, tunable porosity, and stimuli-responsive behavior enable modulation of drug release kinetics, thereby allowing both systemic and local delivery of therapeutic agents. Further, they can also be tuned for controlled and sustained drug delivery of both synthetic drugs and phytochemicals via the skin. Further, due to their structural resemblance to native biological tissues, hydrogels can be engineered to match the mechanical and biological milieu of the cardiovascular microenvironment, making them suitable for internal applications such as myocardial regeneration, and angiogenesis [41, 42].

### 10.5.1 STRUCTURAL COMPOSITION AND CLASSIFICATION OF HYDROGELS

Hydrogels are 3D hydrophilic networks that have the property to absorb and retain large quantities of water or biological fluids while preserving their structural integrity. This is due to the presence of hydrophilic functional groups like hydroxyl, carbonyl, and amide groups. The 3D network-like structure is stabilized either by physical cross-linking or chemical cross-linking. Physical cross-linking can be due to reversible interactions such as hydrogen bonding, ionic interactions, and hydrophobic associations. On the other hand, chemical cross-linking, involving covalent bonds, imparts greater stability and durability [43]. Hydrogels, based on their origin and composition, are broadly classified into natural, synthetic, semi-synthetic, or composite hydrogels. Further, based on cross-linking, these are classified into physical and chemical cross-linked hydrogels [44].

#### 10.5.1.1 Natural Hydrogels

Natural hydrogels are made from materials like chitosan, alginate, and gelatin. These are derived from biopolymers and are inherently biocompatible, biodegradable, and non-immunogenic. These polymers hydrate the stratum corneum and can be formulated to enhance the permeation of drugs and also sustained delivery of both synthetic drugs and herbal bioactives. The cationic nature of chitosan transiently modulates skin barrier properties, improving adhesion. Alginate, on the other hand, provides mild, ionic gelled matrices with high water content. Gelatin contributes to great tissue compatibility [45].

#### 10.5.1.2 Synthetic Hydrogels

Synthetic hydrogels are made from pharmaceutically acceptable polymers, generally categorized under the GRAS category. They show superior control over mesh size, mechanical strength, degradation rate, and drug release kinetics. Further, these synthetic hydrogels produce reproducible and sustained drug release, particularly suitable for CVD applications. Polyethylene glycol (PEG) based hydrogels are widely used under this category due to their inert, non-immunogenic nature and tunable architecture, allowing precise control of both porosity and diffusivity. On the other hand, thermoresponsive polymers (Poly [N-isopropylacrylamide], PNIPAM) enable *in situ* gelling at skin temperature to form surface deposits enabling sustained permeation. Further, biodegradable block copolymer networks can be engineered for prolonged release (24 hours), typically suitable for cardiovascular therapy [46, 47].

#### 10.5.1.3 Semi-Synthetic and Composite Hydrogels

Hybrid hydrogels combine the bioadhesive, biocompatible, and biodegradable properties of natural polymers with reproducible release kinetics of synthetic polymers, making them ideal for long-term usage. Chitosan-PEG, Chitosan-PVA copolymer hydrogels can show superior elasticity, moisture retention, and skin adhesion, supporting prolonged residence and controlled release suitable for cardiovascular applications. Similarly, chemically modified hyaluronic acid hydrogels improve epidermal hydration and transdermal flux, enhancing both dermal permeation and systemic absorption of cardiovascular drugs, including herbal bioactives [48]. Further nanocomposite hydrogels incorporating polymer nanomaterials (such as graphene oxide, silica) provide enhanced mechanical stability, permeation modulation, and oxidative stress protection, improving bioavailability and stability of cardiovascular therapeutics [49, 50].

#### 10.5.1.4 Physically and Chemically Cross-Linked Hydrogels

Physically cross-linked hydrogels are stabilized by reversible ionic associations, hydrogen bonding, or hydrophobic bonding. They are minimally processed transdermal systems. Their stimulus responsiveness allows drug release to adapt dynamically to skin hydration, temperature, and sweat levels. Further, their sol–gel reversibility also enhances safety by preventing skin adherence or irritation, thus making them compatible with chronic therapies. Chemically cross-linked hydrogels, on the other hand, are stabilized by covalent bonding via photo-click chemistry or enzyme-mediated reactions. These provide greater mechanical integrity, occlusivity, and long-wear stability, ensuring zero-order, or near zero-order release, maintaining steady level plasma concentrations of the drug, reducing dosing frequency, and improving patient compliance [51, 52].

### 10.5.2 DRUG ENCAPSULATION AND RELEASE FROM HYDROGELS

Drugs are encapsulated in hydrogel matrices via physical entrapment (drug dispersed within swollen matrix mesh), ionic complexation (electrostatic interaction between drug and polymeric networks), or by covalent conjugation (drug linked to polymer networks by cleavable linkers). The choice of method of encapsulation depends on the drugs chosen and the required pharmacological action [53].

The encapsulated drug from the hydrogel matrix can be released by diffusion-controlled release, swelling-controlled release, chemical-controlled release, and stimulus-responsive release [54].

a. **Diffusion-controlled release:**
Fick's law of diffusion governs drug transport in diffusion-controlled release. The rate of diffusion of the drug from the polymer matrix is governed by mesh size, drug size, and polymer–drug interactions. Further, the cross-linking density governs the flux and helps in maintaining steady-state plasma levels, typically suitable for chronic therapies.

b. **Swelling-controlled release:**
Swellable systems, upon contact with the skin, absorb moisture/sweat and expand, increasing the effective pore size and mobilizing the drug. This mechanism is well-suited for more polar and herbal bioactives, with high-molecular-weight cardiovascular drugs. Recent studies showed that swelling dynamics reshape the polymer geometry and porosity to regulate release.

c. **Chemically-controlled release:**
The release from chemically controlled systems is governed by matrix degradation (hydrolysis or enzyme-mediated) or cleavage of drug–polymer linkers. Enzyme-responsive designs are in demand with closed-loop feedback systems, which enable pathology-linked release. This enables smart and targeted release. These release systems further ensure steady and controlled release for long periods, with less or no irritation on the skin. Many research studies have shown enzyme-degradable hydrogels and the use of drug–polymer linkers.

d. **Stimuli-responsive release:**
These are "smart" release systems that release the drug in response to temperature, pH, redox/ROS level, and light, enabling spatiotemporal control of drug release over oral drug delivery. It also has potential to synchronize circadian rhythms.

### 10.5.3 HYDROGEL-BASED DELIVERY OF CARDIOVASCULAR DRUGS

Hydrogel-based systems have been extensively explored for transdermal delivery of both synthetic and herbal bioactives. Amlodipine-loaded hydrogel matrices showed controlled permeability and prolonged antihypertensive action in *ex vivo* skin models, overcoming the limitations of low oral bioavailability and extensive first-pass metabolism [55, 56]. Metoprolol-loaded hydrogels were studied for triggered drug release with steady-state plasma concentration and improved therapeutic benefits in hypertension and arrhythmia. [57] Atorvastatin- and simvastatin-loaded hydrogels were reported to improve localized LDL modulation, reducing hepatic burden and systemic toxicity [58, 59]. Hybrid systems of nitroglycerine-loaded patches showed vasodilatory effects with reduced dosing frequency and minimal skin irritation.

In addition to synthetic drugs, hydrogel-based drug delivery systems are also explored for improving therapeutic benefits associated with herbal bioactives with cardiovascular applications (Table 10.5). Resveratrol-loaded hydrogel patches showed greater mechanical integrity and prolonged drug release up to 72 hours [60, 66]. Curcumin integrated into composite hydrogel-based microneedles exhibited improved mechanical strength and controlled release behavior [61]. Quercetin encapsulated in GelMA hydrogel microneedles showed efficient skin permeation and significant stress reduction of oxidative stress [62]. Cellulose-based hydrogels were successfully employed for the delivery of berberine, showing its effective drug release, biocompatibility, and feasibility in the management of CVDs [63]. Another self-adhesive hydrogel microneedle platform of ginsenosides and metformin demonstrated ultra-long delivery and potent pro-angiogenic and antifibrotic effects *in vivo*, highlighting its

**Table 10.5** Herbal drugs for CVDs investigated for hydrogel formulations.

| Herbal drug | Hydrogel format | Transdermal evidence | CVD relevance | Source |
|---|---|---|---|---|
| Resveratrol | Hydrogel matrix patch | 72 hours sustained release, High mechanical stability | Antioxidant, endothelial protection | [60] |
| Curcumin | Hydrogel + PLGA microneedle | Stable insertion, controlled drug release | Anti-atherogenic, anti-remodeling | [61] |
| Quercetin | GelMA hydrogel microneedle | Enhanced permeation | vasoprotective flavonoid | [62] |
| Berberine | Cellulose hydrogel | Sustained drug release, Safe transdermal delivery | Antihyperlipidemic, insulin sensitizer | [63] |
| Ginsenoside RK3 | Self-adhesive hydrogel microneedle | >10 days release, proangiogenic, antifibrotic | Anti-ischemic | [35] |
| Puerarin | Electrospun hydrogel membrane | Sustained release, promotes repair | Endothelial protection, anti-ischemic | [64] |
| EGCG | Hydrogel nanocomposite | Improved stability and dermal permeation | Anti-hypertensive, antioxidative | [65] |

importance in ischemic heart disease and vascular remodeling diseases [35]. Collectively, these findings establish hydrogels as promising drug delivery systems in cardiovascular therapy.

### 10.5.4 INJECTABLE HYDROGELS FOR MYOCARDIAL REPAIR

Injectable hydrogels offer excellent therapy for ischemic myocardium by providing mechanical support and controlled delivery of therapeutic moieties. In a first-in-human trial, VentriGel, a cardiac extracellular matrix hydrogel, was injected transendocardially in post-MI patients, showing early signs of functional improvement [67–69]. Alginate-based hydrogels, Algisyl-LVR, were found to be safe in patients with dilated cardiomyopathy, with improvement in heart function in further randomized evaluations. Preclinical studies also showed a reduced left ventricular wall stress and adverse remodeling [70]. Gelatin hydrogels also serve as carriers or depots for biofactors such as basic fibroblast growth factor. Sustained release of biofactors from these gelatin hydrogels improved blood flow and heart function in animal models of chronic myocardial infarction [71]. In another approach, hyaluronic acid hydrogels showed an improvement in the retention and therapeutic efficiency of extracellular vesicles in myocardial infarction, supporting better blood vessel formation and recovery of myocardial tissue [72]. Collectively, injectable hydrogels make a platform for local cardiovascular repair and drug delivery.

### 10.5.5 ADVANTAGES OF HYDROGEL-BASED DRUG DELIVERY

Hydrogel-based drug delivery systems offer multiple advantages for the delivery of herbal drugs via skin for cardiovascular therapy. The high water content, biomimetic structure, resembling extracellular matrix, makes it excellently compatible with skin and enhances patient comfort. By maintaining good hydration, hydrogel enhances the permeation of lipophilic phytoconstituents via the stratum corneum. Further, the mesh size and polymer composition can be precisely adjusted to achieve desired release rates. Hydrogels, additionally, upon using permeation enhancers, lipid carriers, or nanosystems, improve the transdermal flux of herbal drugs. Their painless, noninvasive nature evades first-pass metabolism, offers a safer and more convenient drug delivery system for cardiovascular therapy [73, 74]. In addition, injectable hydrogel systems allow minimally invasive localized therapy to deliver drugs directly to diseased cardiac tissues, whereas stimuli-responsive systems release therapeutic agents in response to microenvironmental changes like pH, temperature, or enzymatic activity [68].

### 10.5.6 CHALLENGES AND LIMITATIONS

Notwithstanding advantages, hydrogel-based delivery of herbal drugs via skin faces numerous challenges, limiting their clinical translation. One key limitation is the inherently low permeability for large, hydrophilic, or poorly water-soluble herbal drugs, limiting their efficient passage via the stratum corneum. This can be tackled by integration of hydrogel systems with chemical permeation enhancers, microneedles, and lipid-based nanocarriers to enhance transdermal permeation. Hydrogels often exhibit inadequate mechanical robustness, which may compromise their integrity during prolonged wear when applied to regions of higher mobility and perspiration, negotiating, negatively affecting drug delivery as well as patient compliance. Use of cross-linked polymer networks or semiocclusive backing layers can overcome this limitation. Furthermore, hydrogel dehydration over time can affect drug release rates, which the use of humectants, glycerol-based water retention systems, or moisture-locking film laminates can mitigate. Further, herbal bioactives like curcumin and resveratrol are chemically unstable in the presence of oxygen and light and require encapsulation to increase stability and shelf life. Finally, the adoption of GMP-compliant manufacturing, employing quality by design (QbD)-based formulation optimization, can avoid batch-to-batch variability [75].

### 10.5.7 FUTURE PERSPECTIVES

The potential of hydrogel-based delivery systems in CVD therapy is moving toward smart, multifunctional, and precision-guided platforms. These hydrogels enable the release of herbal bioactives in response to biological cues. Further, when applied transdermally, in combination with liposomes, phytosomes, or polymeric nanocarriers, they enhance the permeability and bioavailability of phytomedicines such as curcumin, berberine, resveratrol, and ginsenosides. Additionally, hydrogels combined with microneedles enable painless skin permeation, with moisture-retaining and sustained-release properties [76].

In parallel, injectable bioadhesive hydrogels enable the delivery of carriers such as stem cells, exosomes, siRNA, and gene factors, enabling localized, minimally invasive therapy and supporting myocardial repair and vascular regeneration. Going forward, biosensor-enabled hydrogels and AI-assisted dosing feedback systems allow real-time adaptive drug release and further guide toward personalized and self-regulating cardiovascular care [77].

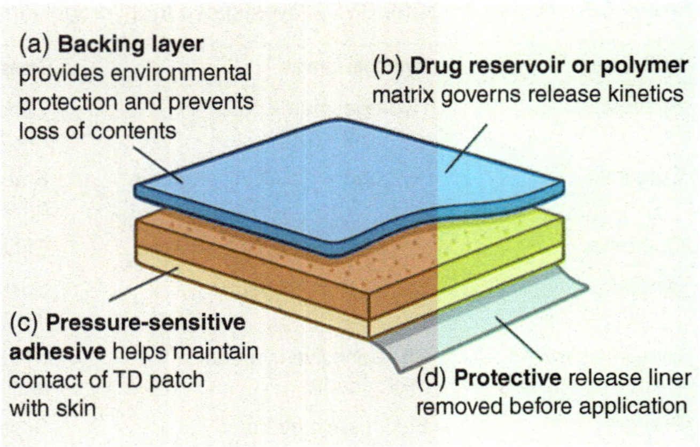


FIGURE 10.3 Components of a transdermal patch.

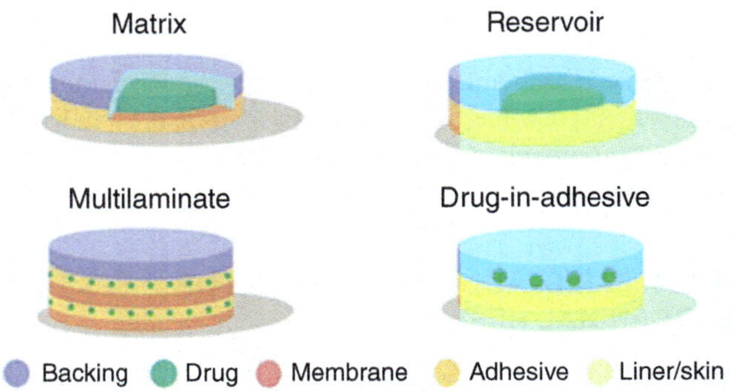


FIGURE 10.4 Types of transdermal patches.

## 10.6 TRANSDERMAL PATCHES IN CARDIOVASCULAR APPLICATIONS

Transdermal (TD) patches are among the most successful and widely accepted forms of noninvasive drug delivery systems, offering numerous benefits over oral and parenteral drug delivery systems, particularly in the delivery of herbal bioactives. These transdermal patches enable controlled and sustained drug delivery across the skin barrier and transport the drug into systemic circulation. Further, they bypass first-pass metabolism and gastrointestinal degradation of drugs, improving their bioavailability and improving patient adherence. Thus, they offer a compelling solution where long-term medication use and consistent plasma levels are critical [78].

### 10.6.1 FUNDAMENTALS OF TD PATCH TECHNOLOGY

TD patches enable drug delivery by facilitating controlled diffusion of active molecules across the stratum corneum into the underlying dermal microcirculation, enabling systemic absorption. A TD patch typically consists of four critical parts or components (Figure 10.3), namely: (a) a backing layer, which provides environmental protection and prevents loss of contents, (b) a drug reservoir or polymer matrix, which governs release kinetics, (c) a pressure-sensitive adhesive that helps in maintaining contact of TD patch with skin, and (d) a protective release liner, which is removed before application [78].

Based on the structural design and release mechanism, transdermal patches are classified into four types, namely, matrix-type patches, reservoir-type patches, drug-in-adhesive patches, and microreservoir patches (Figure 10.4) [78].

- **Matrix-type TD patches:** In these systems, the drug is molecularly dispersed in a polymeric matrix such as PVP or hydroxypropyl methyl cellulose HPMC. These systems show diffusion-controlled release, where the drug gradually migrates from the polymer network into the skin. Due to their simple design, stable release kinetics, and excellent safety profile, matrix patches are widely preferred for chronic cardiovascular therapy and are suitable for both synthetic and herbal bioactives.
- **Reservoir-type TD patches:** These systems consist of a drug contained in a liquid or gel compartment enclosed behind a rate-controlled membrane, allowing precise zero-order release for prolonged durations. Further, these patches also offer precise control over drug release kinetics. However, they have high manufacturing costs and a risk of dose dumping if the rate control membrane is compromised. These are very much suitable for potent cardiovascular drugs where tight plasma-level control is critical.
- **Drug-in-adhesive TD patches:** In this system, the drug is directly incorporated into the pressure-sensitive adhesive layer, which maintains contact with the skin. This design helps in fabricating ultrathin patches with cosmetic appeal, improves patient comfort, and compliance. Due to their ease of fabrication and excellent wearability, they are widely employed for the delivery of both herbal drugs and small molecules.
- **Micro-reservoir TD patches:** In this system, the drug is available as microreservoirs dispersed within a polymeric

matrix. In this system, the polymeric matrix is typically formed by emulsification or coacervation techniques. These systems combine the controlled release precision of reservoir systems and also the robustness and simplicity of matrix systems. The drug from these systems is released in a biphasic manner, with an initial diffusion from microreservoir to polymeric matrix, followed by sustained release from polymeric matrix to skin. Additionally, these systems reduce the risk of dose dumping and also allow tunable pharmacokinetics, thus making it advantageous for chronic CVD therapies.

In addition, to overcome the barrier effect of the stratum corneum to achieve the desired therapeutic level, TD systems employ physical and chemical enhancement techniques. Physical enhancement techniques include iontophoresis, sonophoresis, and microneedle-assisted delivery, which can temporarily disrupt the stratum corneum, enabling permeation of the drug to dermal capillaries for systemic absorption. In contrast, chemical enhancers employ ethanol, terpenes, and nanocarriers like liposomes, ethosomes, and phytosomes in the formulation mixture to improve transdermal permeability of drugs by fluidizing or permeating via lipids of the stratum corneum.

### 10.6.2 MATERIALS USED IN THE FABRICATION OF TD PATCHES

The material selection for the fabrication of TD patches depends on the TD patch design being fabricated. In matrix-type patches, the drug is uniformly mixed with the polymers like HPMC, PVP, PVA, Eudragit variants, or ethylcellulose. These polymers show excellent drug compatibility, flexibility, and belong to the GRAS category, making them suitable for both synthetic and herbal drugs for achieving diffusion-controlled sustained drug delivery systems. In reservoir systems, the rate-controlling release membrane plays the major role, where it is made of materials like ethylene vinyl acetate (EVA), polyurethane, or silica elastomers, offering precise zero-order release. In drug-in-adhesive systems, acrylate, silicone, or polyisobutylene-based pressure-sensitive adhesives (PSAs) are used, into which the drug is directly incorporated. They have been reported to have minimal drug–excipient interactions and suitability for both herbal and aesthetic drugs. Microreservoir systems used polymers like Carbopol, PEG, and EVA-based polymers to incorporate and stabilize microreservoirs of drugs. Additional components like backing layers use polyester/PE and aluminum films, whereas release liners are made of siliconized polyesters [79, 80].

### 10.6.3 FABRICATION OF TD PATCHES

TD patches are fabricated using techniques such as solvent casting and hot-melt extrusion, compression-lamination, and roll-to-roll coating. Among these, solvent casting is widely used for the fabrication of matrix-type and drug-in-adhesive-type TD patches. In this method, the drug is mixed/dispersed into molten polymer or adhesive and is cast onto a Teflon or glass mold. Then, they were dried under controlled temperature and humidity to form a uniform film matrix, which is then laminated with a backing membrane and release liners. In the case of drug-in-adhesive patches, after the drug is mixed with acrylate- or silicone-based pressure-sensitive adhesives, it is then coated onto a backing film using a slot-die coater or knife-over-roll method, compatible with industrial manufacturing. Reservoir-type TD patches are fabricated using heat sealing and laminating techniques, where a drug-loaded gel or liquid formulation is placed between a controlling polymeric membrane, such as EVA or polyurethane, and a backing layer, and sealed. Microreservoir-based systems utilize either emulsification or coacervation techniques, in which the drug is first dispersed as microreservoirs into a polymeric matrix, followed by controlled solvent evaporation and subsequent lamination, film casting onto the backing layer. The microreservoirs of drugs are stabilized using Carbopol, PVP, EVA, and PEG-modified networks and are suitable for both synthetic and herbal drugs. Emerging techniques like 3D printing and roll-to-roll fabrication are gaining attention in recent times for their greater precision and GMP scalability [81–83].

### 10.6.4 DELIVERY OF CVD THERAPEUTICS WITH TD PATCHES

TD patches of both synthetic and herbal cardiovascular drugs are investigated and reported. Synthetic drugs such as nitroglycerin, clonidine, and bisoprolol enable systemic absorption and reduce first-pass metabolism. Nitro-Dur, Transderm-Nitro, and Minitran are commercially available nitroglycerine TD patches commonly used in the management of angina, providing therapeutic effects over 24 hours [84]. Clonidine TD patches are commercially available as Catrapres-TTS and are used in the management of hypertension; these release the drug over seven days. [85] A once-a-day patch of bisoprolol, Brisopatch, is used in the management of hypertension and heart failure [86]. Additionally, nicotine patches like Nicorette InvisiPatch, NicoDerm CQ, and others are used in smoking cessation, helping to mitigate cardiovascular risk associated with tobacco withdrawal [87].

With respect to herbal bioactives, even though there are no Food and Drug Administration (FDA)-approved TD patches, several studies have been conducted to have promising therapeutic effects (Table 10.6). Resveratrol-loaded TD patches using HPMC/PVP as a polymer matrix demonstrated enhanced transdermal permeation and bioavailability [88]. Curcumin-based TD patches have shown effective controlled release and enhanced permeation, making them potentially useful in anti-inflammatory and anti-sclerotic CVD therapy [89]. Quercetin TD patches have shown improved permeation in *in vitro* models and are suitable for once-a-day models, with their endothelial-modulating and vasoprotective actions [90]. Drug-in-adhesives-based TD patches of ginsenoside Rb1confirmed percutaneous absorption from porcine skin models, and potential cardiometabolic applications [91].

**Table 10.6** Herbal drugs for CVDs investigated for transdermal patches.

| Herbal drugs | TD patch platform | Key findings | CVD relevance | Source |
|---|---|---|---|---|
| Resveratrol | Matrix patch (HPMC/ PV + permeation enhancer) | Polymer, permeation-enhancer ratios were optimized, >48-hours release obtained, improved skin permeation | Anti-inflammatory, antioxidant, and endothelial protection | [88] |
| Curcumin | QbD-optimized TD patch | Steady flux and controlled release, improved stability and permeation of curcumin | Anti-inflammatory, anti-atherogenic, antioxidant | [89] |
| Quercetin | Polymeric TD patch | Enhanced percutaneous absorption, 24 hours release | Vasoprotective, antioxidant | [90] |
| Ginsenoside Rb1 | Adhesive TD patch | Optimal absorption through *ex vivo* porcine skin model | Antithrombotic, vasodilatory activity | [91] |
| Puerarin | Electrospun patch | Sustained release of drug >20 days, high biocompatibility | Anti-ischemic, endothelial protective | [64] |
| EGCG | Hydrogel film patch | Stable film with enhanced antioxidant activity, >48-hours release | Inhibits LDL oxidation | [65] |

Electrospun PLLA patches loaded with puerarin demonstrated excellent biocompatibility and showed sustained drug delivery, showing potential in chronic cardiovascular therapies [64]. These findings collectively validate the efficiency of TD patches in cardiovascular therapies.

### 10.6.5 ADVANTAGES IN TD DRUG DELIVERY OF HERBAL CARDIOVASCULAR THERAPEUTICS

Transdermal delivery of herbal bioactives for cardiovascular applications offers several advantages by overcoming the key limitations of oral administration, such as poor intestinal stability, rapid first-pass metabolism, and chemical instability. Phytochemicals like curcumin, resveratrol, quercetin, and ginsenoside, which also suffer from short plasma half-life, can achieve steady-state plasma levels and enhance systemic exposure when delivered via skin. Further, the route is noninvasive, painless, and patient-compliant, making it advantageous for elderly and chronically ill patients with CVD therapies. In addition, the TD route enables controlled or extended release of the drug for prolonged periods of 24 hours and beyond. Thus, reducing the dosing frequency improves adherence. Further, the flexibility in design or fabrication of TD patches enables combination therapy incorporating dual drugs (a synthetic and a herbal), making them much more valuable in chronic CVD therapy [92, 93].

### 10.6.6 CHALLENGES AND LIMITATIONS

Delivery of herbal bioactives via transdermal drug delivery faces several important challenges. Moderately lipophilic and highly potent drugs are ideal for TD patch-based drug delivery. Many herbal extracts and CVD drugs (statins, diuretics) require higher doses than a patch can hold, requiring increased drug concentration, selective purification, and nanoencapsulation techniques. Skin permeability is another major issue, as most of the herbal compounds, such as alkaloids, polyphenols, and saponins, are too large and too polar; their permeability via skin is limited. This necessitates the use of chemical and physical permeation enhancers, which, although they improve drug permeation via skin, can compromise drug stability. Many herbal bioactives are sensitive to heat, light, oxygen, and residual solvents; hence, in fabrication, measures have to be taken to minimize the above exposures. Additionally, patient variability (age, gender, skin condition, or movement) can also affect patch adhesion and drug absorption consistency. Use of flexible hydrogel-based bioadhesive patches can overcome this issue to some extent [79].

Additionally, herbal extracts can show skin irritation and allergic reactions, which necessitate a comprehensive dermal evaluation and adherence to international regulatory standards (FDA, European Medicines Agency (EMA), Ministry of AYUSH (AYUSH) [94]. Moreover, regulatory bodies expect information on stability, permeation, skin safety, and pharmacokinetic evaluation, necessitating the use of an International Council for Harmonisation (ICH) and FDA-aligned formulation development process and GMP-compliant manufacturing, with early integration of *in vitro*, *ex vivo*, and *in vivo* correlation studies for successful clinical translation [95].

### 10.6.7 FUTURE PROSPECTS OF TD PATCH-BASED DELIVERY OF HERBAL DRUGS IN CVDs

The future of herbal TD patches focuses on the development of smart next-generation, highly efficient, personalized platforms that can overcome current limitations of permeability, dose control, and stability. Further, advances in nanotechnology (e.g., Phytosomes, transferosomes, and nanoparticle-based patches) are expected to improve skin permeability and bioavailability of herbal bioactives significantly. In addition, hybrid systems combining TD patch technologies with microneedles and hydrogels are emerging as highly promising strategies for improved permeation, controlled release, and friendly administration [79, 96]. Furthermore, integration of biosensor-enabled systems helps in real-time monitoring and on-demand drug release, which is particularly advantageous in CVD therapy, and helps in preventive and therapeutic care. With rising interest in phytochemicals globally, herbal TD systems are expected to transition from lab to clinical commercialization [96].

## 10.7 COMPARISON OF MICRONEEDLES, HYDROGELS, AND TD PATCHES

From a pharmacodynamic and pharmacokinetic perspective, these three transdermal delivery techniques demonstrate distinct advantages in the delivery of herbal drugs toward CVD applications. Microneedles bypass stratum corneum and provide direct access of drug to the dermis, enabling rapid systemic absorption. Further, the release can be configurable for sustained, immediate, or pulsatile release profiles, making them suitable for emergency cardiovascular conditions such as angina, as well as chronic conditions like hypertension. Hydrogels are biocompatible and excel in sustained, moisture-assisted transdermal drug delivery, improving flux of herbal drugs. Injectable hydrogels on the other hand show immense potential in myocardial tissue repair and healing. TD patches present noninvasive long-term systemic exposure, ideal for chronic maintenance therapy, where stable plasma concentrations are required. In terms of safety and patient compliance, all three platforms are patient-centric [97–99] (Table 10.7).

## 10.8 REGULATORY LANDSCAPE OF HERBAL DRUG-LOADED MICRONEEDLES, HYDROGELS, AND TRANSDERMAL PATCHES

The regulatory pathway of herbal drug-based TDDS (microneedles, hydrogels, and transdermal patches) needs to pass through rigorous global quality frameworks. It must comply not only with conventional pharmaceutical guidelines but also with herbal drug-specific regulations and requirements set by various regulatory agencies. Regulatory agencies like the FDA, EMA, and AYUSH have placed a strong emphasis on source authentication, phytochemical standardization, batch reproducibility, and analytical fingerprinting, as herbal bioactives inherently show greater variability when compared to synthetic drugs. Microneedle patches are evaluated for drug–device compatibility, mechanical robustness, sterility, and dermal biocompatibility. Further, pharmaceutical-related standards related to release kinetics, stability, and pharmacokinetic consistency are also evaluated. Hydrogels are required to demonstrate biocompatibility, predictable release behavior, long-term stability under physiological conditions, and water retention. Whereas, TD patches meet strict standards for component safety, performance, adhesion, dose accuracy, stability, and prevention of dose dumping. They are evaluated under GMP and ICH guidelines, with emphasis on *in vitro* permeation testing, skin irritation studies, and batch reproducibility. Within the intellectual property domain, direct claims on naturally occurring phytochemicals are generally restricted. Hence, a meaningful patent protection, typically focusing on novel design architectures, or process innovations, is required, e.g., nanocarrier-integrated hydrogels of herbal bioactives and microneedle platforms for enhancing permeability. Further, patents also target extraction procedures, purification techniques, or QbD-driven standardization procedures, serving both regulatory and commercial objectives. Despite the commercial success of transdermal systems for synthetic drugs, phytomedicine-based TDDS still face challenges related to extract variability, stability, and GMP standard reproducibility, limiting the commercial success. Further, these systems also involve high manufacturing complexity and regulatory issues. Hence, large-scale adoption is only feasible when it has demonstrated a superior therapeutic advantage over oral herbal supplementation [100–103].

To overcome these translational bottlenecks, collaborative innovation models involving academia, industry, and

**Table 10.7** Comparative evaluation of the three advanced transdermal delivery systems.

| Platform | Release profile | Best suited for | Herbal suitability | Technology readiness |
|---|---|---|---|---|
| Microneedles | Rapid/sustained/pulsatile | Acute use (angina, hypertensive crisis), dose precision | Excellent suitability, bypasses poor permeability of large phenolic herbal drugs like curcumin | Highly translational, already in dermatology and vaccine, CVD trials are emerging |
| Hydrogels | Moisture-assisted sustained release | Chronic therapy, requiring continuous low-dose delivery, high hydration environments | Very high, stabilizes herbal compounds, enhances skin permeation, and reduces irritation. | Preclinical to early clinical stages in CVD |
| Transdermal patches | Controlled delivery with steady-state plasma concentrations | Long-term maintenance therapy (hypertension prevention) | Moderately suitable for potent, lipophilic drugs with low doses, like resveratrol | FDA-approved for synthetic CVD drugs, herbal patches not yet approved |
| Hybrid systems (hydrogel-loaded MN patch) | Dual phase (deep penetration, fast entry, sustained release) | Both acute and chronic cardiovascular conditions | Optimal suitability, combines permeation, protection, and sustained release | Next-generation platforms under active development, high future potential |

translational medicine authorities are increasingly being recognized as critical enablers for clinically viable phytopharmaceutical transdermal platforms.

## 10.9 EMERGING TRENDS AND FUTURE PROSPECTS

The future of phytomedicine-based cardiovascular therapy via skin is moving toward smart and highly personalized technologies. A major shift is seen with smart transdermal patches and wearable microneedle systems, which are no longer just passive drug delivery systems, but now function as response-sensitive platforms capable of releasing herbal bioactives in response to the biological cues (like heart rate, blood pressure, or inflammatory markers). These systems allow dose adjustment in real time, matching therapeutic release with the changing needs of the patient. At the same time, fabrication of microneedles, transdermal patch, or hydrogels can be personalized based on patients' ages, skin type, and disease condition, thereby minimizing variability and increasing patient compliance and therapeutic benefits. Further, integration of AI and machine learning can accelerate the development of phytopharmaceutical-based transdermal systems by predicting skin permeation, ingredient selection, and optimizing herb–drug interaction before the clinical setting (Figure 10.5) [104–107]. However, large-scale production also relies on clinical validation, GMP-ready manufacturing, regulatory approval, and strong IP protection. If the benchmarks are achieved, these systems can mainstream cardiovascular therapy.

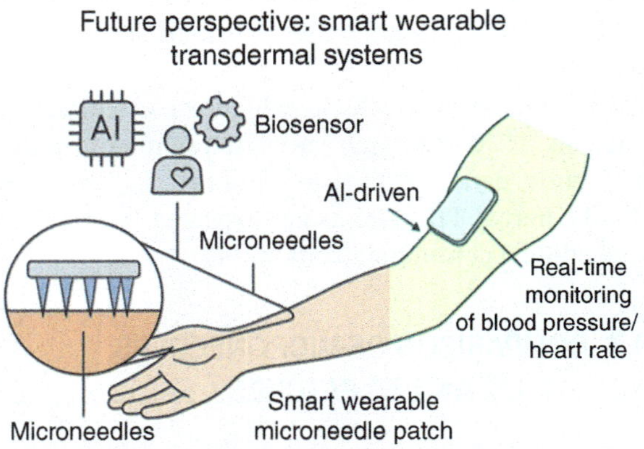


**FIGURE 10.5** AI integrated hybrid TDDS.

## 10.10 CONCLUSION

Traditional herbs hold great potential in the treatment of cardiovascular disorders. However, the clinical translation of these herbal bioactives is hindered by their pharmacokinetic properties. Delivery of these phytochemicals as microneedles, hydrogels, and transdermal patches with phytomedicine can materially improve the therapeutic efficiency of these drugs by addressing the long-standing liabilities of oral delivery, namely poor solubility, instability, extensive first-pass metabolism, and fluctuating plasma exposure. Further, these drug delivery systems are of superior patient compliance compared to oral and parenteral routes. Moreover, these systems can be tuned to meet the chronic therapies. Going forward, with advancement toward smart, hybrid, feedback, and personalized systems, these systems can be tailored for patients' needs to get safer, more effective, and patient-centric cardiovascular therapeutics. Successful clinical translation depends on standardization of herbal bioactives, GMP-compliant manufacturing, regulatory alignment, and strong clinical validation.

## REFERENCES


1. Roth, G.A., Mensah, G.A., Johnson, C.O. et al. (2020). Global burden of cardiovascular diseases and risk factors, 1990–2019: update from the GBD 2019 study. *J. Am. Coll. Cardiol.* 76 (25): 2982–3021.
2. Mensah, G.A., Roth, G.A., and Fuster, V. (2019). *The Global Burden of Cardiovascular Diseases and Risk Factors: 2020 and Beyond*. Washington, DC: American College of Cardiology Foundation.
3. Cicha, I. (2021). The grand challenges in cardiovascular drug delivery. *Front. Drug Deliv.* 1: 784731.
4. Bertol, E. and Favretto, D. (2022). Pharmacokinetics: drug absorption, distribution, and elimination. In: *Karch's Drug Abuse Handbook*, 133–178. CRC Press.
5. Pala, R., Anju, V., Dyavaiah, M. et al. (2020). Nanoparticle-mediated drug delivery for the treatment of cardiovascular diseases. *Int. J. Nanomedicine* 3741–3769.
6. Ita, K. (2017). The potential use of transdermal drug delivery for the prophylaxis and management of stroke and coronary artery disease. *Pharmacol. Rep.* 69 (6): 1322–1327.
7. Iravani, S. and Varma, R.S.J.M. (2022). Advanced drug delivery micro-and nanosystems for cardiovascular diseases. *Molecules* 27 (18): 5843.
8. Shaito, A., Thuan, D.T.B., Phu, H.T. et al. (2020). Herbal medicine for cardiovascular diseases: efficacy, mechanisms, and safety. *Front. Pharmacol.* 11: 422.
9. Ciumărnean, L., Milaciu, M.V., Runcan, O. et al. (2020). The effects of flavonoids in cardiovascular diseases. *Molecules* 25 (18): 4320.
10. Prajapati, A.K. and Shah, G. (2025). Alkaloids and their mechanisms of action in cardiovascular diseases. *Int. J. Drug Discov. Pharmacol.* 4 (3): 100017.
11. Mahomoodally, F. and Ramjuttun, P. (2019). Terpenoids against cardiovascular diseases. In: *Terpenoids Against Human Diseases*, 209–231. CRC Press.
12. Iqbal, I., Wilairatana, P., Saqib, F. et al. (2023). Plant polyphenols and their potential benefits on cardiovascular health: a review. *Molecules* 28 (17): 6403.

13. Ma, X., Lu, J., Gu, X.-R. et al. (2022). Cardioprotective effects and mechanisms of saponins on cardiovascular disease. *Nat. Prod. Commun.* 17 (12): 1934578X221147404.

14. Villaescusa, L., Zaragozá, C., Zaragozá, F., and Tamargo, J. (2023). Herbal medicines for the treatment of cardiovascular diseases: benefits and risks–a narrative review. *Int. J. Cardiol.* 385: 44–52.

15. Mashour, N.H., Lin, G.I., and Frishman, W.H. (1998). Herbal medicine for the treatment of cardiovascular disease: clinical considerations. *Arch. Intern. Med.* 158 (20): 2225–2234.

16. Cheng, Y.-C., Li, T.S., Su, H.L. et al. (2020). Transdermal delivery systems of natural products applied to skin therapy and care. *Molecules* 25 (21): 5051.

17. Karve, T., Dandekar, A., Agrahari, V. et al. (2024). Long-acting transdermal drug delivery formulations: current developments and innovative pharmaceutical approaches. *Adv. Drug Deliv. Rev.* 210: 115326.

18. Yu, Y.-Q., Yang, X., Wu, X.-F., and Fan, Y.-B.J. (2021). Enhancing permeation of drug molecules across the skin via delivery in nanocarriers: novel strategies for effective transdermal applications. 9: 646554.

19. Lopez-Ojeda, W., Pandey, A., Alhajj, M., and Oakley, A.M. (2022). Anatomy, skin (integument). In: *Stat Pearls*. Stat Pearls Publishing.

20. Crasta, A., Painginkar, T., Sreedevi, A. et al. (2025). Transdermal drug delivery system: a comprehensive review of innovative strategies, applications, and regulatory perspectives. 24: 100245.

21. Benet, L.Z., Hosey, C.M., Ursu, O., and Oprea, T.I. (2016). BDDCS, the Rule of 5 and drugability. *Adv. Drug Deliv. Rev.* 101: 89–98.

22. Sparr, E., Björklund, S., Pham, Q.D. et al. (2023). The stratum corneum barrier–from molecular scale to macroscopic properties. *Curr. Opin. Colloid Interface Sci.* 67: 101725.

23. Zhou, R., Yu, J., Gu, Z., and Zhang, Y.J. (2022). Microneedle-mediated therapy for cardiovascular diseases. *Drug Deliv. Transl. Res.* 12 (2): 472–483.

24. Aldawood, F.K., Andar, A., and Desai, S.J.P. (2021). A comprehensive review of microneedles: types, materials, processes, characterizations and applications. *Polymers* 13 (16): 2815.

25. Luo, X., Yang, L., and Cui, Y. (2023). Microneedles: materials, fabrication, and biomedical applications. *Biomed. Microdevices* 25 (3): 20.

26. Zhang, X., Li, M., Gao, Q. et al. (2024). Cutting-edge microneedle innovations: transforming the landscape of cardiovascular and metabolic disease management. *iScience* 27 (9).

27. Panda, A., Sharma, P.K., Shivakumar, H. et al. (2021). Nicotine loaded dissolving microneedles for nicotine replacement therapy. *J. Drug Deliv. Sci. Technol.* 61: 102300.

28. He, J., Zhang, Z., Zheng, X. et al. (2021). Design and evaluation of dissolving microneedles for enhanced dermal delivery of propranolol hydrochloride. *Pharmaceutics* 13 (4): 579.

29. Ita, K., Hatsakorzian, N., and Tolstikov, V. (2013). Microneedle-mediated delivery of atenolol and bisoprolol hemifumarate. *J. Nanopharm. Drug Deliv.* 1 (1): 38–44.

30. Arshad, M.S., Zafar, S., Zahra, A.T. et al. (2021). Fabrication and characterisation of self-applicating heparin sodium microneedle patches. *J. Drug Target.* 29 (1): 60–68.

31. Chaiprateep, E.-O., Sengupta, S., and Keck, C.M. (2025). Microneedle-assisted delivery of curcumin: evaluating the effects of needle length and formulation. *Micromachines* 16 (2): 155.

32. Xing, B., Luo, Q., Gan, T. et al. (2024). Resveratrol-loaded dissolving microneedles: fabrication and *in vitro* evaluation. *Pharm. Front.* 6 (04): e439–e438.

33. Cui, X., Geng, H., Guo, H. et al. (2024). Visualizing the transdermal delivery of berberine loaded within chitosan microneedles using mass spectrometry imaging. *Anal. Bioanal. Chem.* 416 (29): 6869–6877.

34. Anjani, Q.K., Moreno-Castellanos, N., Adhami, M. et al. (2025). Quercetin loaded polymeric dissolving microarray patches: fabrication, characterisation and evaluation. *Drug Deliv. Transl. Res.* 15 (1): 355–371.

35. Wang, Y., Zhong, C., Wang, K. et al. (2025). A self-adhesive ginsenoside Rk3/Metformin-loaded hydrogel microneedle for management of systemic sclerosis. *Gels* 11 (6): 384.

36. Kaur, S.D., Choudhary, S., Sen, S. et al. (2025). Microneedle patches: the next frontier in cardiovascular care. *Drug Deliv. Transl. Res.* 1–16.

37. Avcil, M. and Çelik, A. (2021). Microneedles in drug delivery: progress and challenges. *Micromachines* 12 (11): 1321.

38. O'Connor AC, Beaulieu TJ, Rothrock GD (2016). Economic Analysis of Technology Infrastructure Needs for Roll-to-Roll Manufacturing. (NIST, Gaithersburg, MD) NIST GCR 16-008.

39. Sutar, A.D. and Shukla, R. (2025). Emerging smart microneedle technologies in psoriasis: convergence of nanocarriers, machine learning, and personalized delivery. *RSC Pharm.* 2: 1268–1291.

40. Gupta, J., Gupta, R., and Vanshita, N. (2021). Microneedle technology: an insight into recent advancements and future trends in drug and vaccine delivery. *Assay Drug Dev. Technol.* 19 (2): 97–114.

41. Cao, H., Duan, L., Zhang, Y. et al. (2021). Current hydrogel advances in physicochemical and biological response-driven biomedical application diversity. *Signal Transduct. Target. Ther.* 6 (1): 426.

42. Alex, M., Alsawaftah, N.M., and Husseini, G.A. (2024). State-of-all-the-art and prospective hydrogel-based transdermal drug delivery systems. *Appl. Sci.* 14 (7): 2926.

43. Ho, T.C., Chang, C.C., Chan, H.P. et al. (2022). Hydrogels: properties and applications in biomedicine. *Molecules* 27 (9): 2902.

44. Ahmad, Z., Salman, S., Khan, S.A. et al. (2022). Versatility of hydrogels: from synthetic strategies, classification, and properties to biomedical applications. *Gels* 8 (3): 167.

45. Zhao, L., Zhou, Y., Zhang, J. et al. (2023). Natural polymer-based hydrogels: from polymer to biomedical applications. *Pharmaceutics* 15 (10): 2514.

46. Madduma-Bandarage, U.S. and Madihally, S.V. (2021). Synthetic hydrogels: synthesis, novel trends, and applications. *J. Appl. Polym. Sci.* 138 (19): 50376.

47. Xu, X., Liu, Y., Fu, W. et al. (2020). Poly (N-isopropylacrylamide)-based thermoresponsive composite hydrogels for biomedical applications. *Polymers* 12 (3): 580.

48. Bashir, S., Hina, M., Iqbal, J. et al. (2020). Fundamental concepts of hydrogels: synthesis, properties, and their applications. *Polymers* 12 (11): 2702.

49. Huang, S., Hong, X., Zhao, M. et al. (2022). Nanocomposite hydrogels for biomedical applications. *Bioeng. Transl. Med.* 7 (3): e10315.

50. Liao, X., Yang, X., Deng, H. et al. (2020). Injectable hydrogel-based nanocomposites for cardiovascular diseases. *Front. Bioeng. Biotechnol.* 8: 251.

51. Yang, J., Chen, Y., Zhao, L. et al. (2023). Constructions and properties of physically cross-linked hydrogels based on natural polymers. *Polym. Rev.* 63 (3): 574–612.

52. Bustamante-Torres, M., Romero-Fierro, D., Arcentales-Vera, B. et al. (2021). Hydrogels classification according to the physical or chemical interactions and as stimuli-sensitive materials. *Gels* 7 (4): 182.

53. Vigata, M., Meinert, C., Hutmacher, D.W., and Bock, N. (2020). Hydrogels as drug delivery systems: a review of current characterization and evaluation techniques. *Pharmaceutics* 12 (12): 1188.

54. Ghasemiyeh, P. and Mohammadi-Samani, S. (2019). Hydrogels as drug delivery systems; pros and cons %j trends in pharmaceutical sciences and technologies. *Trends Pharm. Sci.* 5 (1): 7–24.

55. Dobhal, N., Bhatt, J., and Joshi, B.C. (2022). Formulation and characterization of amlodipine loaded in-situ film forming hydrogen for dermal drug delivery. *J. Med. Pharm. Allied Sci.* 11: 4928–4933.

56. Salah, N.M., Elbedaiwy, H.M., Helmy, M.W., and El-Salamouni, N.S. (2024). Topical amlodipine-loaded solid lipid nanoparticles for enhanced burn wound healing: a repurposed approach. *Int. J. Pharm.* 662: 124484.

57. Orduño Rodríguez, A.M., Pérez Martínez, C.J., del Castillo, C.T. et al. (2020). Nanocomposite hydrogel of poly (vinyl alcohol) and biocatalytically synthesized polypyrrole as potential system for controlled release of metoprolol. *Polym. Bull.* 77 (3): 1217–1232.

58. Sharma, S., Kirwale, S.S., Katakia, Y.T. et al. (2023). Development and evaluation of a simvastatin-loaded biopolymeric scaffold for improved angiogenesis and healing of diabetic wounds. *J. Drug Deliv. Sci. Technol.* 87: 104832.

59. Saghafi, F., Ramezani, V., Jafari-Nedooshan, J. et al. (2023). Efficacy of topical atorvastatin-loaded emulgel and nano-emulgel 1% on post-laparotomy pain and wound healing: a randomized double-blind placebo-controlled clinical trial. *Int. Wound J.* 20 (10): 4006–4014.

60. Law, S.K., Liu, C.W.C., Tong, C.W.S., and Au, D.C.T. (2024). Potential of resveratrol to combine with hydrogel for photodynamic therapy against bacteria and cancer—a review. *Biomedicine* 12 (9): 2095.

61. Zhang, Y., Zhou, Z., Liu, N. et al. (2025). Curcumin-loaded PLGA microparticles integrated with ZnO/Gel MA hydrogel microneedles for infectious wound healing and reduction of hypertrophic scars. *J. Nanobiotechnol.* 23 (1): 455.

62. Yi, Y., Yang, Z., Zhou, C. et al. (2024). Quercetin-encapsulated Gel Ma hydrogel microneedle reduces oxidative stress and facilitates wound healing. *Nano TransMed* 3: 100030.

63. Cometa, S., Bonifacio, M.A., Licini, C. et al. (2021). Innovative eco-friendly hydrogel film for Berberine delivery in skin applications. *Molecules* 26 (16): 4901.

64. Zhang, D., Xu, D., Huang, X. et al. (2024). Puerarin-loaded electrospun patches with anti-inflammatory and pro-collagen synthesis properties for pelvic floor reconstruction. *Adv. Sci. (Weinh.)* 11 (21): e2308590.

65. Mehta, C.H., Velagacherla, V., Manandhar, S. et al. (2024). Development of epigallocatechin 3-gallate-loaded hydrogel nanocomposites for oral submucous fibrosis. *AAPS PharmSciTech* 25 (4): 66.

66. Xu, G., Tian, D., Xu, P. et al. (2025). Transdermal delivery of resveratrol by a nanomicelle-loaded enzyme-triggered hydrogel for diabetic wound healing. *ACS Appl. Nano Mater.* 8 (5): 2228–2237.

67. He, S., Zhang, Z., Luo, R. et al. (2023). Advances in injectable hydrogel strategies for heart failure treatment. *Adv. Healthc. Mater.* 12 (19): 2300029.

68. Hoeeg, C., Dolatshahi-Pirouz, A., and Follin, B. (2021). Injectable hydrogels for improving cardiac cell therapy—*in vivo* evidence and translational challenges. *Gels* 7 (1): 7.

69. Zhang, Y., Xu, Y., and Gao, J. (2023). The engineering and application of extracellular matrix hydrogels: a review. *Biomater. Sci.* 11 (11): 3784–3799.

70. Cattelan, G., Guerrero Gerbolés, A., Foresti, R. et al. (2020). Alginate formulations: current developments in the race for hydrogel-based cardiac regeneration. *Front. Bioeng. Biotechnol.* 8: 414.

71. Li, Z., Masumoto, H., Jo, J.I. et al. (2018). Sustained release of basic fibroblast growth factor using gelatin hydrogel improved left ventricular function through the alteration of collagen subtype in a rat chronic myocardial infarction model. *Gen. Thorac. Cardiovasc. Surg.* 66 (11): 641–647.

72. Wu, T. and Liu, W. (2022). Functional hydrogels for the treatment of myocardial infarction. *NPG Asia Mater.* 14 (1): 9.

73. Wahab, S., Ahmad, I., Irfan, S. et al. (2021). Hydrogel: an encouraging nanocarrier system for the delivery of herbal bioactive compounds. *Curr. Nanosci.* 17 (6): 797–807.

74. Liu, B. and Chen, K.J.G. (2024). Advances in hydrogel-based drug delivery systems. *Gels* 10 (4): 262.

75. Lai, W.-F. and Rogach, A.L. (2017). Hydrogel-based materials for delivery of herbal medicines. *ACS Appl. Mater. Interfaces* 9 (13): 11309–11320.

76. Sahu, N., Gupta, D., and Nautiyal, U. (2020). Hydrogel: preparation, characterization and applications. *Asian Pac. J. Nurs. Health Sci.* 3 (1): 1–11.

77. Kováč, J., Priščáková, P., Gbelcová, H. et al. (2023). Bioadhesive and injectable hydrogels and their correlation with mesenchymal stem cells differentiation for cartilage repair: a mini-review. *Polymers* 15 (21): 4228.

78. Bird, D. and Ravindra, N.M. (2020). Transdermal drug delivery and patches—an overview. *Med. Devices Sens.* 3 (6): e10069.

79. Kulkarni, P., Ahmed, K.A., Shirsand, S.B. et al. (2026). Transdermal patches: design, evaluation, and potential applications in modern therapeutics. *Biomed. Mater. Devices* 4: 1609–1627.

80. Kumar, V., Praveen, N., Kewlani, P. et al. (2023). Transdermal drug delivery systems. In: *Advanced Drug Delivery: Methods and Applications*, 333–362. Singapore: Springer Nature.

81. Ashfaq, A., Riaz, T., Waqar, M.A. et al. (2024). A comprehensive review on transdermal patches as an efficient approach for the delivery of drug. *Polym.-Plast. Technol. Mater.* 63 (8): 1045–1069.

82. Cammarano, A., Dello Iacono, S., Meglio, C., and Nicolais, L. (2023). Advances in transdermal drug delivery systems: a bibliometric and patent analysis. *Pharmaceutics* 15 (12): 2762.

83. Villota, I., Calvo, P.C., Campo, O.I. et al. (2022). Manufacturing of a transdermal patch in 3D printing. *Micromachines* 13 (12): 2190.

84. Wong, W.F., Ang, K.P., Sethi, G., and Looi, C.Y. (2023). Recent advancement of medical patch for transdermal drug delivery. *Medicina* 59 (4): 778.

85. Majee, S.B., Gupti, S., Mishra, T., and Bera, R.J. (2025). *In vitro*, *ex vivo* and *in vivo* studies on anti-hypertensive-loaded transdermal and buccal patches. *J. Drug Deliv. Ther.* 15 (3): 142–150.

86. Kiuchi, S., Hisatake, S., Kabuki, T. et al. (2020). Bisoprolol transdermal patch improves orthostatic hypotension in patients with chronic heart failure and hypertension. *Clin. Exp. Hypertens.* 42 (6): 539–544.

87. Olsson Gisleskog, P.O., Perez Ruixo, J.J., Westin, Å. et al. (2021). Nicotine population pharmacokinetics in healthy smokers after intravenous, oral, buccal and transdermal administration. *Clin. Pharmacokinet.* 60 (4): 541–561.

88. Gadag, S., Narayan, R., Nayak, Y. et al. (2023). Design, development and evaluation of resveratrol transdermal patches for breast cancer therapy. *Int. J. Pharm.* 632: 122558.

89. Kriplani, P., Guarve, K., and Singh, B.U. (2021). Formulation optimization and characterization of transdermal film of curcumin by response surface methodology. *Chin. Herb. Med.* 13 (2): 274–285.

90. Kharia, A., Singhai, A., and Gilhotra, R.J. (2020). Formualtion and evalaution of transdermal patch for the treatment of inflammation. *J. Pharm. Sci. Res.* 12 (6): 780–788.

91. Wang, L., Lu, A.P., Yu, Z.L. et al. (2014). The melanogenesis-inhibitory effect and the percutaneous formulation of ginsenoside Rb1. *AAPS PharmSciTech* 15 (5): 1252–1262.

92. Ramadon, D., McCrudden, M.T., Courtenay, A.J., and Donnelly, R.F. (2022). Enhancement strategies for transdermal drug delivery systems: current trends and applications. *Drug Deliv. Transl. Res.* 12 (4): 758–791.

93. Pulipati, S., Puttagunta, S.B., Varshini, S.K. et al. (2025). Exploring the insights and innovations of herbal transdermal patches: A comprehensive review. *IOSR J Dent Med Sci* 24 (3): 64–75.

94. Daniel, A.B., Strickland, J., Allen, D. et al. (2018). International regulatory requirements for skin sensitization testing. *Regul. Toxicol. Pharmacol.* 95: 52–65.

95. Simões, A., Veiga, F., and Vitorino, C. (2024). Question-based review for pharmaceutical development: an enhanced quality approach. *Eur. J. Pharm. Biopharm.* 195: 114174.

96. Mishra, S., Verma, P., Gupta, S. et al. (2022). Nanocarrier and herbal based transdermal patch: an advantage over other drug delivery systems. *Ann. Ayurvedic Med.* 11: 145–156.

97. Waghule, T., Singhvi, G., Dubey, S.K. et al. (2019). Microneedles: a smart approach and increasing potential for transdermal drug delivery system. *Biomed. Pharmacother.* 109: 1249–1258.

98. Labie, H. and Blanzat, M. (2023). Hydrogels for dermal and transdermal drug delivery. *Int. J. Pharm.* 11 (12): 4073–4093.

99. Tiwari, C., Choudhary, M., Malik, P. et al. (2022). Transdermal patch: a novel approach for transdermal. *Drug Deliv.* 12 (6): 179–188.

100. Barkat, M.A., Goyal, A., Barkat, H.A. et al. (2021). Herbal medicine: clinical perspective and regulatory status. *Comb. Chem. High Throughput Screen.* 24 (10): 1573–1582.

101. Joyce, P., Allen, C.J., Alonso, M.J. et al. (2024). A translational framework to DELIVER nanomedicines to the clinic. *Nat. Nanotechnol.* 19 (11): 1597–1611.

102. Gujarathi, N.A., Bakliwal, A.A., Rane, B.R. et al. (2022). Regulatory aspects of drug development for dermal products. In: *Topical and Transdermal Drug Delivery Systems*, 287–310. Apple Academic Press.

103. Paudel, K.S., Milewski, M., Swadley, C.L. et al. (2010). Challenges and opportunities in dermal/transdermal delivery. *Ther. Deliv.* 1 (1): 109–131.

104. Shah SWA, Li, X., Yuan, H. et al. (2025). Innovative transdermal drug delivery systems: benefits, challenges, and emerging application. *BMEMat* 3: e70001.

105. Jeong, W.Y., Kwon, M., Choi, H.E., and Kim, K.S. (2021). Recent advances in transdermal drug delivery systems: a review. *Biomater. Res.* 25 (1): 24.

106. Panchpuri, M., Painuli, R., and Kumar, C. (2025). Artificial intelligence in smart drug delivery systems: a step toward personalized medicine. *RSC Pharm.* 2: 882–914.

107. Zhang, J., Yang, F., Wu, H. et al. (2025). Wearable transdermal drug delivery system controlled by wirelessly powered acoustic waves. *J. Control. Release* 381: 113619.

CHAPTER 11

# Preclinical and Clinical Studies on Herbal Cardiovascular Therapies

**Naga Venkata Lakshmi Sirisha Mulukuri[1], Talluri Sesha Rajeswari[2], Ponakampalli Rambabu[3], and Dasari Santhi Krupa[3]**

[1] *Department of Pharmacognosy, Nitte College of Pharmaceutical Sciences, Nitte (Deemed to be University), Bengaluru, Karnataka, India*

[2] *Ernest Mario School of Pharmacy, Rutgers University, Piscataway, New Jersey, USA*

[3] *Department of Pharmacognosy, Krishna University College of Pharmaceutical Sciences and Research, Machilipatnam, Andhra Pradesh, India*

## 11.1 INTRODUCTION

The frequency of cardiovascular illnesses is significant, particularly in older people. Additionally, people with chronic conditions like diabetes mellitus or impaired kidney function, as well as those with other concomitant conditions, are more likely to have cardiovascular illnesses [1–4]. Increased arterial pressure, which causes hypertension; elevated lipid content, which causes coronary artery disease (CAD); low heart function, which causes heart failure; and abruptly reduced heart blood flow, which can cause stroke, are cardiovascular conditions that significantly impair people's quality of life [5].

As per the WHO data of 2021, disorders related to cardiovascular system are the major etiology behind high mortality rate across the globe that accounts for approximately 179 lakhs deaths per year. So, there is a need to increase awareness, adopt preventive measures, and practice safe and effective treatment methods to safeguard mankind from cardiovascular disorders.

In this modern era, though there are different allopathic medications that majorly focus on symptomatic relief or that target the pathological basis of the CVDs, they have their own drawbacks like unwanted side effects, cost, and some of them demand long-term use of medications. To overcome the existing drawbacks of present treatment methods, there is a need to focus on herbal remedies, which can treat life-threatening cardiovascular disorders that affect the quality of life of mankind [6].

Ancient history reminds the use of conventional systems of healthcare around the world: Ayurveda, traditional Chinese medicine (TCM), and Unani. Traditional healthcare systems focus on herbal medicine that is derived from the use of plant components like leaves, roots, seeds, bark, and flowers. Herbal medicine offers more benefits, as they possess a greater number of bioactive compounds with biological, therapeutic, and medical significance. Majority of the cardiovascular herbs exhibit free radical scavenging property, antiplatelet, lipid-lowering, anti-inflammatory, and vasodilatation properties [4, 6].

In a view to explore and establish herbal medicine for CVDs, there is a need to screen the herbs for activity using preclinical and clinical methods. In this book chapter, we will focus on different existing preclinical and clinical methods that can be selected for screening the herbal medicines and also will discuss about evident scientific studies related to herbs used for CVDs.

## 11.2 PRECLINICAL STUDIES FOR TESTING OF HERBAL MEDICINE IN CARDIOVASCULAR DISORDERS

Rat one-kidney two-clip hypertension model is used to assess how well a substance lowers blood pressure with some herbal extracts. After the induction of anesthesia, in left lumbar region, an incision is made, and the exposed hilum of the left kidney is clipped for about 3–4 hours to ensure the renal artery occlusion. Further, the ganglia are blocked and the renal arterial clip is opened. Animals should be maintained on pentobarbital sodium to maintain spontaneous breathing. The jugular vein is cannulated for drug administration; the carotid artery is used to determine arterial pressure differences (Figure 11.1). These variations are recorded continuously, and the dominant rise in arterial pressure after the opening of the clip, followed by a fall in arterial pressure after the administration of test substances, is noted [1, 2]. Intensity of fall in arterial pressure of the rats is determined for the selected herbal medicine in comparison with the control [3].

In one-kidney one-clip model (Figure 11.2), unilateral nephrectomy was performed, and the renal artery of the remaining kidney was occluded using a clip that leads to increased arterial blood pressure, water, and salt retention

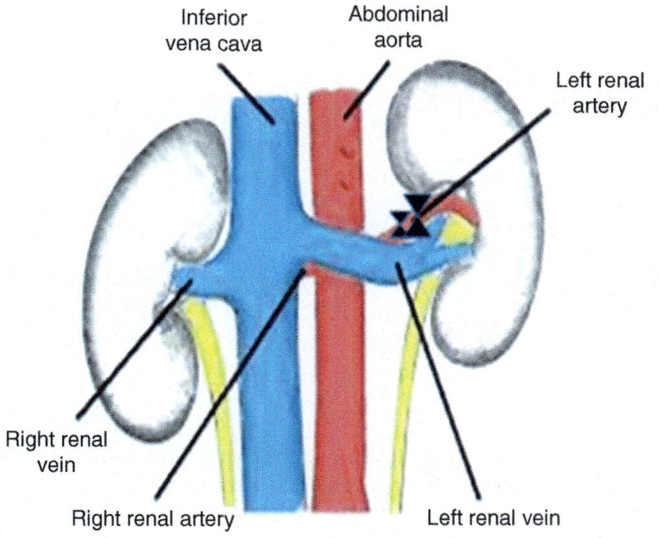


**FIGURE 11.1** One-kidney two-clip model.

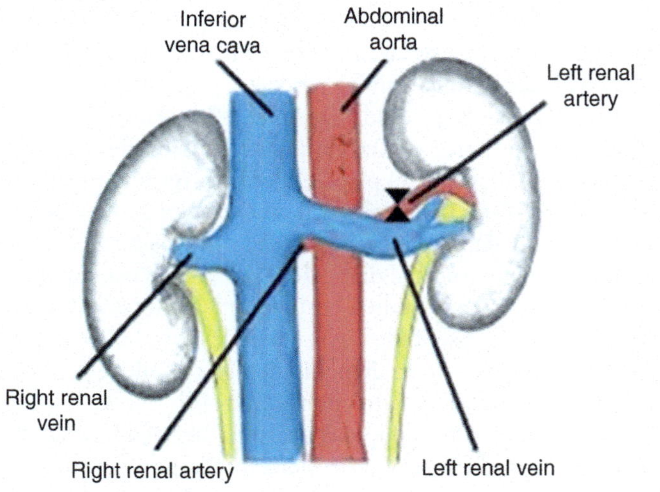


**FIGURE 11.2** One-kidney one-clip model.

that may lead to chronic kidney failure [1]. Vasoactive compounds present in herbal medicine may lead to decrease in blood pressure [1].

*In vivo* pithed rat model is used to assess the effect of herbal medicine on Wistar rats' carotid arterial pressure. Rats are pithed using a steel rod and further provided with ventilation for oxygen support. Carotid artery and jugular vein are cannulated after anaesthetizing the animal. Carotid artery is connected to mercury manometer, and the changes in arterial pressure are recorded in the mercury manometer. Half an hour after pithing, dose-response curves are recorded for test herbal drugs using phenylephrine as standard. Blood from the carotid cannula is also collected, and the blood arterial gas concentration is determined [4, 5].

Male Charles River rats are basically hypertensive in nature. As in renal artery clip method, both the renal arteries are clipped and the open wound is closed. After the initial clipping, hypertension develops in 25 to 30 days. Piezoelectric pulse detector is placed around the proximal tail region to sense the arterial pressure of the rats. Blood pressure of male Charles River rats is monitored for five days. After recording of basal blood pressure on first, third, and fifth day, the effect of test herbal substance and the percentage of fall in systolic pressure are compared using a polygraph [6].

Scientist Dahl had worked to study the role of dietary sodium in human beings in inducing hypertension. The study was conducted in hypertensive S rats that are induced by high salt intake. He found that high sodium-induced hypertension can be decreased by the use of diet including high potassium content and by consuming diet with low levels of salt at the same time. He also states that packed food containing high sodium content produced death in S hypertensive rats [7, 8].

Research carried out by Zicha et al. [9] and Grobe et al. [9] established hypertension by the administration of deoxycorticosteroid acetate (DOCA). This model (Figure 11.3) is based on neurogenic response and also on central nuclei-mediated hypertension. Zicha et al. and Grobe et al., [9] had designed the study in two ways. One way is injecting of DOCA in combination with salt; the second one is injecting of DOCA in combination with salt in uninephrectomy. Salt, one of the commonest causes for the incidence of hypertension in human beings, is also considered in this study. In non-uninephrectomized animals, the rise in blood pressure beyond normal range can be seen within 28 days of DOCA administration. In this study, animals uninephrectomized had shown to induce hypertension within 21 days of treatment. An elevation of blood pressure was observed in two types of rats, and the effect is more in uninephrectomized ones. There was a biphasic response in uninephrectomized rats administered with DOCA in combination with salt (Figure 11.3). Herbal medicine that can act centrally to decrease the blood pressure can be screened by these methods [4, 9–11].

Studies have demonstrated that atherosclerosis may develop in a variety of species, which makes it feasible to get tissues at different stages of the disease as well as the cells required for *in vitro* research. Animal models of atherosclerosis may therefore be able to address the issues of inherent limitations in human research.

Induction of Atherosclerotic disease in different species of animals can be achieved, so it is easy to induce the disease condition and investigate the atherosclerotic disease at different

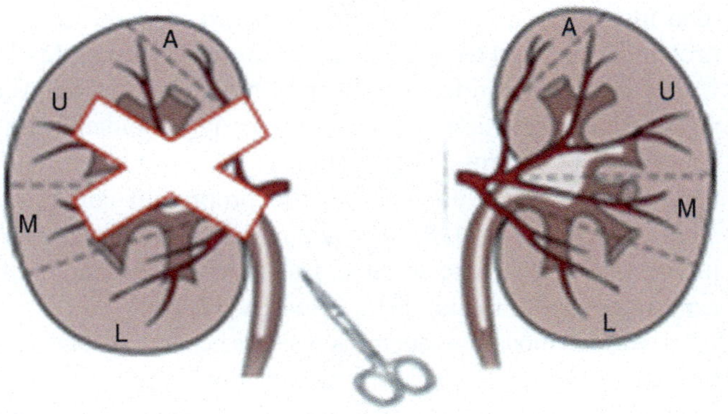


**FIGURE 11.3** Deoxycorticosteroid acetate (DOCA) model.

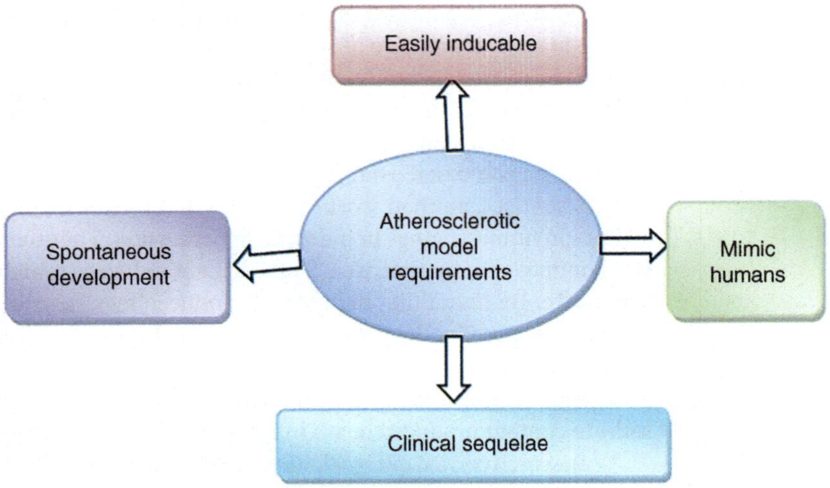


**FIGURE 11.4** Requirements for developing an atherosclerotic animal model.

stages of disease progression; further, the effectiveness of herbal medicine can be evaluated easily in different species of animals.

Ignatowski [12], for the first of its kind, selected rabbits and induced atherosclerosis for conducting research studies; he fed the rabbits with diet rich in protein content [12]. Experimental animals for atherosclerosis research may include small animals like mice, rats, and large animals like dogs [13].

To develop atherosclerotic animal models (Figure 11.4), there are some important requirements to be considered that include ease of induction, atherosclerotic lesion should be same as in humans, atheroma formation should follow the same pathological process as in human beings, and finally, there should be impulsive atherosclerotic lesion formation based on the inducer [14].

Based on the anatomical and physiological relevance and other advantages among different animals, rabbits and mice are the more opted animals for study of atherosclerosis [12, 14, 15]. Thompson developed a genotype inbred mouse (C57BL/6). When this inbred mouse was fed on a diet with high fat/high cholesterol for 25 weeks, there was substantial atheroma formation in all the animals. Paigen B et al., [15], in 1985, tested different genetically modified animals for atheroma formation [15, 16]. Among the tested models, apolipoprotein E knockout ($ApoE^{-}/^{-}$) models were developed. ApoE/LDLR double-KO mice are further modified and showed promising progression in incidence of hyperlipidemia and occurrence of atherosclerotic lesions [17].

Novel studies proved that the proprotein convertase subtilisin/kexin type 9 (PCSK9) adeno-associated virus (AAV) mouse model is a more suitable, fast, flexible, and affordable experimental animal model for research [12, 18].

Animal models of atherosclerosis are generally established by introducing additional risk factors, modifying genes involved in cholesterol metabolism, and accelerating plaque formation through a high-cholesterol or Western-style diet [19, 20].

ApoE3-Leiden, PCSK9-AAV, and ApoE/LDLR double-knockout mice are useful techniques for studying atherosclerosis. Atherosclerotic animal models include mice, rabbits, and some studies include pigs. LDLR-knockout mice and ApoE-deficient mice are the commonly employed models for the study of micro vessel plaque, bleeding, rupture of thrombus, and incidence of myocardial infarction or sudden death. Pigs naturally develop atherosclerosis, which is further accelerated by an atherogenic diet [21–24]. A pig fed even on low-fat chow diet shows limited aortic permeability. Cholesterol level in pigs can rise if the pig is fed with 1.5% cholesterol for 210 days. Sections from hyperlipidemic pig models shows monocyte-based chemoattraction activity [6].

Streptozotocin-induced diabetes in pigs fed on high-fat diet produces atherosclerotic lesions in coronary arteries but shows no effect on blood cholesterol, triglycerides [25, 26]. Atherosclerotic lesions resemble complex coronary lesions with fibrous cap, lipid layer, accumulation of calcium, and bleeding. Inheritance of apoB100 variants shows decrease in LDL clearance [21, 24].

St. Thomas' Hospital (STH) and Watanabe heritable hyperlipidemic rabbits (WHHL) rabbits are the two strain models with hyperlipidemic states. WHHL rabbits resemble human familial hypercholesterolemias, whereas STH rabbits are akin to hypertriglyceridemia and mixed hyperlipidemia in humans [27]. A new model of New Zealand white rabbits possesses hyperlipidemia with reduced high-density lipoprotein (HDL) cholesterol levels. Conversely, abnormal high-level expression of human apoA-I in rabbits results in raised HDL cholesterol levels and decreased atherosclerosis [28–31].

Transwell models are based on interactions between endothelial cells and monocytes that lead to atherosclerosis. Hajishengallis et al., [32–34] observed monocyte adhesion and migration in the presence of chemoattractant-induced inflammation [32–34]. Many *in vitro* models are designed for studying atherosclerotic pathways and to explore new herbal or conventional treatments, including 2D models and 3D models like vessel-on-a-chip and Tissue-Engineered Blood Vessels (TEBVs) model [14, 17, 35].

*In vitro* models of atherosclerosis play a major role to determine the action of herbal medicine against atherosclerotic plaque. Single-cell *in vitro* models are used to understand the mechanisms behind the pathophysiology of atherosclerosis and to estimate drug intake. Two scientists, Schwendeman et al., [19] and Liu et al. [19], designed single-cell systems to determine the uptake of herbal medicine. Schwendeman et al., model is based on human monocytic cell line (THP-1) monocytes differentiated macrophages and the DiD dye-labeled synthetic HDL [19].

The Liu group *in vitro* model is designed based on binding of test substance to umbilical vein endothelial cells or foam cells of humans. Porrini et al., [20] conducted a recent study of polyphenols from herbs using a co-culture inflammatory model made up of human umbilical vein endothelial cell and tumor necrosis factor-alpha (TNF-α) and observed the atherosclerotic plaque incidence. Another study conducted by the Wong group is based on human microvascular endothelial cell co-culture system and is dependent on the efficacy of microparticles on human microvascular endothelial cells [17, 20].

## 11.3 SCIENTIFIC STUDIES ON SOME HERBS USED IN CARDIOVASCULAR DISORDERS

### 11.3.1 HAWTHORN

Hawthorn is the herb used from the ancient times for its heart-protecting properties. Paracelsus [36] used hawthorn berry wine as an herbal medication. Two important natural sources of hawthorn are *Crataegus oxyacantha* and *Crataegus monogyna*. Constituents present in hawthorn include flavonoids, vitexin, hyperoxide, and quercetin that possess free radical scavenging property and action against inflammation. Oligomeric procyanidins will strengthen the blood vessels and improve blood flow. Triterpenes show cardioprotection and anti-arrhythmic action. The proposed mechanism for hawthorn to use as heart-protecting medication includes a rise in contractility of heart muscle that strengthens the heart beat and further increases the cardiac output and working efficiency of the heart. In preclinical studies, hawthorn had shown to increase force of contraction in muscle strip preparation and shortening of human single myocardial cells [36].

#### 11.3.1.1 Preclinical Studies of *Crataegus*

Thiruchenduran Mohana et al., [37] 2015 investigated using Wistar rats to observe the differences between monocyte-to-macrophage differentiation induced by increased cholesterol levels. *C. oxyacantha* containing oligomeric proanthocyanidin was administered to the Wistar rats, and the effect of proanthocyanidin had shown to decrease differentiation between monocyte to macrophage and to prevent atherogenic disturbances, thus making the herb the best option to treat atherosclerosis [37].

Research designed in mice maintained on high-cholesterol diet (HCD) shows that hawthorn with pectin penta-oligogalacturonide (HPPS) had proved its crucial role in maintaining proper metabolism of cholesterol and increasing conversion of bile acids from cholesterol. Results of this study had shown a notable reduction in the levels of liver triglycerides and serum. There was a significant reduction in bile acids in liver and small intestine and a decreased final bile-acid pool when compared with the high-cholesterol diet group. Hepatic farnesoid X receptor (FXR) inactivation and target gene expression were found by molecular research. The final conclusion of the study states that HPPS decreases cholesterol accumulation by increasing liver bile acid synthesis and by increasing fecal excretion of bile acids [38].

*Crataegus* herbal extract releases endothelial nitric oxide and further increases coronary blood flow [39]. Anti-arrhythmic effect after pretreatment with *Crataegus* in a rat ischemic–reperfusion model produced by occluding left coronary artery method had shown a lower incidence of ventricular fibrillation.

#### 11.3.1.2 Clinical Studies of *Crataegus*

In a clinical trial conducted in mild heart failure patients, the study was a placebo-controlled, double-blind study with randomization. When patients were treated with *Crataegus* for 56 days, there was an increase in oxygen uptake, which had also increased the exercise capacity when compared with the placebo group. In another study, *Crataegus* medication was administered to 140 subjects, and their exercise capacity was improved significantly when compared with the placebo group [40].

Research was undertaken on *Crataegus* Extract WS 1442 in chronic heart failure. In the SPICE trail conducted on 2681 patients with systolic heart failure, there was no prominent effect on cardiac mortality and myocardial infarction, but there was a significant reduction in left ventricular ejection failure by 25% and 35% [39].

As per Orhan, Ilkay E et al., [40], *C. oxyacantha* of Rosaceae family is a European Pharmacopeia-recognized medicinal herb. Herbal extracts containing berries or flowers contain constituents such as oligomeric procyanidins. This medicinal herb has been shown to improve cardiac efficiency in heart failure and other CVDs. This hawthorn herb possesses multiple pharmacological properties that include lowering blood pressure, reduction in lipid levels and glucose levels, decreased anxiety, and immune modulation. Bioactive constituents like triterpenes, phenolic acids, fatty acids, and sterols existing in hawthorn herb play a major role in exhibiting increased force of contraction, improved blood flow, enhanced exercise tolerance, blockade of angiotensin-converting enzyme (ACE)-mediated hypertension, and free radical scavenging property, all of which have an impact on cardiac health [40] (Table 11.1).

**Table 11.1** Herbs used for cardiovascular disorders.

| Herb | | Constituents | Uses | References |
|---|---|---|---|---|
| Hawthorn (*Crataegus pinnatifida*) | 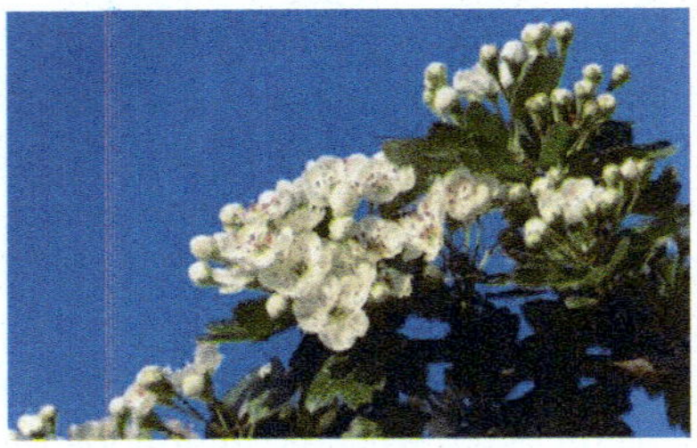<br>*Source:* Didgeman / Pixabay / CC0 | Flavonoids include flavones, flavonols, dihydroflavones, dihydroflavonols, flavanols, and anthocyanins. The glycosidic forms of flavonoids comprise quercetin, apigenin, kaempferol, luteolin, and dihydroflavonoid derivatives | Hypolipidemic, hypotensive, anti-myocardial ischemic, anti-arrhythmic, antithrombotic | [37–40] |
| Garlic (*Allium sativum*) | 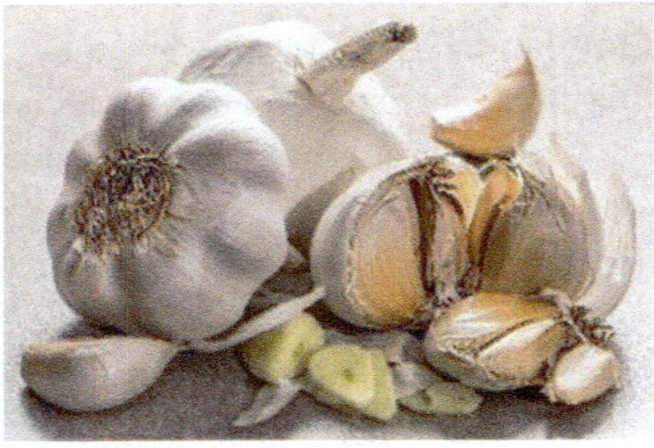<br>*Source:* stevepb / Pixabay / CC0 | *A. sativum* is abundant in sulfurous phytochemicals, including alliin, allicin, ajoenes, and vinyldithiins, along with flavonoids such as quercetin | Antioxidant activity, anti inflammatory, antimicrobial, immunomodulatory | [41–49] |
| Turmeric (*Curcuma longa*) | 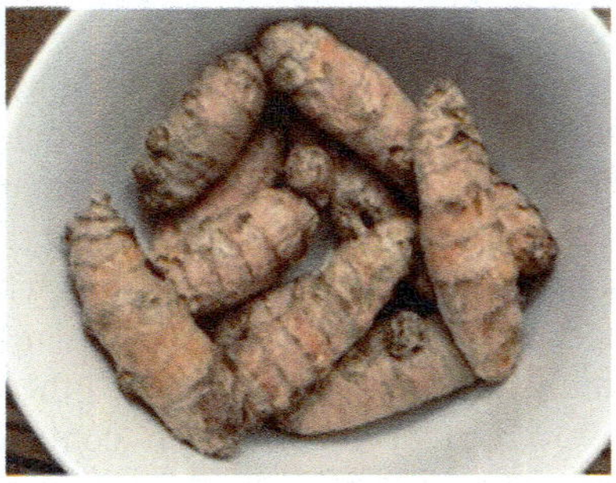<br>*Source:* karenski1 / Pixabay / CC0 | A group of polyphenolic compounds named curcuminoids consist of curcumin, demethoxycurcumin, and bisdemethoxycurcumin | Exhibits anti-inflammatory, anti-HIV, antibacterial, antioxidant, nematocidal, antiparasitic, antispasmodic, and anticancer activities | [37–40] |
| Berberine (*Berberis vulgaris*) | 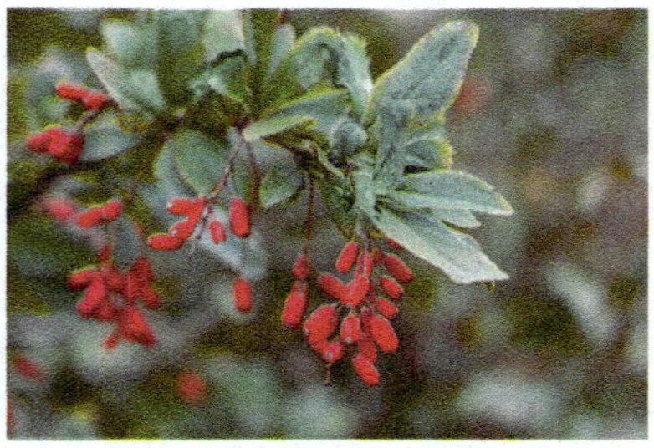<br>*Source:* eliosdnepr / Adobe Stock Photos | Berberine, berbamine, and palmatine | Controls both blood glucose and BP levels.<br>Turmeric normalizes the arterial stiffness and prevents dysfunction of heart ventricles | [50–56] |
| Quercetin | 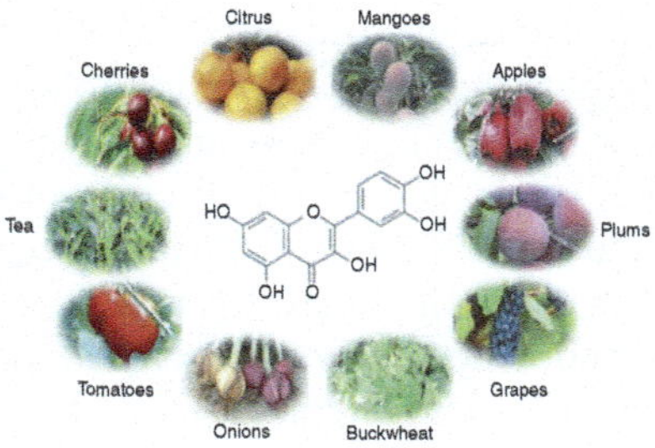<br>*Source:* Goldblatt [2] / John Wiley & Sons / CC BY 4.0 | Flavonoid widely distributed in plants, named as quercetin, demonstrates a range of biological activities | Mechanisms include antioxidant activity, broad-spectrum antibacterial and antiparasitic effects, anticancer and cardiovascular-protective properties, as well as immunomodulatory action | [57, 58] |

*(Continued)*

**Table 11.1** (Continued)

| Herb | Constituents | Uses | References |
|---|---|---|---|
| Catechins (*Camellia sinensis*) 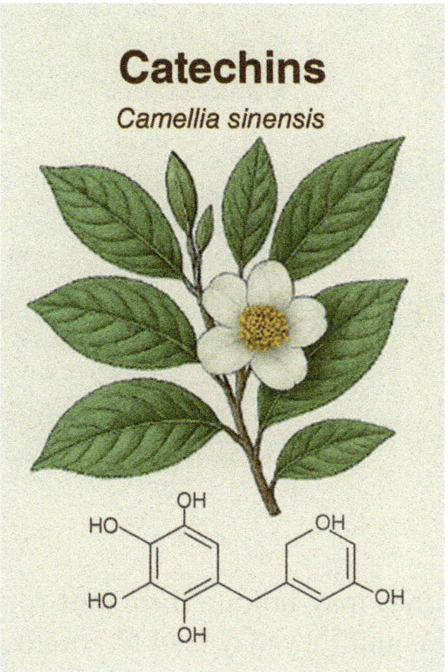  | Polyphenol compounds like flavanols, flavandiols, flavonoids, and phenolic acid catechins, including (−)-epicatechin, epicatechin gallate, epigallocatechin), epigallocatechin gallate), gallocatechin, catechin gallate, and gallocatechin gallate | Antioxidant activity, antimicrobial activity, antiallergenic and anti-inflammatory activities, antiviral and anticancer activities | [59–64] |

## 11.3.2 GARLIC

*Allium sativum* belongs to Alliaceae family. It originated in Asia and spread to china and other regions. Garlic has been used as a traditional medicine since ancient times. Garlic was used for healing during the period of Egyptians, Greeks, and the Roman Empire. Garlic's major benefits include blood pressure- and cholesterol-lowering effects. It blocks platelet aggregation and increases fibrinolysis. Biologically active constituents of *A. sativum* include allyl cysteine sulfoxide, diallyl thiosulfinate, or diallyl disulfide [41].

### 11.3.2.1 Preclinical Studies of Garlic

*A. sativum* consists of hydrogen sulfide and allicin that are released by the action of alliinase on alliin. It is connected with angiotensin II inhibition and blood vessel dilation property, as observed in animal and human cell studies, identifying garlic as an antihypertensive agent. Garlic has been proven to decrease hypoxic pulmonary high blood pressure in the two-kidney one-clip Goldblatt model. Allicin has been reported to show vasodilator properties in a sedated, intact-chest cat model and isolated lung of the rat model [42, 43].

Pedraza-Chaverrí [44] conducted a study based on stimulation of nitric oxide synthase. Normally, repression of nitric oxide (NO) synthesis induces an increase in arterial blood pressure. The inducer may be N-omega-nitro-L-arginine-methyl-ester (L-NAME). Test and control were treated for a period of one month. After one month of administration, NO production was evaluated by estimating the nitrite and nitrate stable end products of nitric oxide in urine samples. The animal group that received L-NAME had shown decrease in $NO_2^-/NO_3^-$ levels, indicating decreased production of nitric oxide, decreased vasodilation, and leading to arterial hypertension [44–46].

Animals fed on garlic had showed an increase in urinary $NO_2^-/NO_3^-$ values, which indicates increased nitric oxide production. Hence, the study concludes that garlic is capable of inhibiting L-NAME-induced arterial hypertension. Animal models had sown garlic to act as both a preventive and therapeutic agent against atherosclerosis, one of the leading causes of mortality. Garlic, by lowering blood cholesterol levels, decreases atherosclerotic plaque formation in vascular walls [43, 47–49]. Early changes in atherosclerotic condition include accumulation of lipids, majorly cholesterol, along with cell proliferation and lipidosis in extracellular matrix. Garlic reduces esters of cholesterol and free cholesterol in atherosclerotic arterial cells after incubating smooth muscle cells in primary culture with garlic powder by its ability to inhibit biosynthesis of triglycerides and cholesterol esters [65, 66].

Garlic extract stimulates hydrolysis of cholesteryl esters, thus reducing their levels and producing anti-atherosclerotic potential. Garlic decreases collagen production and depositions in aorta, thus decreasing the major changes in atherosclerosis making it useful as an antiatherogenic herb [47].

In a study conducted by CS Song [50], 500 mg of garlic extract had shown to produce anticoagulant effect and increase in prothrombin time. Studies also evidenced a decrease in fibrin formation when compared with normal. This effect is more prominent in *in vitro* experiments than in *in vivo* experiments, with the mechanism mediated through precipitation of calcium ions or by fibrin-breaking capacity [50].

### 11.3.2.2 Clinical Studies of Garlic

Javad Kojuri et al., [51] conducted a study on hyperlipidemic patients. Hyperlipidemia is one of the leading causes for atherosclerosis, though there are many allopathic medications that decrease hyperlipidemia; their side effects had led to the use of herbal medicine as a treatment option (Figure 11.5).

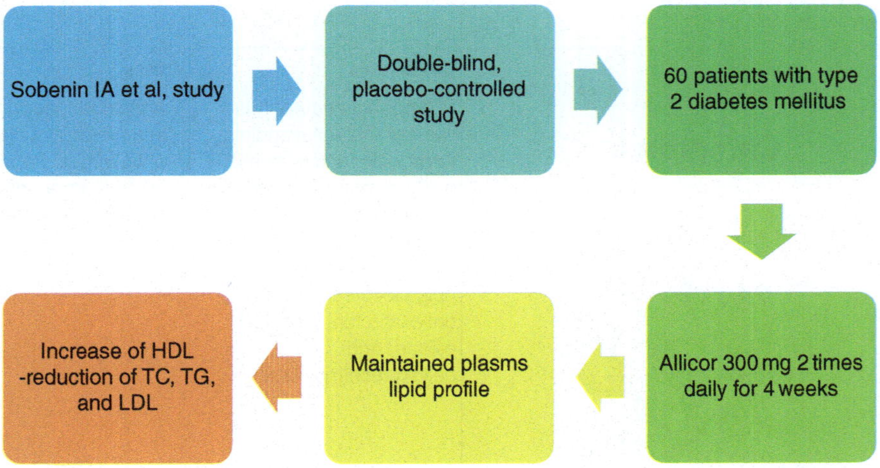


**FIGURE 11.5** Clinical study of garlic by Sobenin et al. [51].

In a study conducted in Shiraz University of Medical Sciences, hyperlipidemic patients were divided randomly into group of 3 groups, which included 50 patients in each group. One group received enteric-coated garlic powder tablet, *Anethum graveolens* tablet, and placebo, respectively, two times a day for each group. The estimated parameters included total cholesterol level, low-density lipoprotein cholesterol, and triglycerides. The garlic-administered group showed reduction in serum cholesterol, decreased triglycerides, and LDL cholesterol; thus, garlic is crucial in controlling the pathology of atherosclerosis [51] (Figure 11.5).

Rizwan Ashraf et al., [49, 50] conducted research to determine the diabetic effect of garlic on hyperlipidemic patients. A total of 70 diabetic hyperlipidemic patients selected from the OPD of the hospital are divided into 2 groups. One group received garlic tablets and the other received placebo for three months. After the study duration, blood samples were analyzed and found to show a marked decrease in serum cholesterol and LDL levels in the garlic-treated group than the other group [49, 50].

## 11.3.3 TURMERIC

Curcumin and its related analogs, hexahydro-analog of curcumin and tetrahydro-analog of curcumin, show a decrease in blood pressure through modulation of signaling pathways like nitric oxide, cyclicGMP, phosphodiesterase, renin, angiotensinogen, and tyrosine kinase [46].

In a study [50, 52], it was detected that turmeric can modulate fat metabolism like production of adipose tissue, breakdown of lipids, and decrease in peroxidation of lipids through altered cell signaling. Curcumin can also alter oxidation of fats, absorption of lipids, metabolism of cholesterol, and is used as a nutraceutical to avoid or treat cardiovascular disorders like CAD and hypertension.

The pathogenesis and clinical manifestation of many metabolic and nonmetabolic diseases are closely involved with dyslipidemia and altered lipid metabolism. Imbalance in lipid metabolism may lead to altered blood cholesterol levels that may initiate thrombus formation in the aorta or arteries, and that may lead to atherosclerosis, which further may lead to cardiovascular disorders like CAD and hypertension. Curcumin is one of the potential bioactive compounds that sets the lipid imbalances through cell-signal modification and prevents the occurrence of cardiovascular disorders like CAD [50, 52].

### 11.3.3.1 Preclinical Studies of Turmeric

Hypercholesterolemia rats are selected and divided into four different groups to determine the effect of turmeric on blood vessels or vascular conditions. Group I receives a standard diet, group II receives a high-cholesterol diet, groups III and IV receive a high-cholesterol diet with turmeric extract. All the treatments were administered for about 28 days orally. Induction of hypercholesterolemia is confirmed based on serum cholesterol levels that are high. The aorta was isolated from the experimental animals, mounted in organ bath, and tested for vasodilation. The animals fed with normal diet showed vasorelaxation or dilation. Animals fed a high-cholesterol diet showed decreased vasorelaxation, and the animals fed a high-cholesterol diet with turmeric extract showed significant vasorelaxation, increased SOD and glutathione values, *hsp70* and *bcl2* increase, and decreased *casp3*. All these changes indicate significant vasorelaxation by turmeric [53].

Turmeric is scientifically *Curcuma longa,* of the Zingiberaceae family. Male Wistar rats are selected for the study, and they should be fed a high-fructose and high-fat diet for about 28 days. The test substance, turmeric extract and the standard drug, captopril, are given every day for two weeks to hypertensive animals. Changes in arterial blood pressure, stiffness of the artery, heart rate, changes in QRS angle of ECG, and nitric oxide (NO) levels are observed. Usually, there may be fall in serum nitric oxide levels in case of high-fructose and high-fat diet, which in turn leads to stiffening of the artery, which further increases arterial resistance and leads to hypertension. In the test group administered with turmeric, the results showed an increase in serum nitric oxide levels, followed by vasodilation and a fall in blood pressure. Turmeric normalizes the arterial stiffness and prevents dysfunction of heart ventricles [50, 54].

#### 11.3.3.2 Clinical Studies of Turmeric

Ferugson et al., [55] investigated that a comparative effect of dietary phytosterols and curcumin. Dietary phytosterols produce an increase in blood cholesterol, whereas turmeric produces a decrease in blood cholesterol levels. This study was a randomized, double-blinded study. Total participants were divided into three groups. One group received placebo, the second group received phytosterols, and the third group received both phytosterols and curcumin. Estimated parameters included LDL cholesterol, fasting total cholesterol, HDL cholesterol, triglycerides, and blood glucose levels. Results of the study indicate a decrease in fasting total cholesterol, LDL cholesterol in the group receiving both phytosterols and curcumin [55]. Yunes Panahi [56] conducted a study in patients with type 2 diabetes (T2D) and cardiovascular diseases or altered lipid metabolism, as there are limited numbers of studies related to altered lipid metabolism in diabetic patients. This study focused on the use of curcumin analogs in the above-mentioned conditions. A total of 118 type 2 diabetic patients were involved in the study. One group received curcuminoids and piperine, and the other group received placebo plus standard. All important parameters linked to lipid metabolism were estimated. Thus, curcuminoids or their supplements can prevent the incidence of CVDs by altering the lipid imbalances, even in comorbid conditions like type 2 diabetes or hyperlipidemia [56].

### 11.3.4 BERBERINE

Berberine shows its effect in altered lipid metabolism through liver LDL-C receptors mediated by extracellular signals. Berberine reduces some transcription factors, including PPAR-γ, acetyl Co-A-related enzymes. It also stimulates adenosine monophosphate (AMP) kinases and inhibits mitogen-activated protein kinase (MAPK) pathway [57].

#### 11.3.4.1 Preclinical Studies of Berberine

Ma Yu-Guang et al., [58] designed a study to check the effect of berberine on BP and vascular protection in rats with diabetes. Streptozotocin was used as a diabetes inducer, and after induction for eight weeks, berberine was administered to diabetic rats. The cerebral artery present in middle region was observed for relaxation in an endothelium-dependent and -independent manner. Major activity of increased conductance calcium-activated potassium channels was observed. Chronic administration of berberine lowers the blood glucose levels and increases dilation of blood vessels in diabetic rats. Berberine also raises the activity of large-conductance calcium-activated potassium channels in vascular smooth muscle cells. So, berberine can be used for controlling both blood glucose and BP levels [58].

Tetrahydroberberine and 8-oxoberberine, both compounds, show altered rhythm of the heart. Berberine may block potassium channels and may stimulate sodium–calcium exchange. It also increases the ventricular action potential duration. Based on all these effects, berberine can be used to treat arrhythmias. Berberine acts on the cardiac muscle, increases the concentration of cyclic adenosine monophosphate (cAMP), and thereby increases the concentration of calcium ions in cardiac muscle. It prevents ventricular fibrillation by altering the potassium channels. It also modifies the sympathetic activity in cardiac muscle [57].

In a study of suprarenal aortic constriction induced by cardiac hypertrophy, berberine increases plasma sympathetic neurotransmitter levels, especially in ventricles of the heart. It shows a positive inotropic effect. A study conducted in dogs evidenced improvement in cardiac output a fall in left vasculogenic erectile dysfunction (VED) after IV administration of berberine [67].

Berberine can act as antagonist on alpha-receptors and inhibits sympathetic vasoconstriction. It can release nitric oxide from vascular smooth muscle endothelium and cause vasodilation. It also acts on potassium channels and calcium channels and finally leads to vasorelaxation [58].

#### 11.3.4.2 Clinical Studies of Berberine

Berberine has also shown to improve heart index and left ventricular ejection fraction and to reduce vascular resistance. Same compound will decrease premature beats that leads to arrhythmias in some clinical trials and also improves the ejection fraction of heart. It also decreases free radical generation, insulin resistance, serum triglycerides, and other parameters linked to cardiovascular disorders [57].

In a clinical trial of 32 patients [57, 58], with increased cholesterol level, berberine was administered twice daily for three months. The compound showed a fall in the cholesterol levels, triglycerides, and LDL-C levels. The study was extrapolated to a large group of 116 patients. All the patients had shown a similar fall in plasma lipid levels and also blood glucose levels. In a controlled study, it was evident that diet and lifestyle modification, along with some natural compounds like berberine, had markedly improved the lipid profile in dyslipidemia patients [57, 58].

### 11.3.5 QUERCETIN

Flavonoids are crucial compounds in our diet that can protect our health through many protective mechanisms. Flavonoids have many health benefits. These compounds are used to reduce blood pressure, inflammation, hyperglycemia, and other blood vessel disorders. Quercetin (Que) majorly blocks lipid peroxidation pathways, increases vasorelaxation, suppresses adhesion molecules, suppresses inflammatory mediators, offers protection through nitric oxide, and prevents aggregation of platelets [59].

Cardiac muscle needs sustainable contractile and electrical activity for its functioning. The energy required for maintaining the functions of the heart is obtained through the biochemical process of oxidative phosphorylation that takes place in mitochondria, which is responsible for 90% of cellular adenosine triphosphate production. Reactive oxygen species are important for communication and also for programmed death of some cells. Pathological mediators like angiotensin II, TNF-α, and catecholamines may disturb the balance and may lead to oxidative stress [60].

#### 11.3.5.1 Preclinical Studies of Quercetin

Nazari et al. [60] designed a study in rats to determine the effect of quercetin. The results of their study indicate sodium channel blockade that led to decreased influx of sodium ions into the cardiac cells and decreased autoregulation of rapid-conducting cells like SA node, AV node, atrial tissue, ventricular tissue, bundle of His, and Purkinje fibers. They had also observed increase in refractory period [60].

Wallace et al. [61] proved the blockade of sodium influx in myocytes of rat ventricles, increased calcium ion conductance, and increased cardiac cell contractility, which evidences que action as an antiarrhythmic agent. Quercetin, by blocking voltage-gated sodium channels, can act as protective against cardiovascular disorders [61].

Balderas E et al. [60, 62] conducted a study on mitoBKC$_a$ channels and observed that quercetin has the capacity to increase mitoBK$_{Ca}$ channel activity and coronary blood vessel relaxation. Their findings also include blockade of hypertrophy induced by phenylephrine through increased opening of mitochondrial ATP-sensitive potassium channels (mitoKATP) channels. This property of que is important for its action against inflammation and cardioprotection [60, 62].

Quercetin acts on ion channels to decrease the influx of calcium ions and efflux of potassium ions. It also inhibits autoregulation and membrane stabilization induced by calcium chloride, thereby exerting a decrease in arrhythmias. If quercetin is added half an hour before induction of oxidative stress by hydrogen peroxide in H9C2 cardiomyocytes, it was observed that que produces an increase in calcium ion concentration and may also lead to cell death. Some studies suggest that quercetin, a polyphenol present in onions, will act against reactive oxygen species. A study by He H et al. states that quercetin blocks dysfunction of mitochondria overload caused by iron in umbilical vein cells, increases viability, and decreases apoptotic cell death [63]. Cardiotoxicity induced by doxorubicin is because of oxidative stress that can be effectively reversed by quercetin [64].

#### 11.3.5.2 Clinical Studies of Quercetin

When quercetin is administered to patients with stage 1 hypertension, there is a marked fall in systolic and diastolic BP and the arterial pressure in the subjects. Obese patients administered quercetin for 42 days showed significant changes in total cholesterol levels and triglycerides [68].

In a study [68] conducted in 85 patients with cardiovascular disorders, 55 patients received Quercetin and others received other drugs used in CVDs. With daily administration of quercetin, there was a dominant decline in interleukin levels and TNF-α.

Quercetin was administered to type 2 diabetic female patients designed in a randomized, double-blinded clinical trial for a duration of 10 weeks. The population was divided into two groups: one group received quercetin, 500 mg capsule every day, and the other group received placebo. Biochemical parameters were evaluated before starting the treatments to the groups and finally after completing the study. Quercetin showed a marked drop in systolic hypertension when compared with the placebo group. The lipid profile of patients (female diabetic subjects), especially HDL, declined; there was also a drop in total cholesterol levels, along with changes in LDL and triglycerides. Quercetin reduced the serum levels of TNF- α and interleukin 6 in patients; this indicates its therapeutic usefulness in cardiovascular disorders and hyperlipidemia.

### 11.3.6 CATECHINS

Catechins include bioactive polyphenolic constituents with varied therapeutic effects, especially in diseases related to the cardiovascular system. They exhibit preservative effect even in ischemia/reperfusion injury of cardiac muscle that generally happens during myocardial infarction and ischemia. Catechin, (−)-epicatechin, and epigallocatechin-3-gallate (EGCG) conserve the myocytes of heart from ischemia, reperfusion, or related structural or chemical modifications. These effects of catechins are essential for increased cell survival, decreasing the size of the infarct, and improving the cardiac function after damage by initiating recovery [69]. Catechins constitute a major group of bioactive compounds in tea, accounting for a substantial proportion of its dry weight, particularly in green and white varieties. Table 11.2 indicates the list of catechins in different varieties of tea.

#### 11.3.6.1 Preclinical Studies of Catechins

Animesh Chowdhury et al., [70] investigated effect of EGCG in elevated serum cholesterol conditions and atherosclerotic plaque formation using a hypercholesterolemic apolipoprotein E–null mouse model. Atherosclerosis was induced in mice by a carotid artery periadventitial cuff injury process. Tests substances were administered to respective groups.

**Table 11.2** Catechins in different varieties of tea.

| | |
|---|---|
| Green tea | Green tea is known for its high catechin content, particularly EGCG (epigallocatechin gallate). The unfermented nature of green tea preserves these beneficial compounds. |
| White tea | White tea, less processed, also contains a good amount of catechins, though generally less than green tea. |
| Oolong tea | Oolong tea is partially oxidized and has low catechin levels compared to green and white tea. |
| Black tea | Black tea is fully oxidized, resulting in a significant decrease in catechin content, with some catechins being converted into other compounds like theaflavins during the oxidation process |

On days 21 and 42, after the start of the experiment, animals were observed for incidence of plaque or atheromatic characters. The results of the study indicated improvement in antioxidant status, decreased inflammation of the blood vessels, and smooth muscle cell replication. EGCG had shown a decrease in atheromatic plaque size by 55% and 73% at 21 and 42 days, respectively [70].

Ramesh et al., [71] assessed the effectiveness of EGCG obtained from *Camellia sinensis*. A significant fall in malondialdehyde (MDA) levels and an increase in antioxidant enzymes and antioxidant profile were observed when compared to rats that received saline treatment. EGCG treatment had corrected the imbalances in serum lipid levels, enhanced antioxidant status in RBCs, and repaired imbalances in the heart tissue, even in rats fed on an atherogenic diet [71]. The EGCG-treated group showed a prominent decrease in bad cholesterol levels and an increase in good cholesterol levels in rats, compared with rats fed a normal diet and rats fed on an atherogenic diet. EGCG had significantly increased the serum cholesterol levels, triglycerides, and lipoprotein cholesterol fractions compared with rats fed on a normal diet. There is variation in malondialdehyde levels and antioxidants enzymes levels in treatment group, atherogenic group and normal group.

Yoshihiro Hotta et al. [72] conducted a scientific study to investigate the catechins isolated from the green tea for their action on the myocardium of the heart and arterial blood pressure. Deviations in the NO and $Ca^{2+}$ contents of the cardiac muscle are determined by using a nitric oxide (NO) electrode and fluorometry, followed by simultaneous recording of pressure developed. There was a dose-dependent influx of calcium ions that led to the development of pressure in the left ventricle. Nitric oxide signaling also increased based on dose of gallocatechin-3-gallate; however, there was no effect on heart rate. Gallocatechin-3-gallate, produced by degradation of epigallocatechin gallate during heating, has a more significant blood pressure-lowering effect than other catechins in experimental rabbits. Each catechin has NO-donating capacity and thus produces NO-mediated relaxation of blood vessels and also offers cardioprotection [72].

An experimental study designed based on Langendorff heart preparation using guinea pig model was conducted to investigate the effect of EGCG or its C-2 epimer, (−)-gallocatechin-3-gallate (GCG) present in green tea. Based on the pressure developed during ischemia/reperfusion in guinea pigs, recovery in control group was 34.4%, whereas recovery of 78.4% was observed in animals receiving EGCG, indicating a marked protective effect on ATP in the tissues. EGCG inhibited calcium excess in mitochondria by altering calcium influx and increasing the acidic nature of the perfusate. EGCG allies the free radicals with high intensity and exhibits antioxidant activity. EGCG or GCG mitigates programmed cell death produced by caspase-3. Thus, EGCG or the C-2 epimer, (−)-gallocatechin-3-gallate (GCG), present in green tea, plays a key role in ischemic heart diseases and protects the heart from free radical- and nitric oxide-mediated damage [73].

In a study involving rats, cardiac hypertrophy was induced through aortic constriction. After three weeks, the heart-to-body weight ratio increased significantly in the constricted group compared with the control group. However, administration of EGCG substantially mitigated this increase, suggesting its potential in alleviating cardiac hypertrophy and improving systolic function [74, 75].

Protecting the heart from remodeling due to excessive pressure is crucial for reducing illness and death. Research has shown that EGCG can help prevent the development of concentric left ventricular hypertrophy caused by pressure overload. In a study on rats with aortic constriction, those who received EGCG treatment had significantly reduced heart weight increases compared to the untreated group. Specifically, EGCG administration led to a substantial decrease in the heart-to-body weight ratio, indicating its potential benefits in mitigating cardiac hypertrophy and improving heart function [74, 75].

#### 11.3.6.2 Clinical Studies of Catechins

In Taiwan city, a clinical study was done to explore the impact of tea consumption in subjects with heart disorders. A total of 1507 human subjects were selected for the study. Subjects who consumed tea daily for the last one year were found to have less incidence of cardiac disorders than the subjects who did not consume tea regularly. A subject who consumed tea daily had 46% less risk of incidence of than others. Similarly, hypertension incidence over the last one year was known to have less incidence of cardiac disorders than the subjects who did not consume tea regularly. The JACC study stated that the rate of occurrence death due to cardiovascular disorders is inversely connected with tea intake. Researchers found that tea intake in a group of 76,979, having age in between 40 and 79 years had strongly decreased deaths due to cardiovascular disorders [69, 76].

A study found that obese women who took green tea extract for 12 weeks saw some pretty impressive results. Their LDL and triglyceride levels dropped, and their HDL levels increased. Plus, they saw boosts in adiponectin and ghrelin, which are hormones that help regulate hunger and metabolism. Although the weight loss was not dramatic, it is still promising. A recent study found that people who drink 1–2 cups of tea per day are 88% less likely to develop diabetes, especially if they are not obese. What is even more impressive is that this benefit applies to people of all ages, regardless of their lifestyle or habits [69].

Research has demonstrated that green tea supplementation can have a profound impact on cardiovascular health. These studies demonstrated that administering green tea at specific dosages can lead to significant reductions in blood pressure and angiotensin II levels. This is accompanied by improvements in the structural integrity of heart cells. The effectiveness of tea in inhibiting ACE activity varies depending on its chemical composition. Notably, certain tea cultivars, such as "Benifuuki," exhibit enhanced ACE-inhibiting properties due to their unique catechin profile. Additionally, teas enriched with gamma-aminobutyric acid (GABA) have been found to offer protective benefits against hypertension in salt-sensitive subjects [77, 78].

### 11.3.7 SILYMARIN

Planning a diet with more plant foods is linked to a decreased incidence of heart-related problems. Plant foods contain flavonoids; these bioactive compounds slow blood clotting, reduce thrombus formation, prevent oxidation of low-density lipoproteins (LDLs), and revitalize endothelial activity. *Silybum marianum* on extraction yields the active constituent *Silybum marianum*. The plant belongs to the Asteraceae family; it is rich in phenolic content [79].

#### 11.3.7.1 Preclinical Studies of Silymarin

Inhibiting lipid peroxidation is one of the suggested methods by which silibinin stabilizes cell membrane permeability and helps the liver maintain levels of glutathione, its own protective antioxidant. Additionally, it has been demonstrated that silibinin enhances clopidogrel's action on atherosclerosis. Three groups of mice on a high-fat diet were given silibinin, clopidogrel, or a combination of the two. Endothelial dysfunction, inflammation, and aortic lesions were all lessened in the mice given silibinin and clopidogrel. Additionally, mice treated with both drugs showed an enhanced antithrombotic efficacy of clopidogrel. Thus, silymarin/silibinin's atheroprotective mechanisms include reduced LDL oxidation and strong antioxidant qualities.

Silymarin demonstrated its strong hypolipidemic action by raising the liver's lipid-metabolizing enzyme levels and lowering the liver's and serum's cholesterol/phospholipid ratio. Triglyceride metabolism through cytochrome P450 family 4 subfamily (CYP4A) is primarily responsible for triglyceride (TG) reduction. Fascinatingly, silymarin increases arachidonic acid levels and improves the transitivity of FXR in a dose-dependent manner. It has been established that FXR is essential for preserving appropriate lipid and glucose metabolism because it regulates the expression of multiple downstream target genes [80, 81].

Research on silibinin/silymarin on hypertension is extremely limited. These studies primarily evaluate hypertension when liver illness is present or when paired with other medications (such tetrandrine). One study investigated the effects of silibinin (300 mg/kg/day) on blood pressure, ventricular hypertrophy, infarct size, and mortality following coronary artery ligation in hypertensive rats [80].

In those rat models, silibinin decreased blood pressure, arrhythmias, left ventricular hypertrophy, and mortality, according to the authors' findings. Rat mortality rates dropped with oral silibinin ingestion, and it reduced blood pressure as effectively as the medication tetrandrine, most likely as a result of its antioxidant properties [82, 83].

Through its underlying mechanisms, silymarin/silibinin may reduce LDL oxidation, a stage in between that leads to the development of atherosclerosis. Excessive production of radical oxygen species (ROS) plays an important role in atherogenesis. When they build up in the arterial wall, LDL oxidation is encouraged, which leads to the development of atherosclerotic plaque, particularly in the early stages. Thus, silymarin/silibinin's atheroprotective mechanisms include reduced LDL oxidation and strong antioxidant quality. However, numerous experimental studies have demonstrated the atheroprotective effects of various antioxidants besides silibinin; there is still disagreement over their therapeutic efficacy [82, 83].

Antioxidants' limited bioavailability has been attributed to the discrepancy, which severely limits their use in atherosclerotic disorders. Silymarin, by acting on specific ABC transporters G5 and G8, modifies the lipid profile in experimental rats that are on high-cholesterol diet [81, 84].

Silibinin appears to be a very powerful antioxidant phytoactive compound. Silymarin and silibinin may enhance vascular function in this situation. Studies on rat models have demonstrated that pulmonary vascular dysfunction can be significantly reduced after eight days of 250 mg/kg/day silymarin and that normal endothelium and vascular elasticity can be recovered following lung ischemia–reperfusion injury in an *ex vivo* model of isolated rat aorta. Additionally, by reducing the levels of asymmetric dimethylarginine (ADMA) in the aorta and plasma, silibinin (20 mg/kg i.p. daily) improves endothelial dysfunction by reversing the inhibition of nitric oxide synthase and thereby increasing NO availability.

Rats have been widely used to study both atherogenesis and myocardial infarction. In myocardial infarction, the primary goal is rapid reperfusion to prevent myocardial necrosis, despite the risk of reperfusion injury, which paradoxically increases cell death. Key mechanisms of reperfusion injury include mitochondrial permeability transition and subsequent cardiomyocyte death, followed by reactive oxygen species release. In a recent study using mice subjected to left anterior descending artery (LAD) ligation, the cardioprotective effects of silibinin were evaluated. Mice were randomly assigned to receive 100 mg/kg silibinin for seven days prior to myocardial infarction or no treatment. Compared with the sham group, silibinin treatment significantly attenuated heart dysfunction induced by ischemia/reperfusion (I/R) injury, as evidenced by higher left ventricular ejection fraction (LVEF) and lower cardiac troponin and B-type natriuretic peptide levels. Another study demonstrated a dose-dependent reduction in infarct size with silymarin treatment (100, 250, and 500 mg/kg). Collectively, these findings confirm the athero- and cardioprotective effects of silibinin.

Numerous researches have also focused on silymarin's hypolipidemic properties. Both a fat-rich diet and N-nitrosodiethylamine (NDEA) can cause hyperlipidemia in rats. Silymarin can dramatically lower total cholesterol triglycerides. Additionally, silymarin appears to raise HDL levels. Notably, an *in vivo* investigation revealed that N-nitrosodiethylamine (NDEA) caused animals' serum levels of phospholipids and free fatty acids to drop after raising their levels of cholesterol and triglycerides. Rats given 1000 mg/l/day of silymarin and NDEA for 16 weeks demonstrated a substantial reduction in triglyceride and cholesterol levels, followed by an increase in phospholipid and free acid levels. Silymarin demonstrated strong hypolipidemic action by raising the liver's lipid-metabolizing enzyme levels and lowering the liver and serum cholesterol/phospholipid ratio. Triglyceride metabolism through CYP4A is primarily responsible for triglyceride (TG) reduction. Interestingly, silymarin raises arachidonic acid levels and dose-dependently enhances the transactivity of FXR.

Two more investigations [81–86] employing rat models have linked silymarin's vasodilator characteristics. When administered at a dose of 200 mg/kg/day for five weeks, silymarin dramatically reduced pulmonary arterial hypertension (PAH) before it progressed to a severe and irreversible state. This effect involves suppression of the C-X-C chemokine receptor type 4/stromal cell-derived factor-1 (CXCR4/SDF-1) chemokine/receptor axis. SDF-1, a stromal cell-derived factor, serves as the ligand for the chemokine receptor CXCR4, and its inhibition may delay pulmonary arteriolar occlusion and vascular remodeling, thereby mitigating pulmonary arterial hypertension.

Silymarin, based on its phenolic content, safeguards the cardiac muscle from free radicals, and in hypertension associated with oxidative stress, prevents plaque formation in the blood vessels and declines the incidence of cardiac toxicity. Basically, oxidative stress is contributed to the pathology and occurrence of many life-threatening CVDs, like increased blood pressure, atheromatic plaque formation in the blood vessels, decreased oxygen supply to the cardiac muscle, and decreased heart function.

#### 11.3.7.2 Clinical Studies of Silymarin

Echocardiographic and electrocardiographic assessments demonstrated that doxorubicin treatment caused a decrease in ejection fraction, tissue Doppler peak mitral annulus systolic velocity, and fractional shortening, along with bradycardia and prolongation of the QT and QRS intervals. Co-administration of silymarin with doxorubicin effectively ameliorated these echocardiographic and electrocardiographic abnormalities. Moreover, silymarin/silibinin co-treatment mitigated doxorubicin-induced histopathological alterations in cardiac tissue. These findings indicate that silymarin/silibinin reduces doxorubicin-induced cardiotoxicity, likely via antioxidant, anti-inflammatory, and anti-apoptotic mechanisms. Silymarin, in particular, scavenges free radicals and protects cardiac tissue from lipid peroxidation [85].

Beyond the clinical trials that were part of the previously stated meta-analyses, other research has looked at the impact of silibinin/silymarin mostly on hyperlipidemia and type 2 diabetes, and with lesser effects on arterial stiffness and renal function.

Vitamins D and E, as well as other herbal ingredients, were given either alone or in conjunction with milk thistle extract (Silybum marinaum extract, silymarin) or silibinin. After using silibinin/silymarin supplements, type 2 diabetes mellitus (T2DM) patients showed notable improvements in their lipid profiles, insulin sensitivity, and glycemic indices in all of those research trials. More research with different target groups showed similar positive results in metabolic parameters: patients with cirrhosis, nonalcoholic fatty liver disease (NAFLD), alcoholic liver disease, and hypertensive diabetic patients [80].

A well-known method called coronary artery bypass grafting (CABG) was used to test silymarin. Silymarin was used as a preoperative treatment for 140 patients undergoing CABG. Values like serum creatinine, LDL, HbA1c, and white blood cell count were found to significantly decline in diabetes patients [80, 86].

### 11.3.8 *GINKGO BILOBA*

*Ginkgo biloba* leaves contain flavonoids and terpenoids. The studies on *G. biloba* leaves are increasing day by day. *Ginkgo biloba* leaf extract (GBLE) is known to act against free radicals and produces anti-inflammatory action. It prevents platelet-activating factor and produces dilation of blood vessels. The leaf extract of GBLE enhances blood supply, releases neurotransmitter, blocks the release of harmful LDLs, and protects the mitochondria from damage due to oxidative stress. In a study conducted in patients with obstructive arteriosclerosis, GBLE showed activity against free radicals and inhibition of lipid peroxidation. This evidence can direct the application of GBLE in the prophylaxis and therapy of heart diseases [87–90].

## 11.4 CONCLUSION

To choose the herb with the highest therapeutic efficacy, develop an appropriate formulation, and suggest clinical usage for the patient's benefit, it is imperative to screen the available herbs for their effectiveness in cardiac problems. Clinical and preclinical data offer evidence-based information on the potential of chosen herbs for medicinal use.

## REFERENCES


1. Goldblatt, H., Lynch, J., Hanzal, R.F., and Summerville, W.W. (1934). Studies on experimental hypertension: I. The production of persistent elevation of systolic blood pressure by means of renal ischemia. *J. Exp. Med.* 59 (3): 347–379.
2. Goldblatt, H. (1947). The renal origin of hypertension. *Physiol. Rev.* 27 (2): 120–165.
3. Page, I.H. (1939). The production of persistent arterial hypertension by cellophane perinephritis. *JAMA* 113: 2046–2048.
4. Folkow, B. (1982). Physiological aspects of primary hypertension. *Physiol. Rev.* 62 (2): 347–504.
5. Chobanian, A.V., Bakris, G.L., Black, H.R. et al. (2003). Seventh report of the joint National Committee on prevention, detection, evaluation, and treatment of high blood pressure. *Hypertension* 42 (6): 1206–1252.
6. WHO (2021). *Cardiovascular diseases (CVDs)*. World Health Organization www.who.int/news-room/fact-sheets/detail/cardiovascular-diseases-(cvds).

7. Dahl, L.K. (1961). Effects of chronic excess salt ingestion. *Am. J. Phys.* 201: 195–198.
8. Dahl, L.K., Heine, M., and Tassinari, L. (1962). Effects of chronic salt ingestion. *J. Exp. Med.* 115: 1173–1190.
9. De Champlain, J. and van Ameringen, M.R. (1980). Role of central catecholamines in DOCA-salt hypertension. *Hypertension* 2 (4): 553–561.
10. Fregly, M.J. (1958). A new method for producing experimental hypertension. *Proc. Soc. Exp. Biol. Med.* 98: 574–578.
11. Young, D.B. and Guyton, A.C. (1987). Neurogenic mechanisms in hypertension. *Hypertension* 9 (2): 121–128.
12. Ignatowski, A. (1909). Influence of animal food on rabbits. *Virchows Arch.* 198: 248–270.
13. Wissler, R.W. (1985). Atherosclerosis models. *Arteriosclerosis* 5: 567–575.
14. Getz, G.S. and Reardon, C.A. (2012). Animal models of atherosclerosis. *Arterioscler. Thromb. Vasc. Biol.* 32: 1104–1115.
15. Paigen, B., Morrow, A., Brandon, C. et al. (1985). Variation in susceptibility to atherosclerosis among inbred strains of mice. *Atherosclerosis* 57: 65–73.
16. Thompson, J.S. (1986). Development of atherosclerosis in mice. *Lab. Invest.* 54: 111–119.
17. Nakashima, Y., Plump, A.S., Raines, E.W. et al. (1994). ApoE-deficient mice develop lesions of atherosclerosis. *Arterioscler. Thromb.* 14: 133–140.
18. Roche-Molina, M., Sanz-Rodriguez, F., Cruz, F.M. et al. (2015). Induction of atherosclerosis by PCSK9-AAV. *Arterioscler. Thromb. Vasc. Biol.* 35: 2132–2142.
19. Schwendeman, A. and Liu, J. (2017). HDL mimetics and atherosclerosis. *Trends Pharmacol. Sci.* 38: 700–714.
20. Porrini, M., Riso, P., Brusamolino, A. et al. (2005). Polyphenols and endothelial inflammation. *J. Nutr.* 135: 2785–2791.
21. Fan, J. and Watanabe, T. (2003). Atherosclerosis in rabbits. *Arterioscler. Thromb. Vasc. Biol.* 23: 1626–1636.
22. Getz, G.S. and Reardon, C.A. (2006). Diet-induced atherosclerosis in pigs. *Curr. Opin. Lipidol.* 17: 631–639.
23. Gerrity, R.G. (1981). Atherosclerosis in pigs. *Am. J. Pathol.* 103: 181–190.
24. Spady, D.K. and Dietschy, J.M. (1985). LDL receptor function. *J. Clin. Invest.* 76: 1113–1122.
25. Dixon, J.L. and Stoops, J.D. (2000). Diabetic atherosclerosis in pigs. *Diabetes* 49: 1657–1665.
26. Gerrity, R.G., Natarajan, R., Nadler, J.L., and Kimsey, T. (2001). Diabetes-induced vascular disease. *Diabetes* 50: 2031–2040.
27. Watanabe, Y. (1980). WHHL rabbit. *Atherosclerosis* 36: 261–268.
28. Kawai, Y. and Morimoto, S. (2004). Hyperlipidemia in New Zealand rabbits. *J. Atheroscler. Thromb.* 11: 217–223.
29. Hoang, A., Murphy, A.J., and Coughlan, M.T. (2009). ApoA-I transgenic rabbits. *Atherosclerosis* 203: 389–395.
30. Fan, J. and Unoki, H. (2012). Transgenic rabbit models. *Thromb. Haemost.* 108: 439–447.
31. Niimi, M. (2011). ApoA-I and atherosclerosis. *Curr. Opin. Lipidol.* 22: 285–292.
32. Weber, C. and Erl, W. (1997). Monocyte adhesion in atherogenesis. *J. Clin. Invest.* 99: 1060–1069.
33. Cybulsky, M.I. and Gimbrone, M.A. (1991). Endothelial adhesion molecules. *Science* 251: 788–791.
34. Ley, K., Laudanna, C., Cybulsky, M.I., and Nourshargh, S. (2007). Leukocyte recruitment. *Nat. Rev. Immunol.* 7: 678–689.
35. Zhang, Y.S. and Khademhosseini, A. (2017). Vessel-on-a-chip. *Science* 356: 3627.
36. Nazhand, A., Lucarini, M., Durazzo, A. et al. (2020). Hawthorn bioactivity. *Antioxidants* 9: 1–25.
37. Mohana, T. and Thiruchenduran, M. (2015). Anti-atherosclerotic effect of *Crataegus*. *J. Ethnopharmacol.* 170: 145–154.
38. Zhu, Y., Liu, Y., Qian, Y. et al. (2019). Hawthorn pectin and cholesterol metabolism. *Food Funct.* 10: 194–204.
39. Holubarsch, C.J.F., Colucci, W.S., and Meinertz, T. (2008). Crataegus WS 1442. *Eur. Heart J.* 29: 141–148.
40. Wang, J., Xiong, X., and Feng, B. (2013). Crataegus in heart failure. *Phytomedicine* 20: 676–681.
41. Ansary, J., Forbes-Hernandez, T.Y., Gil, E. et al. (2020). Garlic and cardiovascular health. *Nutrients* 12: 872.
42. Al-Qattan, K.K. and Thomson, M. (2003). Garlic vasodilation. *Phytother. Res.* 17: 820–823.
43. Banerjee, S.K. and Maulik, S.K. (2002). Garlic and cardioprotection. *Nutr. J.* 1: 4.
44. Pedraza-Chaverrí, J. and Barrera, D. (1998). Garlic and nitric oxide. *Life Sci.* 63: 71–78.
45. Liu, Y., Wang, J., and Zhang, Y. (2022). NO and hypertension. *Hypertens. Res.* 45: 15–25.
46. Ma, L. and Zhu, Y. (2018). Nitric oxide regulation. *Cardiovasc. Drugs Ther.* 32: 325–335.
47. Orekhov, A.N. and Grünwald, J. (1997). Garlic anti-atherosclerotic activity. *Atherosclerosis* 132: 19–27.
48. Sobenin, I.A. and Andrianova, I.V. (2016). Garlic lipid lowering. *Phytomedicine* 23: 1413–1420.
49. Ismail, M.F. and Gad, M.Z. (1999). Garlic and cholesterol. *Br. J. Nutr.* 82: 235–240.
50. Yadollahi, P. and Namazi, S. (2012). Garlic anticoagulant effects. *Phytother. Res.* 26: 1569–1575.
51. Kojuri, J. and Vosoughi, A. (2007). Garlic in hyperlipidemia. *J. Altern. Complement. Med.* 13: 113–116.
52. Yang, Y. and Kim, Y.J. (2024). Curcumin and lipid metabolism. *Nutrients* 16: 210.
53. Kam, A. and Li, K.M. (2012). Turmeric vasorelaxation. *Br. J. Pharmacol.* 165: 2403–2415.
54. Patonah, A. and Suhartono, E. (2021). Curcumin antihypertensive effect. *Clin. Exp. Hypertens.* 43: 29–36.
55. Ferguson, J.J.A. and Stojanovski, E. (2018). Curcumin and cholesterol. *J. Nutr.* 148: 192–200.
56. Panahi, Y. and Khalili, N. (2017). Curcuminoids in diabetes. *Phytother. Res.* 31: 1836–1844.
57. Xia, Y. and Luo, H. (2015). Berberine cardiovascular effects. *Am. J. Chin. Med.* 43: 1–20.
58. Ma, Y.G. and Liang, L. (2017). Berberine vascular protection. *Cardiovasc. Diabetol.* 16: 15.
59. Yang, D. and Wang, T. (2020). Quercetin cardiovascular protection. *Oxid. Med. Cell. Longev.* 2020: 1–15.
60. Nazari-Khanamiri, F. and Ghasemnejad-Berenji, M. (2023). Quercetin ion channels. *Life Sci.* 314: 121295.
61. Wallace, C.H.R. and Baczkó, I. (2006). Quercetin antiarrhythmic effects. *Br. J. Pharmacol.* 147: 70–82.
62. Balderas, E. and Zhang, J. (2019). MitoBKCa and quercetin. *Cardiovasc. Res.* 115: 1246–1258.
63. He, H. and Wang, L. (2019). Quercetin mitochondrial protection. *Free Radic. Biol. Med.* 134: 552–561.
64. Dulf, F.V. and Vodnar, D.C. (2024). Quercetin cardiotoxicity reversal. *Antioxidants* 13: 112.
65. Botham, K.M. and Wheeler-Jones, C.P.D. (2013). Cholesterol metabolism. *Atherosclerosis* 231: 1–12.
66. Malekmohammad, K. and Rafieian-Kopaei, M. (2021). Garlic bioactivity. *J. Herb. Med.* 26: 100417.
67. Hong, Y. and Hui, S.C. (2003). Berberine in heart failure. *J. Cardiovasc. Pharmacol.* 41: 407–414.
68. Salehi, B. and Machin, L. (2020). Clinical effects of quercetin. *Crit. Rev. Food Sci. Nutr.* 60: 335–357.
69. Li, S. and Lo, C.Y. (2013). Catechins and cardiovascular protection. *J. Nutr. Biochem.* 24: 1417–1426.

70. Chowdhury, A. and Sarkar, J. (2016). EGCG anti-atherosclerotic effects. *Atherosclerosis* 251: 422–430.
71. Ramesh, E. and Geraldine, P. (2009). EGCG and antioxidant defense. *Phytomedicine* 16: 492–498.
72. Hotta, Y. and Igarashi, K. (2006). Catechins and NO. *J. Cardiovasc. Pharmacol.* 47: 476–483.
73. Hirai, M. and Hotta, Y. (2007). EGCG ischemia-reperfusion. *Am. J. Physiol. Heart Circ. Physiol.* 292: H1147–H1155.
74. Hao, J. and Kim, C.H. (2007). EGCG cardiac hypertrophy. *Am. J. Phys.* 292: H1427–H1434.
75. Hao, J. and Shen, W. (2007). EGCG ventricular remodeling. *J. Mol. Cell. Cardiol.* 43: 485–494.
76. Kuo, K.L. and Wu, C.C. (2009). Tea intake and mortality. *J. Am. Coll. Cardiol.* 54: 1501–1509.
77. Kurita, I. and Maeda-Yamamoto, M. (2010). Tea ACE inhibition. *Food Chem.* 120: 385–390.
78. Tadano, T. and Hotta, Y. (2010). GABA-tea antihypertensive effect. *J. Agric. Food Chem.* 58: 913–917.
79. Maron, D.J. (2004). Flavonoids and cardiovascular disease. *J. Nutr.* 134: 3189S–3191S.
80. Kadoglou, N.P.E. and Vraka, C. (2022). Silymarin cardiovascular effects. *Nutrients* 14: 1234.
81. Krečman, V. and Štrukelj, B. (1998). Silymarin pharmacology. *Planta Med.* 64: 479–484.
82. Taleb, S. (2018). Oxidative stress and atherosclerosis. *Nat. Rev. Cardiol.* 15: 337–352.
83. Toghroli, M. and Alizadeh, M. (2024). Antioxidant bioavailability. *Clin. Nutr.* 43: 101–110.
84. Li Volti, G. and Salomone, S. (2011). Silymarin endothelial protection. *Br. J. Pharmacol.* 163: 1522–1536.
85. Singh, S. and Prakash, J. (2023). Silymarin cardiotoxicity protection. *J. Ethnopharmacol.* 302: 115889.
86. Voroneanu, L. and Covic, A. (2017). Silymarin in CABG patients. *Int. Urol. Nephrol.* 49: 1301–1309.
87. Dubey, A.K. and Shankar, P.R. (2004). Ginkgo antioxidant effects. *Indian J. Pharmacol.* 36: 191–198.
88. Noor-E-Tabassum and Khan, M.R. (2022). Ginkgo and oxidative stress. *Biomed. Pharmacother.* 148: 112746.
89. Biernacka, J. and Zielińska, M. (2023). *Ginkgo biloba* cardiovascular protection. *Phytother. Res.* 37: 2214–2226.
90. Liu, J., Li, H., and Shi, M. (2016). Foam cell models. *Biochim. Biophys. Acta* 1861: 1403–1414.

CHAPTER 12

# Toxicological and Pharmacokinetic Considerations in Herbal Medicine

Madhavi Latha Samala[1], Anu Pravallika Janipalli[1], Gowri Gollu[2], and Nalini Mathala[3]

[1] *Department of Pharmaceutics, Aditya College of Pharmacy, Surampalem, Andhra Pradesh, India*

[2] *Department of Pharmaceutical Analysis, Raghu College of Pharmacy, Visakhapatnam, Andhra Pradesh, India*

[3] *Department of Pharmacology, Raghu College of Pharmacy, Visakhapatnam, Andhra Pradesh, India*

## 12.1 INTRODUCTION

According to World Health Organization, approximately 80% of the populations in developing countries rely on these herbal preparations. Herbal medicines are isolated from plants and plant parts, including leaves, flowers, fruits, barks, seeds, and roots. They have been widely used in the treatment and management of a variety of cardiovascular diseases (CVDs) because of their ability to exhibit a wide range of therapeutic benefits such as antioxidant, diuretic, vasodilatory, lipid-lowering, antihypertensive, anti-inflammatory, and antiproliferative properties [1]. Herbal medicines have been known for their long-term disease prevention capability. Their trending use in CVDs is further supported by clinical and pharmacological evidence and traditional knowledge of their properties [2]. Besides these benefits, they show challenges associated with their safety, therapeutic potential, and prediction of pharmacokinetic behavior. Herbal preparations are of natural origin and have a long history of application in traditional systems of medicine. So, herbal medicines are believed to be generally harmless and are used for self-medication, neglecting the need for medical supervision. However, some herbal compounds may produce harmful physiological effects on overconsumption or when used with other medicines. For instance, ephedra and its alkaloid ephedrine may cause hypertension, stroke, and myocardial infarction [3]. Over consumption of licorice may induce excess mineralocorticoids, which result in hypokalemia and hypertension. Aconite alkaloids are reported to cause arrhythmias [4]. There is less awareness of toxicity, adverse effects, and safety associated with herbal preparations, which should be raised among the public. Several factors may result in herbal toxicity, including complexity of constituents, presence of contaminants, adulterants, interactions with co-administered drugs, and clinical implications [5]. Hence, the study of toxicological and pharmacokinetic properties is necessary for applying traditional knowledge of herbal medicines in safe, effective, modern cardiovascular therapy.

### 12.1.1 COMPLEXITY OF HERBAL CONSTITUENTS

Conventional formulations consist of a single, well-characterized active compound responsible for its therapeutic property, and their safety, efficacy, and pharmacokinetic behaviors are well defined by preclinical and clinical studies. Herbal formulations consist of complex bioactives like alkaloids, flavonoids, glycosides, and terpenoids, that may interact actively within the body and these interactions may influence pharmacokinetic properties of concurrently administered drugs, which may further cause disturbances in therapeutic efficacy and toxicity profile. Herbal medicines often cannot be completely characterized due to lack of standardized evaluation procedures for identifying the specific component responsible for its therapeutic efficacy, leading to complicated safety assessment, and have been employed in therapy based on historical use but not on the standard clinical findings. Chemical finger printing, a technique for identifying the unique chemical composition of a compound, is not fully established for most of the bioactives [6]. Herbs like ginseng, bilberry, echinacea, turmeric, St. Johns' wort, and valerian root contains a variety of compounds, and the specific component responsible for their therapeutic potential is not fully understood [7].

### 12.1.2 NEED FOR INTEGRATED TOXICOLOGICAL AND PHARMACOKINETIC EVALUATION

For a drug to be acceptable therapeutically, it should have a clear safety profile. Toxicological evaluation is beneficial in identifying adulterants, contaminants, toxins, and associated adverse effects resulting from the use of unstandardized herbal formulations [8]. Presence of these toxins and adulterants in cardiovascular herbal products may lead to serious cardiovascular risks. Preclinical safety and toxicity evaluation has to be done by performing various toxicological and genotoxicity assessments. Pharmacokinetic evaluation includes assessment of absorption, distribution, metabolism, and excretion (ADME) patterns of herbal formulations, which help in predicting their pharmacological actions, therapeutic efficacy, and safety profile. Pharmacokinetic evaluation also provides for optimizing dose, estimating frequency and duration of administration, and is thereby necessary for fixing dosage regimens. In cardiovascular therapy, herbal medicines are widely used along with conventional medications, resulting in herb–drug interactions. Pharmacokinetic evaluation also enables in predicting these interactions and ensures safe combination therapy. In view of cardiovascular health management, even minor changes in pharmacodynamic balance can result in serious consequences. Hence, understanding safety and pharmacokinetic properties of each component is essential. Therefore, toxicological and pharmacokinetic data has to be integrated in the evaluation of herbal formulations for ensuring scientific use and clinical and regulatory compliance [5]. Toxicological and pharmacokinetic data are linked with one another. Toxic effects of a drug depend on the concentration and tissue distribution characters of the drug. For example, occurrence of hepatotoxicity with use of high concentrations of *Piper methysticum* and green tea extracts for long periods in people with high mass index [9]. So, integration of pharmacokinetic and toxicological data finds use in modeling dose–response relationships, detecting ideal therapeutic windows, and predicting drug accumulation, and concurrently allowing for rational formulation design and regulatory evaluation.

## 12.2 TOXICOLOGICAL CONSIDERATIONS IN HERBAL MEDICINE

Although herbal medicines are often perceived as safe and have a long history of usage, extensive studies and immense research on these medicines indicate that several factors can cause toxicity, including plant components or their metabolites with toxic potential, adulteration, herb–drug interactions, contamination with microorganisms, and environmental pollutants [10].

### 12.2.1 TYPES OF TOXICITY

The toxicity levels are different from case to case and are influenced by duration of administration, dosage, and individual susceptibility, as discussed in the following sections.

- **Acute toxicity:** Assessments of herbal extracts and bioactive ingredients are essential to determine the potential hazards associated with short-term exposure. Such studies typically involve administration of a single or limited dose within a brief period, usually within 24 hours, to determine critical information on immediate toxic effects [11]. The obtained data are critical for determining safe dosage ranges, guiding clinical utilization, and regulatory safety evaluations [12]. Acute studies determine relative acute toxicities by various routes of exposure, as well as the possibility to produce local effects, including irritation and sensitization.
- **Sub-chronic toxicity:** Refers to harmful effects resulting from repeated exposure to a substance over an intermediate period, typically ranging from 28 to 90 days. These studies act as a bridge between acute and chronic toxicity evaluations, revealing dose–response relationships, organ-specific susceptibility, and early pathogenic manifestations. In herbal toxicology, sub-chronic studies help to determine no observed adverse effect levels (NOAELs) and to identify biochemical and histopathological changes associated with repeated use [13].
- **Chronic toxicity:** Defined as deleterious effects resulting from prolonged or repeated exposure to a substance, typically ranging from 6 to 24 months. These studies estimate the risk of carcinogenicity, reproductive and developmental toxicity, and systemic organ damage on prolonged usage.

#### 12.2.1.1 Organ-Specific Toxicity of Herbal Medicines

**Hepatotoxicity:** Herbal-induced hepatotoxicity is the most significant adverse outcome associated with herbal medicines, ranging from mild transaminase elevation to acute liver failure. As the liver is the major site for biotransformation, it is mainly susceptible to damage from reactive metabolites, particularly when herbs are given in higher doses or for longer periods.

For example, green tea (*Camellia sinensis*) extracts are extensively promoted on their anti-oxidant potential, weight-management properties, and cardiovascular protective effects. These properties are largely attributed due to the presence of bioactive compounds like catechins, particularly epigallocatechin gallate. Although, moderate consumption is generally safe, higher doses of green tea extract have been increasingly associated with herb-induced livery injury [14].

- **Nephrotoxicity:** The kidneys are highly vulnerable to toxic injury because of their high metabolic activity, high rate of blood perfusion, large endothelial surface area, and large fraction of cardiac output. Susceptibility is further enhanced by active uptake of substances by tubular cells and low pH of urine. In addition, the renal tubules are engaged in active transport and concentrate substances, which increases local concentration of the herbal toxins and can directly damage tubular cells [15]. For example, aristolochic acids, a group of toxins occurring in the species of *Aristolochia* and *Asarum,* exert chronic nephrotoxic effects, leading to end-stage renal failure and an elevated incidence of with upper tract urothelial carcinoma [16].
- **Neurotoxicity:** Several cardiotonic drugs can exert neurotoxic effects on both central and peripheral nervous systems, with clinical manifestations ranging from mild headaches and dizziness to seizures or psychosis. The risk is especially significant with long-term use, excessive dosing, or improper processing of herbs. For example, *Digitalis purpurea* (foxglove) is a cardiotonic herb that contains potent cardiac glycosides such as digoxin and digoxin, which are effective in heart failure and arrhythmias. Owing to its narrow therapeutic index, glycoside accumulation can lead to neurotoxicity, arrhythmias, and gastrointestinal disturbances [17].

### 12.2.2 CONTAMINANTS AND ADULTERANTS

Although herbal products are considered as natural remedies, they are susceptible to contamination and adulteration at various stages, including farming, harvesting, processing, storage, and distribution. Both pose significant clinical and toxicological risks to consumers due to lack of standardized manufacturing practices, insufficient regulatory monitoring, and inadequate quality control. Contaminants may be introduced unintentionally through environmental exposure, improper handling, or poor agricultural practices. These contaminants or pollutants can exert acute or chronic harmful effect depending on the intensity and duration of exposure. Adulterants are substances that are not listed, but which are added deliberately for economic gain or therapeutic effect.

- **Heavy metals:** Herbal plants may absorb toxic heavy metals, which are poisonous, such as lead, arsenic, cadmium, and mercury from contaminated soil, irrigation water, and atmospheric sources. Prolonged exposure to these metals in herbal plants can cause severe health consequences like neurotoxicity, hepatotoxicity, nephrotoxicity, and an elevated risk of carcinogenesis [18].
- **Pesticides:** The extensive use of pesticides in herbal agriculture leads to residual deposits in the finished product. These residues may disturb endocrine function, damage neurological development, and also have the potential to cause long-term toxicities [19]. Several commonly used medicinal plants have been reported to contain residual pesticides, resulting in significant toxicological concerns. For example, green tea contain residues of chlorpyrifos and triazophos, which can lead to hepatotoxicity and neurotoxicity. In the same way, *Curcuma longa* (turmeric) may carry endosulfan and malathion residues, posing risks of nephrotoxicity [20].
- **Microbial contamination and mycotoxins:** Herbal products are highly susceptible to microbial contamination, which often raises from inadequate hygiene during processing, careless handling, and unsuitable storage conditions. Among these contaminants, fungi, especially *Penicillium* and *Aspergillus* species, produce ochratoxins that exert nephrotoxic, hepatotoxic, and carcinogenic properties [21]. Hawthorn fruit (*Crataegus fructus*) is vulnerable to fungal proliferation by *Aspergillus* and *Penicillium* species, which leads to the production of ochratoxin, posing possible potential toxicological hazards [22].
- **Intentional and unintentional adulteration:** Herbal medicines are often prone to both intentional and unintentional adulteration, which can adversely influence their safety, therapeutic efficacy, and quality. Intentional adulteration refers to the deliberate incorporation of substances, such as synthetic drugs, low-cost plant materials, or artificial colorants into herbal formulations to enhance their apparent effectiveness or profitability. In contrast, unintentional adulteration arises accidentally during cultivation, harvesting, processing, or storage. Both forms reduce the therapeutic effectiveness and also cause severe health impacts in consumers.

### 12.2.3 HERB–DRUG INTERACTIONS

Patients suffering with CVDs generally receive multiple medications, including herbal medicines. In such patients, herb–drug interactions are being the most considerable pharmacological and toxicological challenge that needs to be addressed for their safe clinical use [23]. Herbal medicines interact with conventional drugs either pharmacokinetically or pharmacodynamically when administered simultaneously, leading to a range of toxicities and reduced therapeutic efficacy [24]. Many of the cardiovascular drugs exhibit a narrow therapeutic index, so even minor changes in pharmacokinetic concentrations can result in significant clinical issues. A thorough understanding of mechanisms involved, preventive measures of herb–drug interactions, and their clinical significance is necessary for employing herbal remedies in cardiovascular therapy.

#### 12.2.3.1 Mechanisms of Herb–Drug Interactions

Herb–drug interactions are classified into two types: pharmacokinetic interactions and pharmacodynamic interactions.

**12.2.3.1.1 Pharmacokinetic Interactions** These affect ADME of drugs. Pharmacokinetic interactions involve modulation of metabolizing enzymes, drug transporter proteins, and plasma protein binding. Herbal constituents exhibit enzyme induction or inhibition that may lead to specific change in plasma concentrations [23]. Human cytochrome P450 (CYP450) is the most influenced enzyme. Permeability glycoprotein (P-gp) is an ATP-dependent efflux transporter that helps in the excretion of drugs by reducing their absorption in the intestine. Herbal constituents like curcumin, ginsenosides, and green tea catechins have been found to inhibit P-gp, resulting in toxicity because of increased absorption of co-administered drugs [25]. Several experimental and clinical findings confirmed the occurrence of herb–drug interactions across various classes of cardiovascular drugs that involve CYP family and transporter proteins. For instance, St. John's wort activates pregnane X receptor and induces CYP3A4 enzyme (which metabolizes 50% of medications oxidatively) and efflux drug transporter P-gp. It reduces blood cyclosporin concentrations and may result in heart transplant rejection [26]. St. John's wort also induces other cytochrome enzymes, including CYP3A4 and CYP2C9, and increase metabolism of cardiovascular drugs like statins, calcium channel blockers, and warfarin. As more metabolizing enzymes are induced, plasma drug concentrations, and consequently therapeutic efficacy, tend to decrease [27]. Another study reported inhibition of CYP3A4 enzyme by 47% within four hours after ingestion of grapefruit juice, altering the metabolism of calcium channel blockers like felodipine, amiodarone, and nifedipine, leading to arrhythmias and hypotension [28]. Grapefruit juice also inhibits CYP2C6, CYP2D6, CYP2J2, and drug transporter proteins such as P-gp and organic anion transporter polypeptide (OATP) proteins that improve drug efflux/influx in enterocytes. However, the bioavailability of digoxin is not affected by grapefruit juice, even though it is a strong substrate for P-gp [29]. Green tea catechins were reported to inhibit CYP3A and P-gp in the intestine. Effect of green tea on CYP 450 forms increases exposure to some drugs like simvastatin, sildenafil, and tacrolimus. Similarly, its effect on transporter proteins of OATP family reduces the exposure to drugs like rosuvastatin and nadolol [30]. In a four-week clinical study, it was found that International Normalized Ratio (INR) and peak plasma concentrations of warfarin have decreased after administration of American ginseng, as it induces CYP3A4, leading to a decreased anticoagulant effect of warfarin [31]. Verapamil, a calcium channel blocker, is a strong P-gp inhibitor and shows a tendency to interact with herbs. Garlic, yarrow, and turmeric were found to inhibit P-gp during absorption. With concurrent administration of herbs and calcium channel blockers, adverse reactions like turmeric-induced diarrhea, dizziness, constipation, and palpitation have been observed [32]. In assessing drug safety and efficacy, plasma protein binding is one of the important parameter to consider. Drugs generally bind to human serum albumin, the most abundant plasma protein, which has a large number of binding sites. Herbal constituents may displace the co-administered drug from the binding site on plasma proteins, which increases free drug concentration leading to toxicity. A study developed analytical methods for calculating specific binding parameters between different types of active herbal constituents and plasma proteins [33]. Albumin is the primary binding site for 99% of warfarin. Herbs like willow bark, ginseng, green tea, and garlic exhibit competitive binding to albumin and may inhibit protein binding of warfarin and increase its free fraction in plasma leading to hemorrhage [34].

**12.2.3.1.2 Pharmacodynamic Interactions** The interactions occur when the effect of one drug is influenced by co-administration of another drug and are known as pharmacodynamics interactions. Herbal actives and the drugs directly compete for a particular binding site or target and interfere with physiological mechanisms. These include synergistic or antagonistic effects that alter the drug's pharmacological action at the target site [35].

- **Additive effects:** A synergistic effect is observed to occur between *Gingko biloba* and antithrombic agents [35]. Antiplatelet activity is produced by garlic and ginger. So, when co-administered with vitamin K antagonists like warfarin, antithrombotic agents like clopidogrel, and other cardiac drugs like aspirin, they produce an additive effect leading to excessive bleeding [34, 35]. *Crataegus oxyacantha* (hawthorn), used as a cardiotonic, in combination with digoxin increases the effects of antihypertensive drugs like ACE inhibitors and beta-blockers, causing hypotension and dizziness [36]. Yohimbine causes arrhythmias in patients on digoxin by inducing sympathetic effects [37].
- **Antagonistic effects:** In cardiac therapy, caffeine, when co-administered with adrenergic agents, antithrombic agents, and anti-arrhythmics, exhibits competitive adenosine antagonistic activity, leading to hypertension, myocardial infarction, and bleeding risk. So, excessive intake of caffeine in cardiac patients is to be monitored; otherwise, it may cause tachyarrhythmias, insomnia, and angina pectoris [38]. Yohimbine interacts with various cardiovascular drugs like antihypertensives (clonidine, methyldopa) by acting as an antagonist for $\alpha_2$-adrenergic receptor inhibition. High doses may lead to cardiac ischemia [37].

Hence, careful study and monitoring of pharmacokinetic and pharmacodynamic interactions are necessary to ensure safe and concomitant clinical use of herbal remedies in cardiovascular therapy.

### 12.2.4 ALLERGIC AND IDIOSYNCRATIC REACTIONS

Allergic and idiosyncratic reactions are rare but remain a major concern while using herbal medicines in CVD management because they are unpredictable and may result in serious consequences. It is important to understand these reactions for ensuring patient safety and preventing life-threatening events. These are dose-independent and the proper mechanism involved is unknown. Individual immune responses to some herbal constituents and contaminants may be involved. A complete medication history of the patients is required for designing herbal medicine-integrated dosage regimen in cardiovascular patients [39].

#### 12.2.4.1 Allergic Reactions

Plant proteins, polysaccharides, and secondary metabolites that act as allergens may trigger immune-mediated responses. After exposure to these allergens, they induce type I (immunoglobulin E–mediated) or type IV(T-cell–mediated) immune-specific hypersensitivity reactions [40]. These allergies may result in major cardiovascular risks like anaphylaxis, hypotension, and tachycardia [41]. Serious allergic reactions that become life-threatening are known as anaphylactic shock, which may be caused by active constituents themselves or contaminants in the formulation [42]. Type I hypersensitivity reactions involve mast cell degranulation, histamine release, and vasodilation, leading to systemic anaphylaxis, hypotension, and arrhythmias. T-cell-mediated immune injury is caused by type IV hypersensitivity responses, resulting in delayed allergic myocarditis [43].

#### 12.2.4.2 Idiosyncratic Reactions

Idiosyncratic reactions are also immune-mediated responses that are rare and unpredictable. These occur due to genetic polymorphisms in metabolizing enzymes, reactive metabolite formation, or abnormalities in activation of immune system. No specific immunological mechanisms are involved [44]. These reactions result in unusual cardiovascular damage because of their ability to cause disturbances in mitochondrial function, modulations of ion channels, and endothelial damage.

Various herbal agents have proven to exhibit allergic and idiosyncratic reactions with cardiovascular drugs [40]. Mechanisms involved in producing these adverse reactions are histamine-mediated vasodilation, immune cell activation, genetic susceptibility, and reactive metabolite formation. Typical examples of herbal agents involved in these reactions are presented in this section. Herbs can release reactive metabolites during their cardiac or hepatic metabolism. These metabolites interact with cardiac proteins by forming covalent compounds, thereby resulting in direct cardiac toxicity or initiating immune responses. Kavalactones of *P. methysticum* like methysticin cause hepatotoxicity by forming reactive metabolites and also by depleting glutathione [45]. Kava is used as muscle relaxant, and it has proven to cause cardiac ischemia and sudden death in sportsmen in Australia [46]. Gingko extracts are commonly used for enhancing circulation and memory power. Gingko may cause mild to severe allergic reactions, including itching, difficulty in breathing, heart palpitations, and cross-reactivity with related herbal compounds [47]. Sulphur-containing compounds in garlic produce allergic reactions by causing mast cell activation and release of histamine and leukotrienes. These substances may lead to mild allergic dermatitis and rhinitis or to severe hypotension through vascular dilatation. Anaphylactic shock may also occur in severe cases, which reduces cardiac output and total block of circulatory system [48]. A case report has shown the development of respiratory allergy associated with skin and blood pressure issues after ingestion of locally made Asian ginseng syrup within three minutes in Bangkok by a 20-year-old male medical student [49]. Detoxifying enzymes like CYP2D6, NAT 2 (N-acetyltransferase 2), and GSTM1 (glutathione S-transferase Mu 1) are responsible for metabolism of cardiac agents. Any genetic polymorphism in these enzymes may increase the risk of developing idiosyncratic reactions in a person by influencing metabolism and excretion patterns [50]. Aristolchic acid causes idiosyncratic vasculitis. Continuous exposure to this drug causes fibrotic lesions and ischemia. Immediate reactions result in inflammation in vascular muscles and the myocardium [9].

### 12.2.5 INDIVIDUAL SUSCEPTIBILITY AND RISK FACTORS

The pharmacological and toxicological effects of herbal medicine may vary among individuals. This interindividual variability results from the intrinsic interaction of physiological, genetic, and environmental factors that influence pharmacokinetics, encompassing ADME, along with the pharmacodynamic response of herbal substances. A thorough understanding of these factors is crucial for optimizing the safety and efficacy of herbal therapies and for anticipating possible adverse reactions and herb–drug interactions.

- **Physiological factors:** Changes in the pharmacological and toxicological responses of herbal medicines are significantly influenced by physiological variables like age, sex, and body composition. Infants and children, owing to immature hepatic and renal detoxification systems, are mainly vulnerable to contaminants such as pesticides, aflatoxins, and heavy metals [51]. Conversely, elderly individuals commonly experience reduced metabolic and excretion efficiency and altered cardiac physiology, which collectively intensify their sensitivity to toxic herbal glycosides or herb–drug interactions [52]. Moreover, sex-specific differences in the activity of drug-metabolizing enzymes, especially in the CYP450 super family, might be the causes of the variability in metabolism and systemic responses to herbal compounds.
- **Genetic factors:** Genetic factors largely contribute to the individual responses and play a key part in determining the safety and efficacy of herbal medicines. Polymorphic forms of CYPP450, especially CYP3A4, CYP2C9, and CYP2D6, can markedly alter the metabolism of herbal compounds, resulting in either decreased therapeutic benefits or increased toxicity. As an example, CYP2D6 variability may influence the metabolism of alkaloid-rich compounds, heightening the risk of neurotoxic effects [53].
- **Pathological conditions:** The presence of underlying pathologies can profoundly alter the toxicological response of herbal medicines. Individuals with hepatic impairment, exhibit reduced biotransformation, rendering them especially susceptible to the hepatotoxicity of substances, especially pyrrolizidine alkaloids [54]. On the contrary, renal insufficiency diminishes the clearance of heavy metals and other slowly excreted metabolites, leading to enhanced nephrotoxicity. Individuals with preexisting CVD conditions face additional hazards, as overconsumption of cardiotonic herbs like *Convallaria majalis* and *D. purpurea* may trigger arrhythmias and overt cardiotoxic risks [55].
- **Maternal and neonatal considerations:** The periods of pregnancy and lactation are times of heightened physiological vulnerability, during which exposure to herbal medicines may pose significant maternal, fetal, or neonatal risks. During gestation, large number of phytochemicals readily crosses the placenta, potentially exerting teratogenic, embryotoxic, or fetotoxic effects [56]. In lactating women, phytoconstituents may be secreted into breast milk, exposing neonates, whose detoxification systems are immature, to potential risks [57]. The herbs, comprising volatile oils and alkaloids, may damage gastrointestinal activity, neurological development, or overall infant safety [58]. These considerations underscore the need of careful risk–benefit assessment and cautious use of herbal medicines during pregnancy and breastfeeding.

### 12.2.6 TOXICOLOGICAL TESTING METHODOLOGIES (*IN VITRO, IN VIVO, IN SILICO*)

Toxicological testing involves various experimental models, including *in vitro*, *in vivo*, and *in silico* methods, to provide better understanding and prediction of mechanisms involved, dose–response relations, and organ-specific toxicity [59].

#### 12.2.6.1 *In Vitro* Toxicology Testing

It involves testing medicines on isolated cells and tissues under controlled laboratory conditions without influencing the physiology of body. *In vitro* assays can detect mechanisms of toxicity at the cellular and molecular levels [60]. Cytotoxicity assays involving techniques like MTT (3-[4,5- dimethylthiazol-2-yl]-2,5-diphenyl tetrazolium bromide) assay and lactate dehydrogenase release tests are used for evaluating cell viability and membrane integrity after interacting with herbal drug extracts. Using human cardiomyocytes, *C. sinensis* tea extracts can be screened to detect safe dosage limits and any oxidative stress profiles, thereby employing the extract in cardiac therapy [61]. Genotoxicity can be detected by micronuclear assays and chromosomal aberration tests. Genotoxic evaluation is necessary for predicting carcinogenic risks associated with continuous herbal usage. The genotoxic potential of amiodarone, an antiarrhythmic drug, was assessed by monitoring the difference in the chromosomal aberrations in different rat models [62]. Organ-specific toxicity can be assessed using hepatocyte cultures, cardiomyocyte models, and renal proximal tubule cells. Human-induced pluripotent stem cell-derived cardiomyocytes offer a new drug-screening and diagnostic method for determining the effects of herbal drugs on electrophysiology of heart [63].

#### 12.2.6.2 *In Vivo* Toxicological Testing

It involves evaluation of systemic, organ-specific, and chronic toxic effects of chemicals and herbal preparations in whole living animals, like laboratory mouse and rat models, under physiological conditions [64]. They are essential for developing dose–response relationship, target organ toxicity, and $LD_{50}$ values, which cannot be determined by *in vitro* toxicity studies. Cardiovascular toxicity testing was performed using rodent electrocardiographic studies and echocardiography to predict vascular changes, after exposing to herbal products [65]. Toxic effects of *Ephedra* alkaloids on the heart, like increase in heart rate and blood pressure, was determined by using animal models [3].

#### 12.2.6.3 *In Silico* Toxicological Testing

It involves the use of mathematical algorithms, machine learning, and chemiinformatics to screen herbal toxicity early by considering physical properties, chemical structure, and pharmacological activity while minimizing animal use. Quantitative structure activity relationship models, ADMET prediction platforms like ADMET predictor™, Swiss ADME, and pkCSM are used to estimate ADME properties of multicomponent herbal drug effectively. Many herbal compounds with cardioprotective potential have been screened using molecular docking and network pharmacology [66].

By combining findings from *in vitro, in vivo,* and *in silico* models, toxicological evaluation of herbal preparations can be performed more efficiently and robustly, ensuring their safe and clinical use in cardiovascular health [67]. The sequential steps in assessing herbal toxicity are shown in Figure 12.1.

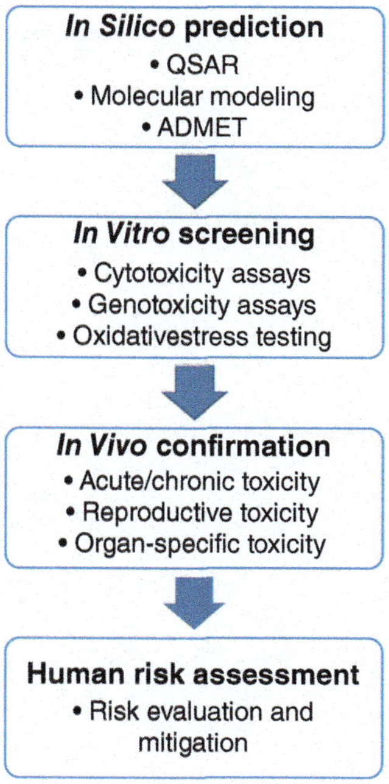


**FIGURE 12.1** Sequential approach to herbal toxicity assessment.

## 12.3 PHARMACOKINETIC CONSIDERATIONS OF HERBAL MEDICINE

### 12.3.1 PHARMACOKINETICS OF HERBAL MEDICINES

Most of the biologically active components of herbal extracts, containing flavonoids, terpenoids, tannins, and carotenoids, are polar and exhibit poor GI penetration due to their large chemical sizes. Bioavailability and tissue penetration through lipophilic membranes are lower for herbal medicines [2].

In the following sections, the pharmacokinetic considerations and bioavailability of various bioactive compounds are discussed.

### 12.3.2 FLAVONOIDS

Flavonoids are prevalent polyphenolic chemicals in many foods produced by the secondary metabolism of plants. Flavonoids are classified based on their skeletal structures such as glycosides, which includes: (1) flavones (like luteolin and apigenin), (2) flavanols are natural compounds found in fruits and vegetables such as myricetin and quercetin, (3) fruits like oranges which contain flavanones (naringenin and hesperidin), (4) epicatechin and catechins are flavanols which are present in apples and berries, (5) isoflavones (daidzein and genistein) are phytoestrogens whose function is similar to human estradiol function, and (6) at last anthocyanidins (pelargonidin and cyanidin), which are the colored flavonoids found in grapes, berries, and other fruits and vegetables. These six primary categories of flavonoids structures are presented in Figure 12.2

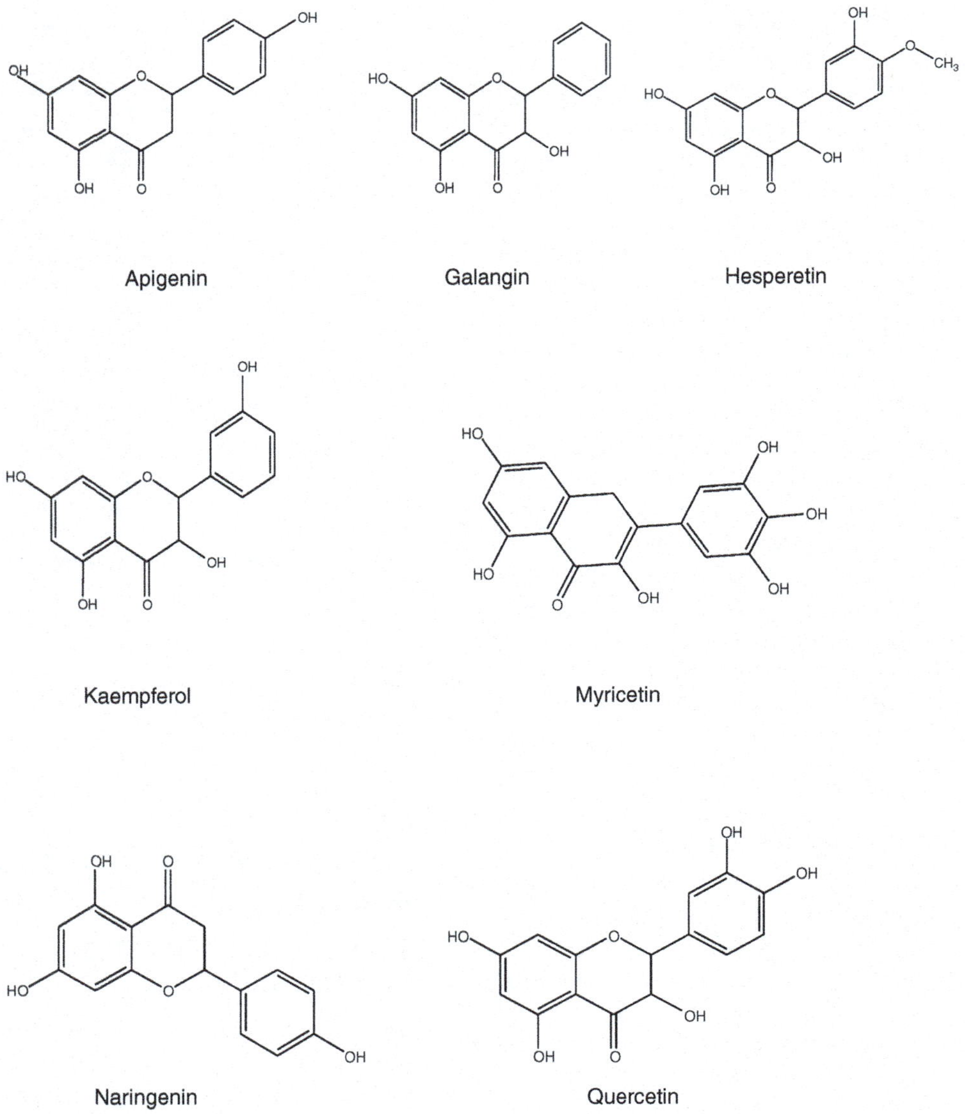


**FIGURE 12.2** Chemical structures of flavonoids.

- **Pharmacokinetic and bioavailability considerations of flavonoids:**

  The majority of flavonoids that human's intake are obtained from the diet. The possible cardioprotective effects of flavonoids depend on the absorption and movement of flavonoid metabolites from the gut into the bloodstream. The main site for flavonoid absorption is the gastrointestinal tract. Intestinal permeability, intestinal microbes, and molecular structures all have a significant impact on absorption [68]. The chemical structure indicates that flavonoids have high lipophilicity. As a result, they are poorly soluble, which makes many common flavonoids less bioavailable. Many flavonoids exist in glycosylated macromolecules; therefore, glycosidases synthesized from gut microorganisms are required to decompose them into phenolic acids or glycosides for absorption. The pharmacokinetics of flavonoids are represented in Table 12.1. Flavonoids are absorbed and transported throughout the body via the transporter families that transport organic anions (OAT), such as MFS (major facilitator superfamiliy), SLC22A (solute carrier 22A), and other sub-classes of SLC22A, which are involved in distribution and excretion of anions from the body [86]. Past research on apigenin has demonstrated that 5–10% of apigenin can be absorbed after administration. Similarly, quercetin, whose structure is bound to glycosides, shows improved bioavailability to almost more than 50%. Distribution of flavonoids occurs by binding to serum albumin.

The metabolism of flavonoids occurs via glucuronide conjugation and methylation. After entering the bloodstream, herbal drugs undergo phase II metabolic reactions by liver enzymes, including CYP450 and their subclasses CYP1A2 and CYP3A4, which mediate the oxidative demethylation reactions for many flavonoids However, many approaches have been evaluated to improve the bioavailability of flavonoids. It has frequently been discovered that dietary flavonoids, either alone

**Table 12.1** Bioavailability of various herbal active constituents in treating cardiovascular diseases.

| Compound | Typical oral bioavailability | Cardiovascular area focused | General delivery systems |
|---|---|---|---|
| **Flavonoids** | | | |
| Quercetin [69, 70] | Poor solubility, rapid metabolism through glucuronidation, sulfation, and methylation. Oral bioavailability is low (<10%) | Atherosclerosis, hypertension, endothelial dysfunction | Liposomes, inclusion complexes, nanoparticles |
| Naringenin [71, 72] | Low solubility, poor water solubility, and extensive first-pass metabolism. Oral bioavailability (15%) | Lipid metabolism, endothelial dysfunction, anti-inflammatory in atherosclerosis | Nano particles, complexation, Lipid based and polymer based formulations |
| Hesperidin [73, 74] | Appreciable solubility. Limited intestinal absorption due to p-glycoprotein efflux and rapid elimination. Oral bioavailability (20%) | Vascular endothelial dysfunction, anti-inflammatory in cardiovascular disorders | Complexation, micronization, eutectic mixtures |
| Kaempferol [75, 76] | Very low oral bioavailability (2%) due to extensive first-pass metabolism | Anti-atherosclerosis | Nanoparticles, phospholipid complexation, solid dispersion |
| Apigenin [77, 78] | Poor solubility, oral bioavailability (20–30%) | Anti-inflammatory, limited effect | Nanoparticles, Bio SNEDDS[a], encapsulation |
| **Terpenoids** | | | |
| Pinene [79] | Poor oral bioavailability (10–20%), rapid absorption, extensively metabolized through oxidation reaction | Vasorelaxant, hypotensive effects | Microencapsulation and liposomes |
| Myrcene [80] | Low oral bioavailability (5–10%), rapid first-pass metabolism | Mild vasorelaxant and anti-inflammatory effects in myocardial ischemia | Liposomes |
| Artemisinin [81] | Very low bioavailability (10–15%) due to rapid metabolism | Protects myocardium | Liposomes and solid-based dispersions |
| **Carotenoids** | | | |
| Β-Caryophyllene [82] | Poor solubility. enhanced moderate bioavailability (35–40%) through Β-Caryophyllene-Self Emulsifying Drug Delivery Systems (BCP-SEDDS) formulations | Antihypertensive and cardioprotective effects in ischemic conditions | Lipophilic, nanoemulsions, BCP-SEDDS |
| β-Carotene [83] | Absorption ranges from 5% to 10%, depends on dietary fat intake | Reduces low-density lipoprotein (LDL) oxidation, improves endothelial function | Emulsified form and micellar form |
| Astaxanthin [84] | Highly lipophilic, low bioavailability (10–12%) | Enhances lipid profiles and improves endothelial function | Nano formulations, oil-based capsules, and sustained-release formulations |
| β-Cryptoxanthin [85] | Comparatively high absorption | Reduces atherosclerotic markers | Liposomes |

[a] Bio SNEDDS: Bio-self emulsifying novel drug delivery system.

or in combination, can change the pharmacokinetic profile of other medications. Antihypertensive drugs like lisinopril and captopril and other cardiac drugs such as digoxin with a low therapeutic index have shown altered pharmacokinetic profiles due to interaction with flavonoids [69, 87].

Thus, to improve the bioavailability of flavonoids, numerous strategies, including intraportal drug delivery during surgery and drug delivery using novel nanomaterials, have been assessed to increase the bioavailability of flavonoids, as shown in Table 12.1. Relevant research on the delivery of flavonoids by nanomaterials in CVDs has to be established.

### 12.3.3 TERPENOIDS

Terpenoids are five-carbon isoprene unit naturally occurring organic compounds that are derived from plants. The stability and reactivity of terpenoids depend on 2-methyl groups attached to two double bonds [88]. Terpenes, including

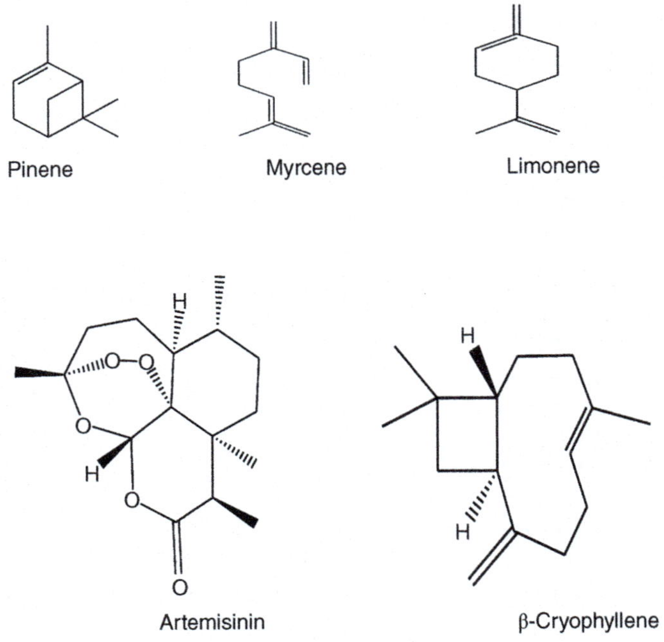


**FIGURE 12.3** Chemical structures of terpenoids.

pinene, myrcene, limonene, terpinene, p-cymene, artemisinin and β-caryophyllene, are commonly available as terpenoids in dietary sources, which are also available as essential oils, as shown in Figure 12.3 and Table 12.1.

According to several researchers' reports, terpenoids may have therapeutic uses in the management of diseases related to heart and blood vessels, like myocardial infarction, hypertension, thrombosis, and other cardiac disorders, by regulating the mechanism of mitogen-activated protein kinase (MPAK) pathway and modulating inflammation and apoptosis.

The mechanism of terpenoids, such as β-caryophyllene, artemisinin, and pinene as, cardioprotective herbal medicines occurs by inhibiting the NLRP3 inflammasome, i.e., NOD-nucleotide-binding oligomerization domain, LRR leucine-rich repeat NLR protein-containing family, which prevents inflammation associated with hypertension, myocardial infarction, atrial fibrillation, and heart failure. Terpenoids have several characteristics that need to be controlled to increase their effectiveness in preventing CVDs: poor dissolution, decreased biological availability, decreased cellular uptake, and significant inconsistency associated with their high volatility [89]. Due to these properties of terpenoids, discussing the kinetic parameters is considerable to improve the potency and therapeutic effect of terpenoids in the prevention of CVDs.

- **Pharmacokinetic consideration of terpenoids:** Terpenoid bioavailability refers to the penetration of the required dose of herbal drug into cardiac cells to produce cardioprotective effects. Terpenes are highly lipophilic; therefore, aqueous solubility is less in the gut lumen, so to improve the bioavailability lipid-phase incorporation is an important consideration during dosing of terpenes. The kinetics of terpenoids are shown in Table 12.1. In the human body, terpenoids undergo changes due to enzymatic actions and pH conditions in cardiomyocytes, liver, and other tissue cells.

Terpenoids are mostly available as essential oils due to their lipophilic nature. Terpenoids are highly permeable through the skin. Through the oral route, terpenoids have a minimum rate of absorption through upper gastrointestinal tract; through the inhalation route, maximum absorption happens to lungs, which are readily available to systemic circulation and to target cells. Metabolism of terpenoids occurs in the liver, as many of these essential oils undergo only one phase of reactions, either phase I or phase II. For example, camphor was metabolized to 5-exo-hydroxycamphor by phase II reactions. Compounds that were excreted as glucuronides are menthol and peppermint oil, which are excreted through kidneys. Terpenoids have a short elimination, and the clearance rate is high; therefore, accumulation of metabolites is impossible. Terpenoids are eliminated from the body by renal excretion through kidneys, along with elimination via the lungs through exhalation, and also through the skin [90].

Essential oils of terpenoids are used to increase the bioavailability of other drugs, such as galangal essential oil added to flurbiprofen microemulsion gel, an anti-inflammatory drug, to increase the bioavailability, similarly ligustrazine, an antiplatelet aggregation drug, is used to increase the transdermal absorption of ligustrazine. Different terpenoids have different pharmacokinetics, especially absorption and metabolism, based on their lipophilicity, molecular weights, solubility, and different GI tract sites for drug absorption and intestinal pH. Certain terpenoids are administered as transdermal routes other than oral and inhalation.

From the above evidence, terpenoids have been formulated as cardioprotective drugs, based on the fact that these days researchers' interest in traditional herbal and plant-based medicines, even in the face of advancements in synthesis of chemical elements through the development of contemporary synthetic therapies, continues to grow. Even though drugs for CVDs are abundant, the desire for new, safe, less–cost, and more potent drugs is increasing. Hence, more research and clinical studies has to be reported for herbal medicines in CVD.

### 12.3.4 CAROTENOIDS

Carotenoids represent a category of natural, fat-soluble pigments predominantly located in edible plant parts, including flowers and roots. Researchers have identified almost 600 carotenoids compounds, of which nearly 50 carotenoid compounds can be consumed through human diet. Lycopene, α-carotene, zeaxanthin, β-cryptoxanthin, β-carotene, and lutein, found in tomato, grape fruit, and carrots, are most common carotenoids. Their main function is as provitamin vitamin A, contributing to the synthesis of vitamin A [91]. Several case studies have reported that carotenoids have a protective role against CVDs by reducing inflammation such as inhibition of nonthrombogenic circulating cells, inhibition of NF-κB pathway, which triggers the up regulation of vascular cell adhesion molecules.

- **Pharmacokinetics and bioavailability considerations of carotenoids:**
  Carotenoids are nonpolar compounds with high lipophilicity, which results in minimal absorption. Therefore, carotene compounds are administered as micelles and, in the stomach, as components of bile pigments. Carotenoids are then transported as micelles to enterocytes, where absorption takes place through passive process of diffusion or transport by receptor assistance. Carotenoid distribution occurs through transporters like SR-B1 (Scavenger Receptor Class B1), NPC1L1 (Niemann–Pick C1-Like1), and CD36 (Cluster of Differentiation 36) [82]. At least 40% of the carotenoids that are consumed are unaltered because of metabolic activities.

The distribution of carotenoids takes place by the incorporation of carotenoids into chylomicrons, followed by transport into the lymphatic system. Carotenoids are distributed to different organs and stored in lipophilic compartments of cells or tissues. Plasma protein binding of carotenoids is unknown. Pharmacokinetics of carotenoids are shown in Table 12.1. Carotenoids are significantly less concentrated in plasma than the primary lipids. Studies conducted *in vivo* have shown that HDL has about 0.05 carotenoid molecules per particle, while LDL has about one carotenoid molecule. Almost 75% or carotenoids bind to LDL, and only a less percentage bind to HDL. Depending on the particular carotenoid, the human body has an uneven distribution of carotenoids. Carotenoids are preferentially absorbed by specific tissues, and they typically concentrate in peripheral body organs like eyes, adipose tissue, skin, and adrenal glands.

Metabolic pathways of carotenoids were unknown, as specific carotenoids follow specific metabolic pathways. Lycopene, a carotenoid, shows varied concentration of 2,6-cyclolycopen-1,5, diols and other oxygenated metabolites. Chemical structure of carotenoids were shown in Figure 12.4. *In vivo* oxidation lead to epoxides, which are transferred to 5,6-dihydroxy-5,6-dihydrolycopene, which has a physiological function in human cells. Lipid metabolism is involved in the metabolic pathways of carotenoids, such as lipolysis and autophagy, which are involved in the pathogenesis of several diseases. Therefore, carotenoids in LDL lipoproteins can reduce the risk of myocardial infarction and other risks of carcinogenesis in adults [83, 91].

Even though carotenoids are beneficial in the treatment of CVDs due to their less adverse effects, more availability, and less expensive, more research on bioavailability, therapeutic window calculations, and pharmacokinetic parameters assessment through clinical studies must be done in future.

## 12.4 CONCLUSION

Toxicological and pharmacokinetic considerations are essential requirements and form the basis for the safe and effective use of herbal medicines in the treatment of CVDs. Phytomedicine's complex nature demands toxicological evaluation to detect intrinsic phytotoxins, contaminants, and adulterants that could compromise patient safety. Pharmacokinetic profiling also required to determine how herbal constituents are absorbed, distributed, metabolized, and excreted. The chapter emphasizes toxicological and pharmacokinetic considerations of flavonoids, terpenoids, and carotenoids. These insights are critical for predicting herb–drug interactions, ensuring dose optimization, and establishing regulatory standards. With regard to CVDs, patients are highly vulnerable and often on multiple medications. Advanced tools of *in silico* modeling can be integrated with *in vitro* and *in vivo* studies to provide more precise toxicity prediction and risk assessment of herbal medicines. Hence, rigorous toxicological and PK evaluations are indispensable for integrating herbal therapies responsibly into modern clinical practice.

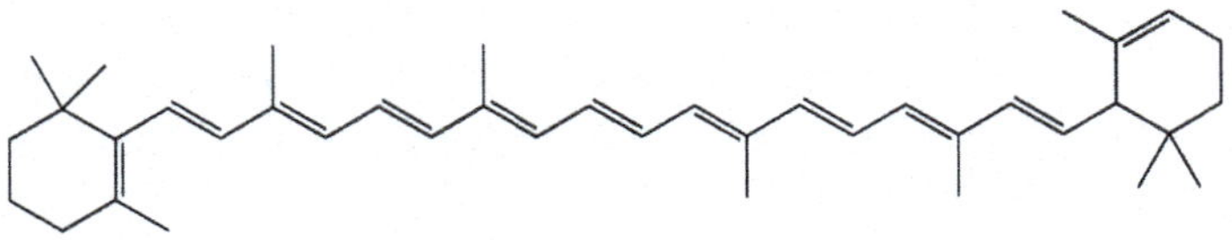

α-Carotene

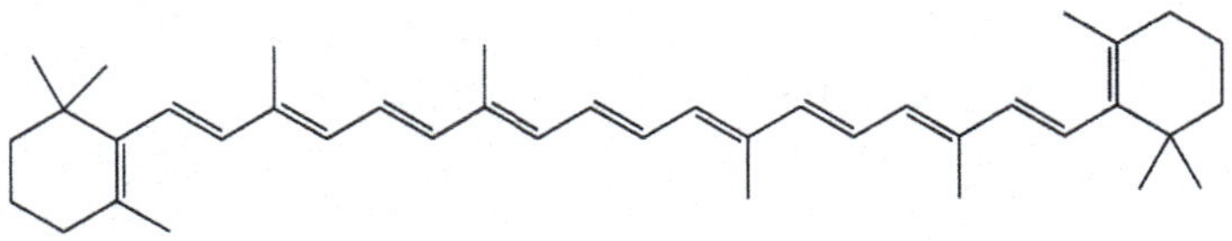

β-Carotene

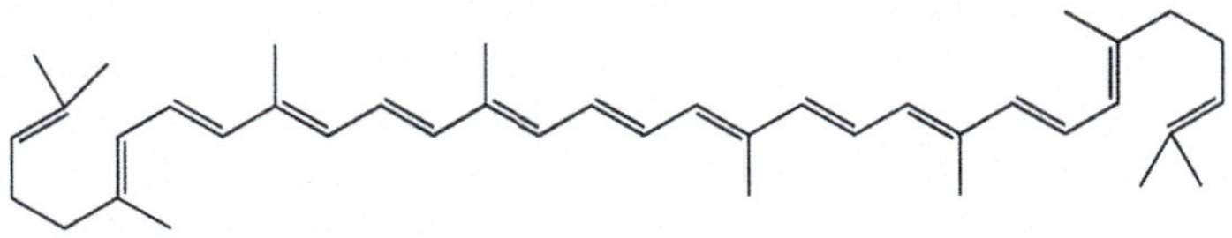

Lycopene

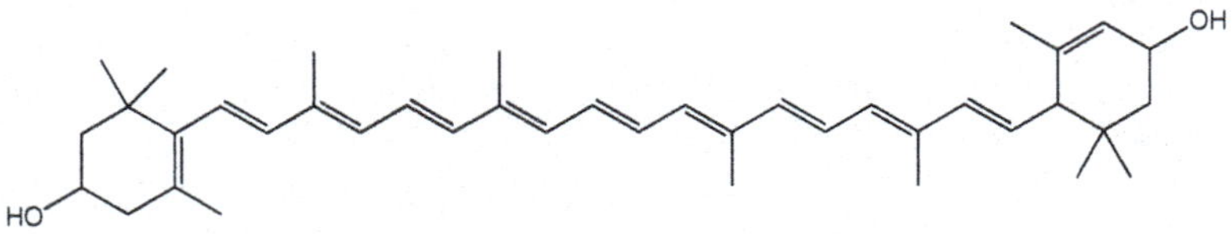


Lutein

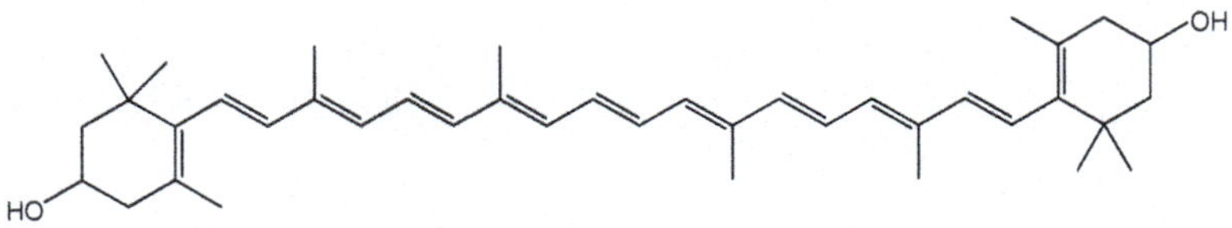


Zeaxanthin

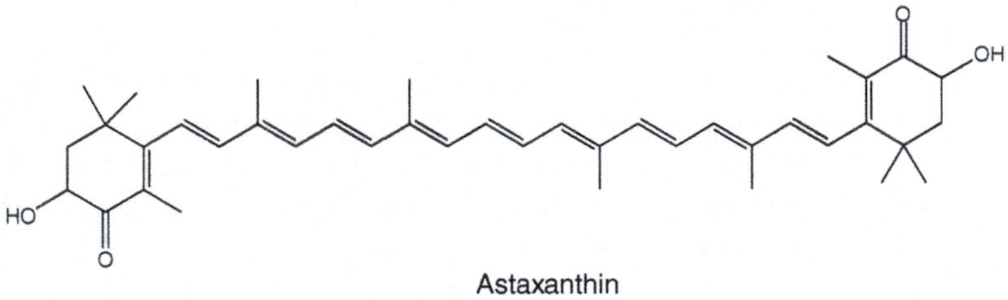


Astaxanthin

**FIGURE 12.4** Chemical structures of carotenoids.

## REFERENCES


1. Perez-Vizcaino F, Duarte J. Flavonols and cardiovascular disease. *Mol. Aspects Med.* 2010; 31(6): 478–494. https://doi.org/10.1016/j.mam.2010.09.002.Epub.
2. Shaito A, Thuan DTB, Phu HT, Nguyen THD, Hasan H, Halabi S, Abdelhady S, Nasrallah GK, Eid AH, Pintus G. Herbal medicine for cardiovascular diseases: efficacy, mechanisms, and safety. *Front. Pharmacol.* 2020; 11: 422. https://doi.org/10.3389/fphar.2020.00422.
3. Haller CA, Benowitz NL. Adverse cardiovascular and central nervous system events associated with dietary supplements containing ephedra alkaloids. *N. Engl. J. Med.* 2000; 343 (25): 1833–1838. https://doi.org/10.1056/NEJM200012213432502.
4. Chan TY. Aconitum alkaloid poisoning related to the culinary uses of aconite roots. *Toxins (Basel)* 2014; 6(9): 2605–2611. https://doi.org/10.3390/toxins6092605.
5. Saad B, Azaizeh H, Abu-Hijleh G, Said O. Safety of traditional Arab herbal medicine. *Evid. Based Complement. Alternat. Med.* 2006; 3(4): 433–439. https://doi.org/10.1093/ecam/nel058.
6. Neergheen-Bhujun VS. Underestimating the toxicological challenges associated with the use of herbal medicinal products in developing countries. *BioMed Res. Int.* 2013; 2013: 804086. https://doi.org/10.1155/2013/804086.
7. Barnes J, Anderson LA, Gibbons S, Phillipson JD. *Echinacea* species (*Echinacea angustifolia* (DC.) Hell., *Echinacea pallida* (Nutt.) Nutt., *Echinacea purpurea* (L.) Moench): a review of their chemistry, pharmacology and clinical properties. *J. Pharm. Pharmacol.* 2005; 57(8): 929–954. https://doi.org/10.1211/0022357056127.
8. Saper RB, Kales SN, Paquin J, Burns MJ, Eisenberg DM, Davis RB, Phillips RS. Heavy metal content of Ayurveda herbal medicine products. *JAMA* 2004; 292 (23): 2868–2873. https://doi.org/10.1001/jama.292.23.2868.
9. Debelle FD, Vanherweghem JL, Nortier JL. Aristolochic acid nephropathy: a worldwide problem. *Kidney Int.* 2008; 74(2): 158–169. https://doi.org/10.1038/ki.2008.129.Epub.

10. Ekor, M. (2014). The growing use of herbal medicines: issues relating to adverse reactions and challenges in monitoring safety. *Front. Pharmacol.* 4: 177.
11. Eldesoqui, M., Ahmed, M.E., Abdel-Kareem, M.A. et al. (2023). Curcumin mitigates malathion-induced renal injury: suppression of apoptosis and modulation of NF-κβ/TNF-α and Nrf 2, and HO-1 signaling. *Meta* 13 (11): 1117.
12. Singhuber, J., Zhu, M., Prinz, S., and Kopp, B. (2009). Aconitum in traditional Chinese medicine—a valuable drug or an unpredictable ris? *J. Ethnopharmacol.* 126 (1): 18–30.
13. Morimoto, M., Tatsumi, K., Yuui, K. et al. (2021). Convallatoxin, the primary cardiac glycoside in lily of the valley (*Convallaria majalis*), induces tissue factor expression in endothelial cells. *Vet. Med. Sci.* 7 (6): 2440–2444.
14. Teschke, R. and Eickhoff, A. (2015). Herbal hepatotoxicity in traditional and modern medicine: actual key issues and new encouraging steps. *Front. Pharmacol.* 6: 72.
15. Jha, V. and Rathi, M. (2008). Natural medicines causing acute kidney injury. *Semin. Nephrol.* 28 (4): 416–428.
16. Han, J., Xian, Z., Zhang, Y. et al. (2019). Systematic overview of aristolochic acids: nephrotoxicity, carcinogenicity, and underlying mechanisms. *Front. Pharmacol.* 10: 648.
17. Wang, Z., Han, H., Wang, C. et al. (2021). Hepatotoxicity of pyrrolizidine alkaloid compound intermedine: comparison with other pyrrolizidine alkaloids and its toxicological mechanisms. *Toxins* 13 (12): 849.
18. Ernst, E. (2002). Toxic heavy metals and undeclared drugs in Asian herbal medicines. *Trends Pharmacol. Sci.* 23 (3): 136–139.
19. Sajad, M., Shabir, S., Singh, S.K. et al. (2024). Role of nutraceutical against exposure to pesticide residues: power of bioactive compounds. *Front. Nutr.* 17 (11): 1342881.
20. Chen, L., Mo, H., Zhao, L. et al. (2017). Therapeutic properties of green tea against environmental insults. *J. Nutr. Biochem.* 40: 1–3.
21. Opuni, K.F., Kretchy, J.P., Agyabeng, K. et al. (2023). Contamination of herbal medicinal products in low-and-middle-income countries: a systematic review. *Heliyon* 9 (9): e19370.
22. Yu, J., Guo, M., Jiang, W. et al. (2022). Illumina-based analysis yields new insights into the fungal contamination associated with the processed products of *Crataegi fructus*. *Front. Nutr.* 9: 883698.
23. Surana AR, Agrawal SP, Kumbhare MR, Gaikwad SB. Current perspectives in herbal and conventional drug interactions based on clinical manifestations. *Futur. J. Pharm. Sci.* 2021; 7: 103. https://doi.org/10.1186/s43094-021-00256-w.
24. Jyothi MV, Ashok Babu VL, Wagh VD, Rasheed A, Dayaramani R, Panigrahy UP, Wal P, Gunjal SD. Herbal interactions with cardiac medications: a comprehensive review of potential interactions between herbal drugs and commonly prescribed cardiac medications. *Curr. Drug Saf.* 2025; 20(2): 94–119. https://doi.org/10.2174/0115748863289321240424063819.
25. Zhou S, Lim LY, Chowbay B. Herbal modulation of P-glycoprotein. *Drug Metab. Rev.* 2004; 36(1): 57–104. https://doi.org/10.1081/dmr-120028427.
26. Tirona RG, Bailey DG. Herbal product-drug interactions mediated by induction. *Br. J. Clin. Pharmacol.* 2006; 61(6): 677–681. https://doi.org/10.1111/j.1365-2125.
27. Izzo, A.A. and Ernst, E. (2009). Interactions between herbal medicines and prescribed drugs: an updated systematic review. *Drugs* 69 (13): 1777–1798. doi: 10.2165/11317010-000000000-00000. PMID: 19719333.
28. Bailey DG, Dresser GK. Interactions between grapefruit juice and cardiovascular drugs. *Am. J. Cardiovasc. Drugs* 2004; 4(5): 281–297. https://doi.org/10.2165/00129784-200404050-00002.
29. Becquemont, L., Verstuyft, C., Kerb, R. et al. (2001). Effect of grapefruit juice on digoxin pharmacokinetics in humans. *Clin. Pharmacol. Ther.* 70 (4): 311–316.
30. Werba JP, Misaka S, Giroli MG, Shimomura K, Amato M, Simonelli N, Vigo L, Tremoli E. Update of green tea interactions with cardiovascular drugs and putative mechanisms. *J. Food Drug Anal.* 2018; 26 (2): S72–S77. https://doi.org/10.1016/j.jfda.2018.01.008.
31. Yuan CS, Wei G, Dey L, Karrison T, Nahlik L, Maleckar S, Kasza K, Ang-Lee M, Moss J. Brief communication: American ginseng reduces Warfarin's effect in healthy patients: a randomized, controlled trial. *Ann. Intern. Med.* 2004; 141(1): 23–27. https://doi.org/10.7326/0003-4819-141-1-200407060-00011.
32. Prieto-Garcia JM, Graham L, Alkhabbaz O, Mazzari ALDA. Potential pharmacokinetic interactions of common cardiovascular drugs and selected European and Latin American herbal medicines: a scoping review. *Plants (Basel)* 2023; 12(3): 623. https://doi.org/10.3390/plants12030623.
33. Jiao Q, Wang R, Jiang Y, Liu B. Study on the interaction between active components from traditional Chinese medicine and plasma proteins. *Chem. Cent. J.* 2018; 12(1): 48. https://doi.org/10.1186/s13065-018-0417-2.
34. Ackermann RT, Mulrow CD, Ramirez G, Gardner CD, Morbidoni L, Lawrence VA. Garlic shows promise for improving some cardiovascular risk factors. *Arch. Intern. Med.* 2001; 161(6): 813–824. https://doi.org/10.1001/archinte.161.6.813.
35. Czigle S, Nagy M, Mladěnka P, Tóth J; OEMONOM. Pharmacokinetic and pharmacodynamic herb-drug interactions-part I. Herbal medicines of the central nervous system. *PeerJ* 2023; 11: e16149. https://doi.org/10.7717/peerj.16149.PMID.
36. Tankanow, R., Tamer, H.R., Streetman, D.S. et al. (2003). Interaction study between digoxin and a preparation of Hawthorn (*Crataegus oxyacantha*). *J. Clin. Pharmacol.* 43 (6): 637–642.
37. Fasinu PS, Bouic PJ, Rosenkranz B. An overview of the evidence and mechanisms of herb-drug interactions. *Front. Pharmacol.* 2012; 3: 69. https://doi.org/10.3389/fphar.2012.00069.
38. Hamad AKS. Caffeine and arrhythmias: a critical analysis of cardiovascular responses and arrhythmia susceptibility. *J. Saudi Heart Assoc.* 2024; 36(4): 335–348. https://doi.org/10.37616/2212-5043.1402.
39. Ventura MT, Boni E, Cecere R, Buquicchio R, Caloiguiri GF, Martignago I, Incorvaia C, Ridolo E. Importance of hypersensitivity in adverse reactions to drugs in the elderly. *Clin. Mol. Allergy* 2018; 16(7). https://doi.org/10.1186/s12948-018-0083-x, 7
40. Bose S, Das PP, Banerjee S, Chakraborty P. A comprehensive review on natural products caused allergy and its mechanism. *J. Herb. Med.* 2023; 42(3): 100778. https://doi.org/10.1016/j.hermed.2023.100778.
41. Liperoti R, Vetrano DL Bernabei R, Onder G. Herbal medications in cardiovascular medicine. 2017; 69 (9): 1188–1199. https://doi.org/10.1016/j.jacc.2016.11.078, *J. Am. Coll. Cardiol.*
42. Guo YJ, Wang DW, Meng L, Wang YQ. Analysis of anaphylactic shock caused by 17 types of traditional Chinese medicine injections used to treat cardiovascular and cerebrovascular diseases. 2015; 2015: 420607. https://doi.org/10.1155/2015/420607, *BioMed Res. Int.*
43. Marwa K, Goldin J, Kondamudi NP. Type IV hypersensitivity reaction. [Updated 2025 May 4]. In: *Stat Pearls [Internet]*. Treasure Island, (FL): Stat Pearls Publishing. 2025 Jan-. Available from: https://www.ncbi.nlm.nih.gov/books/NBK562228.
44. Uetrecht J, Naisbitt DJ. Idiosyncratic adverse drug reactions: current concepts. *Pharmacol. Rev.* 2013; 65(2): 779–808. https://doi.org/10.1124/pr.113.007450.

45. Zhou P, Gross S, Liu JH, Yu BY, Feng LL, Nolta J, Sharma V, Piwnica-Worms D, Qiu SX. Flavokawain B, the hepatotoxic constituent from kava root, induces GSH-sensitive oxidative stress through modulation of IKK/NF-κB and MAPK signaling pathways. *FASEB J.* 2010; 24 (12): 4722–4732. https://doi.org/10.1096/fj.10-163311.
46. Clough AR, Wang Z, Bailie RS, Burns CB, Currie BJ. Case-control study of the association between kava use and ischaemic heart disease in Aboriginal communities in eastern Arnhem Land (Northern Territory) Australia. *J. Epidemiol. Community Health* 2004; 58(2): 140–141. https://doi.org/10.1136/jech.58.2.140.
47. Kochibe N. Allergic substances of *Ginkgo biloba*. In: Hori T, Ridge RW, Tulecke W, Del TP, Trémouillaux-Guiller J, Tobe H. (eds) *Ginkgo biloba A Global Treasure*. Springer, Tokyo. 1997. 281-292. https://doi.org/10.1007/978-4-431-68416-9_23.
48. Mulrow C, Lawrence V, Ackermann R, Ramirez GG, Morbidoni L, Aguilar C, Arterburn J, Block E, Chiquetti E, Gardener C, Harris M, Heidenreich P, Mullins D, Richardson M, Russell N, Vickers A, Young V. Garlic: effects on cardiovascular risks and disease, protective effects against cancer, and clinical adverse effects: summary. 2000. In: *AHRQ Evidence Report Summaries*. Rockville, (MD): Agency for Healthcare Research and Quality. Available from: https://www.ncbi.nlm. nih.gov/books/NBK11910/.
49. Wiwanitkit, V. and Taungjaruwinai, W. (2004). A case report of suspect ginseng allergy. *Med. Gen. Med.* 6 (3): 9.
50. Ahmed S, Zhou Z, Zhou J, Chen SQ. Pharmacogenomics of drug metabolizing enzymes and transporters: relevance to precision medicine. *Genom. Proteom. Bioinf.* 2016; 14(5): 298–313. https://doi.org/10.1016/j.gpb.2016.03.008.
51. Hauptman, M. and Woolf, A.D. (2017). Childhood ingestions of environmental toxins: what are the risks? *Pediatr. Ann.* 46 (12): e466–e471.
52. Agbabiaka, T.B., Spencer, N.H., Khanom, S., and Goodman, C. (2018). Prevalence of drug–herb and drug–supplement interactions in older adults: a cross-sectional survey. *Br. J. Gen. Pract.* 68: e711–e717.
53. Don, C.G. and Smieško, M. (2020). *In silico* pharmacogenetics CYP2D6 study focused on the pharmacovigilance of herbal antidepressants. *Front. Pharmacol.* 11: 683.
54. Stickel, F. and Shouval, D. (2015). Hepatotoxicity of herbal and dietary supplements: an update. *Arch. Toxicol.* 89 (6): 851–865.
55. Botelho, A.F., Pierezan, F., Soto-Blanco, B., and Melo, M.M. (2019). A review of cardiac glycosides: structure, toxicokinetics, clinical signs, diagnosis and antineoplastic potential. *Toxicon* 158: 63–68.
56. Ernst, E. (2002). Herbal medicinal products during pregnancy: are they safe? *BJOG* 109 (3): 227–235.
57. Sim, T.F., Sherriff, J., Hattingh, H.L. et al. (2013). The use of herbal medicines during breastfeeding: a population-based survey in Western Australia. *BMC Complement. Altern. Med.* 13 (1): 317.
58. Shan, Q., Yu, W., Xu, Q. et al. (2024). Detoxification and underlying mechanisms towards toxic alkaloids by Traditional Chinese medicine processing: a comprehensive review. *Phytomedicine* 129: 155623.
59. Jităreanu A, Trifan A, Vieriu M, Caba I-C, Mârțu I, & Agoroaei L. Current trends in toxicity assessment of herbal medicines: a narrative review. *Processes* 2023; 11(1): 83. https://doi.org/10.3390/pr11010083.
60. Eisenbrand G, Pool-Zobel B, Baker V, Balls M, Blaauboer BJ, Boobis A, Carere A, Kevekordes S, Lhuguenot J-C, Pieters R, Kleiner J. Methods of *in vitro* toxicology. *Food Chem. Toxicol.* 2002; 40 (2–3): 193–236. https://doi.org/10.1016/S0278-6915(01)00118-1
61. Priyadarshi S, Valentine B, Han C, Fedorova OV, Bagrov AY, Liu J, Periyasamy SM, Kennedy D, Malhotra D, Xie Z, Shapiro JI. Effect of green tea extract on cardiac hypertrophy following 5/6 nephrectomy in the rat. *Kidney Int.* 2003; 63(5): 1785–1790. https://doi.org/10.1046/j.1523-1755.2003.00914.x.
62. Almeida MR, de Oliveira Lima E, da Silva VJ, Campos MG, Antunes LM, Salman AK, Dias FL. Genotoxic studies in hypertensive and normotensive rats treated with amiodarone. *Mutat. Res.* 2008; 657(2): 155–159. https://doi.org/10.1016/j.mrgentox.2008.09.005.
63. Khan JM, Lyon AR, Harding SE. The case for induced pluripotent stem cell-derived cardiomyocytes in pharmacological screening. *Br. J. Pharmacol.* 2013; 169(2): 304–317. https://doi.org/10.1111/j.1476-5381.2012.02118.
64. Pawar, B., Gupta, T., Vasdev, N. et al. (2023). Chapter 1 – Understanding pharmacotoxicology. In: *Advances in Pharmaceutical Product Development and Research, Essentials of Pharmatoxicology in Drug Research* (ed. R. Tekade), 1–28. Academic Press https://doi.org/10.1016/B978-0-443-15840-7.00025-7.
65. Rokutan H, Anker SD, Springer J. *In vivo* models of cardiac diseases: application to drug development and screening. *Expert Opin. Drug Discov.* 2010; 5(1): 65–78. https://doi.org/10.1517/17460440903460299.
66. Zarenezhad E, Hadi AT, Nournia E, Rostamnia S, Ghasemian A. A comprehensive review on potential *in silico* screened herbal bioactive compounds and host targets in the cardiovascular disease therapy. 2024; 2024: 2023620. https://doi.org/10.1155/2024/2023620, *BioMed Res. Int.*
67. Moumou M, Tayebi A, Hadini A, Noman OM, Alhalmi A, Ahmoda H, Amrani S, Harnafi H. Combining *in vitro*, *in vivo*, and *in silico* approaches to explore the effect of *Ceratonia siliqua* and *Ocimum basilicum* rich phenolic formula on lipid metabolism and plasma lipoprotein oxidation in mice fed a high-fat diet: a follow-up study. *Metabolites* 2025; 15(1): 36. https://doi.org/10.3390/metabo15010036.
68. Ross, J.A. and Kasum, C.M. (2002). Dietary flavonoids: bioavailability, metabolic effects, and safety. *Annu. Rev. Nutr.* 22: 19–34. https://pubmed.ncbi.nlm.nih.gov/12055336/.
69. Chen, P., Chen, F., Guo, Z.L. et al. (2023). Recent advancement in bioeffect, metabolism, stability, and delivery systems of apigenin, a natural flavonoid compound: challenges and perspectives. *Front. Nutr.* 10: 1221227. https://pmc.ncbi.nlm.nih.gov/articles/PMC10410563/.
70. Sasaki, G.Y., Vodovotz, Y., Yu, Z., and Bruno, R.S. (2022). Catechin bioavailability following consumption of a green tea extract confection is reduced in obese persons without affecting gut microbial-derived valerolactones. *Antioxidants (Basel)* 11 (12): 2490. https://pubmed.ncbi.nlm.nih.gov/36552698/.
71. Zaheer Y, Ali MA, Rehman M, Iftikhar M, Anwar S, Ali A, Mobeen A, Iqbal M, Iqbal S, Younis MR, An R, Dong J, Ihsan A. Naringenin loaded solid lipid nanoparticles alleviate oxidative stress and enhance oral bioavailability of naringenin. *Colloids Surf. B Biointerfaces* 2025; 247: 114423. https://doi.org/10.1016/j.colsurfb.2024.114423.
72. Shulman, M., Cohen, M., Soto-Gutierrez, A. et al. (2011). Enhancement of naringenin bioavailability by complexation with hydroxypropyl-β-cyclodextrin. *PLoS One* 6 (4): e18033. https://doi.org/10.1371/journal.pone.0018033 PLoS One 2012; 7(10). 10.1371/annotation/c5a7bd78-0cd2-4575-a9fe-6729b2c2a217.
73. Wdowiak, K., Walkowiak, J., Pietrzak, R. et al. (2022). Bioavailability of hesperidin and its aglycone hesperetin-compounds found in citrus fruits as a parameter conditioning the pro-health potential (neuroprotective and antidiabetic activity)—mini-review. *Nutrients* 14 (13): https://pubmed.ncbi.nlm.nih.gov/35807828/.
74. Crescenti A, Caimari A, Alcaide-Hidalgo JM, Mariné-Casadó R, Valls RM, Companys J, Salamanca P, Calderón-Pérez L, Pla-Pagà L, Pedret A, Delpino-Rius A, Herrero P, Samarra I, Arola L, Solà R, Del Bas JM. Hesperidin bioavailability is increased by the presence of 2S-diastereoisomer and micronization—a randomized, crossover

and double-blind clinical trial. *Nutrients* 2022; 14 (12): 2481. https://doi.org/10.3390/nu14122481.

75. Chen M, Xiao J, El-Seedi HR, Woźniak KS, Daglia M, Little PJ, Weng J, Xu S. Kaempferol and atherosclerosis: from mechanism to medicine. *Crit. Rev. Food Sci. Nutr.* 2024; 64(8): 2157–2175. https://doi.org/10.1080/10408398.2022.2121261.
76. Barve, A., Chen, C., Hebbar, V. et al. (2009). Metabolism, oral bioavailability and pharmacokinetics of chemopreventive kaempferol in rats. *Biopharm. Drug Dispos.* 30 (7): 356–365. https://pubmed.ncbi.nlm.nih.gov/19722166/.
77. Bhattacharya, M. and Mandal, S. (2025). Medical and biological role of apigenin: a comprehensive review. *Pharm. Res.-Mod. Chin. Med.* 14: 100576. https://www.sciencedirect.com/science/article/pii/S2667142525000053.
78. Hsu SJ, Chung HC, Chang CH, Liao YC, Liu TW, Lin SM, Lee CK. Rapid evaluation of apigenin bioavailability and hypouricemic bioactivity by targeted metabolomics study in enterohepatic microenvironment mimetic cell culture model. *Food Res. Int.* 2025; 209: 116281. https://doi.org/10.1016/j.foodres.2025.116281.
79. Silva, M.L., Bernardo, M.A., Singh, J., and de Mesquita, M.F. (2022). Cinnamon as a complementary therapeutic approach for dysglycemia and dyslipidemia control in type 2 diabetes mellitus and its molecular mechanism of action: a review. *Nutrients* 14 (13): 2773. https://www.mdpi.com/2072-6643/14/13/2773.
80. Gonçalves T, Almeida A, Pontes L, Oliveira J, Feitosa M, Júnior J, Veras R, Medeiros I. Monoterpenes in vascular function: a review of bioactivity and mechanisms of action. *Int. J. Mol. Sci.* 2025; 26 (18): 9243. https://doi.org/10.3390/ijms26189243.
81. Fu, C., Shi, H., Chen, H. et al. (2020). Oral bioavailability comparison of Artemisinin, Deoxyartemisinin, and 10-Deoxoartemisinin based on computer simulations and pharmacokinetics in rats. *ACS Omega* 6 (1): 889–899. https://pubmed.ncbi.nlm.nih.gov/33458540/.
82. Mödinger Y, Knaub K, Dharsono T, Wacker R, Meyrat R, Land MH, Petraglia AL, Schön C. Enhanced oral bioavailability of β-caryophyllene in healthy subjects using the VESIsorb® formulation technology, a novel self-emulsifying drug delivery system (SEDDS). *Molecules* 2022; 27(9): 2860. https://doi.org/10.3390/molecules27092860.
83. Liu, X., Wang, N., and Gao, Z. (2022). β-Carotene regulates glucose transport and insulin resistance in gestational diabetes mellitus by increasing the expression of SHBG. *Clin. Exp. Pharmacol. Physiol.* 49 (12): 1307–1318. https://doi.org/10.1111/1440-1681.13712.
84. Odeberg, J.M., Lignell, Å., Pettersson, A., and Höglund, P. (2003). Oral bioavailability of the antioxidant astaxanthin in humans is enhanced by incorporation of lipid based formulations. *Eur. J. Pharm. Sci.* 19 (4): 299–304. https://pubmed.ncbi.nlm.nih.gov/12885395/.
85. Burri, B.J., La Frano, M.R., and Zhu, C. (2016). Absorption, metabolism, and functions of β-cryptoxanthin. *Nutr. Rev.* 74 (2): 69–82. https://pubmed.ncbi.nlm.nih.gov/26747887/.
86. Mansuri, M.L., Parihar, P., Solanki, I., and Parihar, M.S. (2014). Flavonoids in modulation of cell survival signalling pathways. *Genes Nutr.* 9 (3): 400. https://pmc.ncbi.nlm.nih.gov/articles/PMC4026439/.
87. Hu, L., Luo, Y., Yang, J., and Cheng, C. (2025). Botanical flavonoids: efficacy, absorption, metabolism and advanced pharmaceutical technology for improving bioavailability. *Molecules* 30 (5): 1184. https://pmc.ncbi.nlm.nih.gov/articles/PMC11902153/.
88. Kawada, T., Goto, T., Takahashi, N., and Hirai, S. (2010). Various terpenoids derived from herbal and dietary plants function as PPAR modulators and regulate carbohydrate and lipid metabolism. *PPAR Res.* 2010: 483958. https://pmc.ncbi.nlm.nih.gov/articles/PMC2896613/.
89. Alves-Silva, J.M., Zuzarte, M., Marques, C. et al. (2016). Protective effects of terpenes on the cardiovascular system: current advances and future perspectives. *Curr. Med. Chem.* 23 (40): 4559–4600. https://pubmed.ncbi.nlm.nih.gov/27604093/.
90. Silva EAP, Carvalho JS, Guimarães AG, Barreto RSS, Santos MRV, Barreto AS, Quintans-Júnior LJ. The use of terpenes and derivatives as a new perspective for cardiovascular disease treatment: a patent review (2008–2018). *Expert Opin. Ther. Pat.* 2019; 29(1): 43–53. https://doi.org/10.1080/13543776.2019.1558211.
91. Kotake-Nara, E. and Hase, M. (2020). Effect of dispersed form on the bioavailability of β-carotene from daily intake in humans. *Biosci. Biotechnol. Biochem.* 84 (12): 2545–2557. https://www.tandfonline.com/doi/pdf/10.1080/09168451.2020.1803728.

CHAPTER 13

# Frameworks for Regulations, Standardization, and Authentication of Cardiovascular Herbal Drugs

Kumar CSP[1], Surya Prakasarao Kovvasu[2], and Gummadi RamaKrishna[1]

[1] Department of Pharmaceutics, School of Pharmacy, Aditya University, Surampalem, Andhra Pradesh, India

[2] College of Pharmacy, Western University of Health Sciences, Pomona, CA, USA

## 13.1 INTRODUCTION

The global health landscape is bearing a high responsibility in CVDs such as angina pectoris, coronary artery disease (CAD), congestive heart failure, myocardial infarction, and ischemic artery disease. All of these diseases are among the most life-threatening conditions in people; therefore, there are many options for managing these CVDS. Allopathic approaches, traditional, and combined approaches are applicable in the CVD management; among these approaches, the traditional approach is majorly adapted nowadays because of their clinical effectiveness. Herbal preparations/formulations are applicable in traditional practice because phytochemical constituents are efficient and effective in their therapeutic activity. The therapeutic activity of these phytochemicals may be discovered or undiscovered, but they are desperately useful in effective management of CVDs. Especially, these preparations consist of cardiovascular (CV)-effective constituents such as antioxidants, anti-inflammatory, vasoactive, and hypolipidemic agents, and are key for CVD management. Because of the abundant availability of herbs as resources for such phytochemical agents, herbal preparations for CVD management are highly utilized globally. Nevertheless, the approval of herbal preparations are limited because of regulatory incompliance, different dosages for same herbal preparation across various regions countries, and noncompliance with ordinary regulatory framework, there is a great necessity for framing, regulating, and directing an internationally harmonized regulatory framework to get globally unique herbal formulations for effective medical management. This harmonized regulatory framework gives direction on identification, isolation, characterization, quantification, and authentication of phytochemical constituents in herbal preparations to avoid adulteration. Adulteration affects the therapeutic activity of herbal preparation; hence, these regulation frameworks give directions on resource identification to identify and get the right therapeutic effect out of phytochemical constituents.

We require great knowledge on regulatory frameworks of the World Health Organization (WHO), European Medical Agency (EMA), United States Food and Drug Administration (USFDA), and AYUSH to get harmonized directions on authentication of phytochemical resource, identification and characterization of phytochemical constituents, manufacturing facilities, herbal preparation specifications, evaluation specifications, marketing, and post-marketing studies.

By identifying and accurately estimating phytochemical agents, we can develop approaches for consistency, reliability, and modern quality control of herbal preparations. Modern authentication techniques, such as DNA barcoding and metabolomic finger printing, are used for authentication and quality control of phytochemical constituents. For the safety, efficacy, and quality of herbal preparations, we should examine the regulatory guidelines, authentication methods, and conformation procedures.

Finally, the collaboration between traditional medical knowledge and modern quantification knowledge only enables the success of CV herbal preparations. With the review of global regulatory framework in time, enhanced research and development of herbal preparations is possible [1–3].

## 13.2 REGULATORY FRAMEWORKS FOR HERBAL CARDIOVASCULAR DRUGS

### 13.2.1 WORLD HEALTH ORGANIZATION GUIDELINES

WHO supports the development and promotion of phytochemical preparations through its directions, and it is a global central authority. The advancement of global public health, prevention of pathological exacerbation, and enhancement of global health are supported by the WHO, a specific organization of the United States (US). The recommendations of WHO are drawn through careful procedures, and this direction is supported by rigorous, evidence-based research. The organization delivers a broad range of policies on different facets of health, from contagious and long-term ailments to psychological care/health, physical safety, and Medicare systems. The WHO also supports the prevention and management of major disorders such as COVID-19, HIV/AIDS, malaria, and tuberculosis by releasing protocols. In addition, it provides proof-based instructions pertained to nutrition, immunization, hygiene practices, antimicrobial use, and maintenance of air and water quality.

Medical practitioners, legislators, and central government are helped by WHO guidance in framing sound recommendations to strengthen prophylaxis and public health measures. Economically backward nations with poor healthcare settings require WHO recommendations and sound proof-backed policy guidance to develop their infrastructure. WHO regularly updates its articles for maintaining the significance and precision, for incorporating current scientific outcomes, and responding to current universal health issues. Global health initiatives remain contemporary through continuous alignment with updated WHO standards. The WHO provides research-driven frameworks that foster effective and equitable medical care nationwide, anchoring global health policies through its regulations [4–6].

### 13.2.2 UNITED STATES FOOD AND DRUG ADMINISTRATION

Regulations of phytochemical constituents in the United States are basically covered under Dietary Supplement Health and Education Act (DSHEA), enacted in1994 and monitored by the USFDA. According to these regulations phytochemical preparations are usually classified as dietary supplements; hence, phytochemical preparations are required to adhere to USFDA regulations. When phytochemical preparations are intended for use as botanical drugs, they should adhere to the Botanical Drug Development Guidance, which dictates the processes and documentation required for regulatory criteria.Manufactures/scientists seeking market approval for phytochemical preparations have to perform clinical studies and submit clinical data to demonstrate therapeutic efficacy and safety. In addition to that, they have to submit chemistry, manufacturing, and controls (CMC) document along with safety data with respect to phytochemical preparations. Phytochemical preparations must meet stringent USFDA regulations for quality, efficacy, and safety before they enter into the market. Through crystal clear guidelines, USFDA encourages and controls phytochemical preparations within stringent regulatory framework. USFDA encourages new establishments in the phytochemical manufacturing domain, new medical care, and therapeutic safety through its perception and directs phytochemical preparation safety systems through its guidelines. It resolves global health needs by working dynamically to harmonize all regulations beyond the national regulations to provide safe, efficacious, and qualitative phytochemical preparations. It stands as a major regulatory body among all national regulatory bodies through its evidence-based and crystal clear regulatory system. In addition to that, USFDA regulates the safety of food, drug, and health devices and examines their quality, safety, and efficacy. It plays an important role in approving new medicines and vaccines, validation of clinical protocols, and post-marketing studies for new drug products [7–9].

### 13.2.3 EUROPEAN MEDICINES AGENCY

EMA is a key agency in regulating phytochemical preparations in the European region; the herbal medicinal product committee (HMPC) especially looks after the regulation of phytochemical preparations in the Europe continent and plays an important role in validation of the quality, safety, and efficacy of phytochemical preparations. HMPC prepares and publishes monographs, which consists of detailed reviews on herbal constituents, and also explain the traditional and sustained therapeutic applications of the herbal constituents that are present in the monograph. This monograph remains as references for quality, safety, and efficacy of herbal preparations of respective nations, and also remains as references for different manufacturers and regulatory bodies. By these regulations as evidence-based evaluations, EMA encourages safe and efficacious utilization of herbal therapeutics, ensures belief, and secures public health. By its regulations, EMA maintains balance between scientific authentication and the esteem of traditional medical practice. Its transparency and systemic evaluation approach strengthen reliability and encourage responsible validation of phytochemical preparations in healthcare systems. EMA, through its stringent regulation policies, contributes to developing new herbal formulations with great regulatory compliance. Through stringent evaluation approaches, EMA completely examines therapeutic effects, safety data, and quality control data of herbal preparations. EMA enables all the herbal formulations to be marketed with sound quality through stringent evaluation approaches and makes them effective and efficacious therapeutically. Beyond regulation framing, it concentrates on transparency and data transfer of herbal preparations. It gives the evidence-based information on advantages and hazards and enables the consumers to take extensive decisions on herbal preparations. Directions on medical–herbal reactions, contraindications, and adverse effects are incorporated in the EMA regulatory framework.

Finally, through commitment on transparency, scientific rigor, and people education it encourages safe, efficacious and right utility of herbal preparations throughout Europe [10–12].

### 13.2.4 INDIAN MINISTRY OF AYUSH

AYUSH is a ministry of India; it plays key role in framing, regulating, and encouraging the regulatory framework for traditional practices such as Unani, Siddha, and Homeopathy. AYUSH formulates specifications through preparing official pharmacopoeia and formulary and gives directions on quantity, purity, and quality of traditional medical preparations. It protects consistency in manufacturing facilities by applying current Good Manufacturing Practices (GMP), and through that, it protects against criticism, adulteration, and decline in quality of therapeutics. AYUSH's regulatory framework covers manufacturing of various herbal preparations; among those, CV-related formulations are also covered. For example Arjuna-related preparations, especially applicable for CVDs; for such preparations, stringent reviews were performed to protect quality and therapeutic accuracy. Along with regulations, AYUSH encourages research and development (R&D) in traditional medical care systems, especially through clarification of therapeutic effects, therapeutic confirmation, and investigation of abilities of new clinical approaches. Through these acts, AYUSH strengthens scientific evidence-based traditional medical approaches and integrates them into standards-based health systems. AYUSH is responsible for registration and approval of all marketed traditional medicine in India and protects consumers from duplicate and poor-quality traditional preparations by allowing products that adhere to quality and regulatory specifications. Through the programs and approaches, AYUSH protects not only India's cultural and medical inheritance but also plays important role in enhancement of quality in national health care systems. It enhances economy for the herbal industry by focusing on quality guarantee, authentication, and current Good Manufacturing. Especially, it shows economic influence on CV health industry by availing reliable, safe, and efficacious preparations.

Finally, AYUSH regulatory frameworks have strengthened the reliability and consistency of the Indian traditional medical system. AYUSH can enhance the production of traditional medical preparations by improving its regulatory systems and research approaches; by that, it brings product quality and global recognition and helps in public health and wealth [13–15].

## 13.3 STANDARDIZATION APPROACHES FOR HERBAL CARDIOVASCULAR DRUGS

### 13.3.1 EVALUATION OF DRUGS MACROSCOPICALLY AND MICROSCOPICALLY

Primary techniques for the evaluation of herbal materials macroscopically and microscopically are identification, validation, and quality assessment. Examining the features such as color, texture, odor, size, and shape comes under macroscopic evaluation. This serves us to understand the possible features such as deterioration, issues in handling, and possible pollutants in the crude drug. By examining microscopically, we can understand the internal and microscopic structures of the plant such as its xylem and phloem vessels, trichomes, and fibers. This reveals the anatomy of the plant we are handling. This is the difference between macroscopic and microscopic evaluation. By this watchful observation of all these diagnostic and anatomical characters, researchers can understand quality, material source, and possible adulterants. Notably, these evaluations help researchers develop and standardize novel herbal formulations beyond their traditionally use. It enables the researchers to analyze variations in crude materials and refine the processing techniques to ensure similarity and repeatability of the final product through these morphological observations. It helps both consumer and the manufacturer by the optimization of the consistency and efficacy of the final herbal product. It also plays a key role in the safety of public health. These systemic techniques are the basic for the formation of the collection of crude drug and its processing and manufacturing. Manufacturers can produce proper extraction and storage techniques for the preservation of active phytochemicals. It helps its safety and integrity. Because of this uniformity, the safety and consistency are improved between different batches. It ensures that it reaches the pharmacopoeial and regulatory standards. If modern analytical techniques like microscopy, chromatography, and spectroscopy are included in the evaluation process, they will give us the absolute picture of the whole herbal product. The assurance of quality, authenticity, and safety of the product is increased by this multidisciplinary approach. It is possible for manufacturers to develop high-quality herbal formulations by adopting this setting, which is compatible with international standards. These can meet the consumer expectations and ensure the safety of the consumer [16–18].

### 13.3.2 CHROMATOGRAPHIC TECHNIQUES

Methods like thin layer chromatography (TLC), high performance liquid chromatography (HPLC), gas chromatography (GC), and high performance thin layer chromatography (HPTLC), are the best tools used for evaluating herbal medicines. Uniformity between the batches is increased; thereby, product quality is increased by these techniques. They optimize the accurate separation, qualification, and identification of these phytochemical compounds. Through this profiling, producers can authenticate herbal preparations, confirm their purity, and identify any possible adulteration. These analytical techniques strengthen assurance and build faith in the presence of specific therapeutic components in phytochemical products and are therefore important for process of standardization and quality validation in herbal product manufacturing. This increases the faith in the consumer. These techniques also play a key role in the research and product development beyond their use as tools in quality assurance. Researchers are able to discover novel phytoconstituents, study their pharmacological actions, and investigate their potential therapeutic applications by observing the chemical profiles. With these Insights obtained from such analyses, it will lead to the design of novel formulation and the enhancement of existing products. Thereby, they increase the innovation in herbal sector. The value of the chromatographic analysis in safety, stability, and degradation studies is critical for determining storage requirements and shelf life of the herbal products. Changes in composition over time and their monitoring will help ensure that products hold on to their efficiency and safety throughout their intended lifespan. Apart from getting their detailed chemical picture, these evaluations promote transparency during the process of manufacturing and regulation. They help manufacturer to show compliance to rigorous quality standards and serve as a main factor to build up their trustworthiness with health authorities and consumers [19–21].

### 13.3.3 SPECTROSCOPIC METHODS

For herbal formulations, spectroscopic analytical approaches such as UV–visible spectroscopy, Fourier transform infrared (FTIR) spectroscopy, nuclear magnetic resonance (NMR) spectroscopy, and mass spectroscopy (MS) play a key role in the comprehensive chemical profiling. The structural depiction of chemical components can be done by these techniques through their distinctive spectral fingerprints. It enhances the researchers' ability to gain valuable knowledge about distinctive chemical compounds and possible adulteration and enables them to enhance quality control. For producing therapeutically consistent herbal products, such kind of knowledge is necessary. For examining the stability and deterioration of herbal products, spectral analysis is important apart from their use in regular analysis. The change in the spectral patterns over time makes it feasible to detect degradation patterns and helps enhance product storage conditions. By the combination of spectroscopic data with the chemometric tools such as principal component analysis (PCA) and partial least squares discriminant analysis (PLS-DA), data explanation is enhanced. Identification of invisible correlations, such as classification of complex mixtures, and prediction of quality parameters, is enabled by this combination. These methods make them particularly dominant when only small or limited samples are present because of their nondestructive nature. The combination of spectroscopic and chromatographic systems like HPLC or GC, spectroscopy gives a complete view of the herbal formulation's whole chemical landscape. The quality, safety, and regulatory compliance are guaranteed by the application of spectroscopic analysis. These methods will help in making dependable and effective herbal medicines that promote consumer confidence and public health by explaining the chemical and structural features of active compounds.

In summary, spectroscopic tools help as necessary tools in herbal product assessment, facilitating qualitative and quantitative evaluation, verifying authenticity, and detecting adulterants. Every spectroscopic method gives clear information: UV–visible spectroscopy approximates compound concentration, IR detects functional groups, NMR discovers molecular structure, and MS explains molecular mass and fragmentation patterns. These techniques provide a precise, nondestructive, and efficient means to ensure the standardization and therapeutic reliability of herbal medicines [22–24].

### 13.3.4 STANDARDIZATION BY USING MARKERS

Standardization by markers is a systemic technique to guarantee that the herbal medicine is trustworthy. It is done by spotting and quantifying chemical molecules, which are normally called markers. These markers indicate their pharmacological ability, and they are used as reference chemicals. For example allicin in *Allium sativum* or arjunolic acid in *Terminalia arjuna*. By this method, producers can spot these bioactive chemicals and estimate their concentration. This concentration is directly proportional to the product's effectiveness [25]. For the batch-to-batch uniformity, this method plays a key role. It guarantees that the product meets the consistent quality and potency at any time during production. It plays a vital role in maintaining regulatory standards and provides measurable standards for product authentication. It correlates both therapeutic ability and chemical composition and provides reliability of the formulation and dose accuracy. It connects orthodox knowledge and scientific chemical analysis and ensures that herbal medicine can still be used along with modern medicine and it is dependable. Finally, this technique provides a strong foundation for proficient validation for herbal drug development and quality assurance.

## 13.4 METHODS FOR AUTHENTICATION

### 13.4.1 PHARMACOGNOSTICAL ANALYSIS

For verifying the purity of the crude herbal material, pharmacognostical evaluation is necessary, and it is done by well-established techniques like morphological, anatomical, and histologist evaluation. It is done to verify the primary plant sources based on their structural and morphological features. Authenticity, quality, and purity of the herbal drugs, along with the detection of adulteration and contamination, ensured by this pharmacognostical evaluation. To reach the pharmacognostical standards for raw herbal drugs, this process integrates macroscopic, microscopic, and phytochemical assessment. The product quality could not be compromised, so the researchers keenly observe the plant morphology, tissue organization, and cellular features. This will help detect the inconsistencies in the product. This phase is necessary for maintaining integrity and dependability of herbal products.

Standardized methods in approved well-known pharmacological guidelines give an accurate way to provide precision in the process of analysis. The reproducibility of the result mainly depends on the analyst and the accuracy of the reference sample. Modern analytical techniques like chromatography and spectroscopy are integrated with traditional knowledge for understanding product composition. This is integration will provide strong quality assurance methods. Researchers can analyze the pharmacological ability of the drugs by precisely identifying plant species. More than its role in the quality control, it will help in the development of new herbal formulations. More than this, these evaluations, help in the conservation of therapeutically useful plants and herbs. Ultimately, this ensures that products are safe, effective, and genuine with standardization achieved through pharmacognostical evaluation, which remains the keystone for the herbal product. Amalgamation of scientific analytical methods with conventional diagnostic methods serves a diverse approach for the maintenance of quality standards in herbal medicine production [26–28]

### 13.4.2 TECHNIQUES IN MOLECULAR ANALYSIS

For precise identification and confirmation of herbal raw materials, effective molecular analytic methods like DNA barcoding, random amplified polymorphic DNA (RAPD) analysis, and internal transcribed spacer (ITS) sequencing are used. The identification of herbal materials, identification of adulteration, and classification of species are done by these powerful DNA-based approaches. The quality assurance of herbal formulations is achieved by these genetic markers, and researchers can determine the botanical origin of the crude drug material and build up the total quality and authenticity. The major advantage of these methods is that the correct plant species can be identified using DNA barcoding, even after the loss of observable morphological characters during processing. This area is the place where the conventional methods fail. We can still get the knowledge of the original plant material even after extraction by these methods. For tracing the integrity of the product after the production, these molecular methods are applied at various stages of manufacturing. The researchers can analyze the product quality and detect the unintended materials in the product by the help of these methods because of their capability to detect the adulterants and confirm declared plant species. It protects consumers from the toxic or low-quality products through genetic observation. This helps in improving the integrity, safety, and efficiency of the herbal drugs. More than that, it helps in the analysis and development of new herbal formulations. These methods also help in the development of novel genetic references and databases of the medicinal plants. It accelerates the development of these databases and their role in quality control and herbal medicine standardization. These modern methods not only build up regulatory standards and consumer safety but also help in the innovation and the development of safe and standard herbal products. In the end, the molecular analytical methods herbal medicine have changed the industry in the way products are produced and evaluated [29].

### 13.4.3 CHEMOMETRIC AND METABOLOMIC PROFILING

Chemometric and metabolomic profiling uses advanced tools to separate different plant species and variants when the morphological characters are not enough for detection. It uses advanced statistical and analytical methods. The process involves large-scale analysis of the phytochemical constitutes of plant material and through research. By evaluating the biomarker signatures and metabolic patterns, they help in the validation of plant species, quality assurance, and adulteration in herbal formulations. By evaluating complex chemical fingerprints of extracts of herbal drugs, chemometric and metabolic profiling serve as powerful strategies for clarifying and conforming herbal drugs. Practically, these advanced methods depend on analyzing the datasets by using high-end statistical models or machine learning algorithms. The data is obtained from advanced technological instrumentation techniques like MS and NMR spectroscopy to generate detailed chemical profiles.

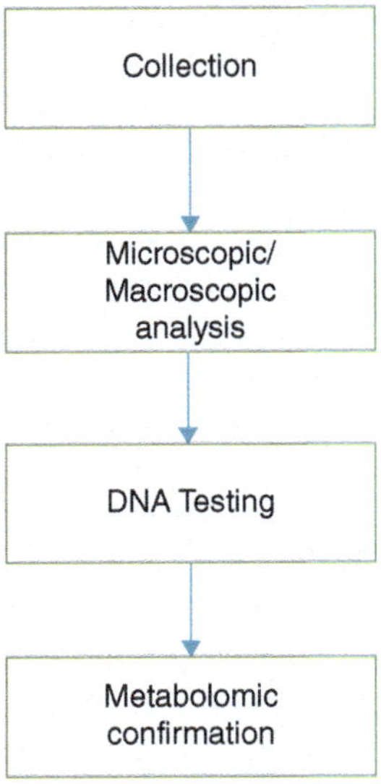


**FIGURE 13.1** Authentication process for herbal cardiovascular drugs.

Distinctive markers and distinctive characteristic patterns among different plant variants are disclosed by this evaluation. Fine differences in the formulation, which help to indicate the adulteration or degradation, are identified by applying these methods in quality control. Standardization protocols, uniformity of the formulation, and analytical methods in herbal drug evaluation are achieved by employing this approach. Discovery of new biomarkers, clarifies and amplifies the process of authentication. It makes a way for developing better standardization protocols for production and quality control. By integrating analytical tools such as DNA barcoding and chromatographic methods, chemometric and metabolomic profiling offer a complete framework for clarification. This combination increases accuracy and trustworthiness of the evaluation methods. Scientists and manufacturers can guarantee the purity, reliability, and genuinity of the herbal products by adopting these modern bioanalytical techniques. Consumer satisfaction with herbal formulations and the growth in the herbal drug industry are achieved by adopting these chromatographic methods and chemometric and metabolomic profiling techniques [30, 31]. The following is the authentication process for herbal cardiovascular drugs as shown in Figure 13.1.

## 13.5 CASE STUDIES

### 13.5.1 *TERMINALIA ARJUNA*: A CARDIOPROTECTIVE HERB

In the Ayurvedic system *T. arjuna* is a well-known medicinal plant for its effects on heart like cardioprotective and cardiotonic actions. Arjunolic acid, which is extracted from the bark, is the chief phytoconstituent marker, and its concentration is normally present in the range of 5% in standardized extracts. Its therapeutic benefits in cardiovascular disorders, including angina pectoris and congestive heart failure, are supported by a large amount of pharmacological and clinical studies. *T. arjuna* is considered a powerful additional agent for the treatments of cardiac disorders because of its medicinal activity and safety profile. *T. arjuna* can be considered for modern cardiovascular therapy because of its strong activity.

*T. arjuna* also has anti-inflammatory, antioxidant, and antimicrobial activities. Along with cardioprotective activity, they collectively increase the cardioprotective benefits of this drug. Endothelial activity, control of lipid metabolism, and reduction in oxidative stress can be achieved by these properties, so comprehensive cardiovascular activity is maintained. Because of its ability to regulate most physiological pathways, it increases its potential in the treatment of many cardiac conditions.

Modern research has also investigated the collective effect of *T. arjuna* extract along with established cardiovascular agents. This investigation revealed the collective effect increases potential and decreases adverse reactions, making it a supportive therapeutic agent. This kind of collective effect provides the potential for making treatment better and decreases the potential risk of side effects.

The investigation for the mechanistic pathways and molecular targets has increased because of the increasing interest in *T. arjuna* research. Modern research tries to find the accurate biochemical pathways and targets; because of this, a new natural-based approach for CVD management is made. *T. arjuna* is highly considered as an integrative and evidence-based cardiac care option, which provides a secure and effective alternative along with conventional pharmacotherapy [32, 33].

### 13.5.2 *ALLIUM SATIVUM* (GARLIC)

*Allium sativum*, commonly known as garlic, is a part of the most researched medicinal herbs because of its exceptional antihypertensive, hypocholesterolemic, and antithrombotic effects, and it is well recognized. It is normally made into capsules or tablets, and the concentration of allicin is used as a standard, as it is the main bioactive compound used for its medicinal activity. Because of differences in conventional medical systems, legal status, and manufacturing practices across various nations, the classification and oversight of these drug products vary.Even with these differences, the garlic-based formulations are well accepted around the world because of their cardiovascular properties, supported by the scientific evidence showing its role as an agent regulating cardiovascular health.

The effects like protection by decreasing blood pressure, serum cholesterol, and platelet aggregation are considered as the primary pharmacological effects of allicin derived from derived from garlic. Different mechanisms, such as angiotensin-converting enzyme (ACE) inhibition, increased nitric oxide bioavailability, and enhancement of vascular relaxation are considered the primary effects of allicin. The anti-inflammatory activity derived from antioxidant activity also helps in maintaining cardiovascular health. Antimicrobial, antiviral, and anticancer properties are also exhibited by garlic. These immunomodulatory and anti-inflammatory effects make garlic helpful in the management of cardiovascular health and other conditions.

Diverse regulatory standards around the world increase the necessity for similar and good quality control protocols and consistent manufacturing procedures to ensure the safety and efficacy of garlic formulations. GMPs and analytical verification of allicin content and product purity acceptance can ensure consumer confidence and satisfaction. With extensive research support, therapeutic versatility, and favorable safety, garlic remains a key ingredient in nutritional foods and nutraceuticals that offers, potential cardiovascular benefits and other chronic disorders [34, 35].

### 13.5.3 *GINKGO BILOBA*

In Europe and China, *Ginkgo biloba* is widely used medicinal herb and is widely regarded both conventional and modern herbal medicine. The primary alkaloids present in the *G. biloba* are ginkgolides and bilobalide, which are used to quantify concentrations in standard preparations. The primary therapeutic activity of *G .biloba* is improving peripheral blood circulation and reducing platelet aggregation. The European Medicine Agency (EMA) admits the traditional use of *G. biloba*, showing its potential in promoting cardiovascular health. *G. biloba* is still researched for its potential in supporting cardiovascular wellness and enhancing cognitive performance because of its vasoactive and antioxidant properties. Because of this performance, it is aligned with regulatory standards and supported by clinical evidence.

Neuroprotective and cognition-enhancing abilities are also possessed by *G. biloba* along with its cardiovascular action. Increased cerebral blood flow and management of oxidative stress are also achieved by *G. biloba*, making a way for its use in improving memory and mental clarity. Many studies have indicated this activity; yet, we need more studies like well-controlled clinical trials to conclude its effect on neural activity.

*G. biloba* is commercially available in various dosage forms like capsules, tablets, and herbal teas. Consumers are encouraged to buy standardized products with ginkgolide and bilobalide content to guarantee the safety of the costumer and efficacy of the product. People with the preexisting medical conditions are advised to see medical advice and consume standardized-quality products.

Finally, *G. biloba* is a natural medicine with well-proven benefits for both cardiovascular and cognitive health. Guided by scientific evidence and responsible use, as well as product quality and medical supervision, therapeutic effects can be increased and risks reduced.Consumers can include *G. biloba* into their health schedule by informed decision-making [36,37]. Refer Table 13.1 for herbal drugs commonly used and their marker compounds.

**Table 13.1** Common herbal cardiovascular drugs and their marker compounds.

| Herb | Active marker compound | Pharmacological action |
|---|---|---|
| *Terminalia arjuna* | Arjunolic acid | Cardioprotective |
| *Allium Sativum* | Allicin | Hypolipidemic |
| *Gingko Biloba* | Ginkgolides | Antiplatelet, vasodilatory |

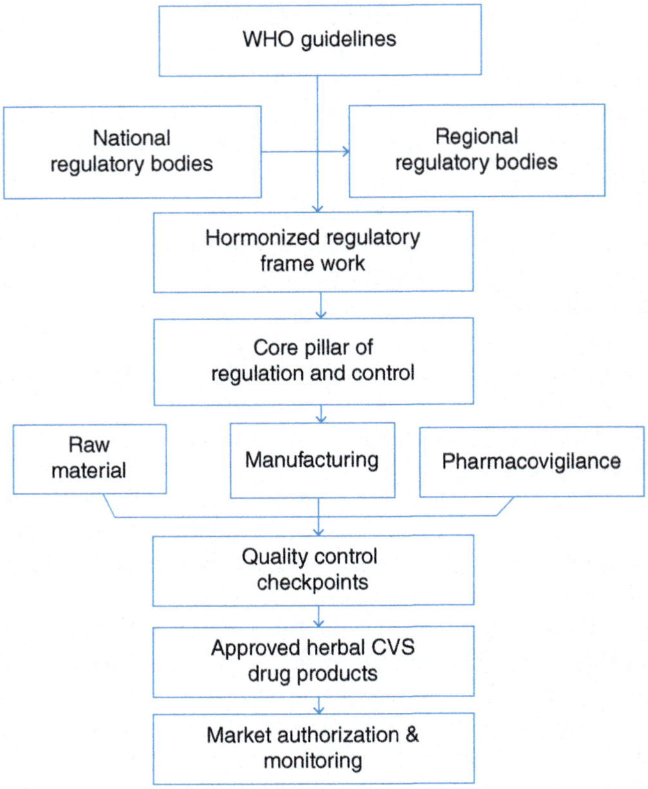


**FIGURE 13.2** Proposed framework for harmonized regulation of herbal cardiovascular drugs.

## 13.6 CHALLENGES AND OPPORTUNITIES

The herbal regulatory system remains a critical system because different regions and different nations are following different specifications for the same herbal preparations. Hence, all continents should follow a uniform regulatory framework to ensure the safe and effective use of herbal formulations. Approval and coordination of herbal preparations are obstructed because of the lack of uniform categorization, manufacturing quality parameters, clinical conformation at the global level. It is urgently needed to strengthen the pharmacovigilance system to observe and evaluate the herbal preparation's safety and therapeutic efficacy. Data exchange and collaboration between government and private industries may encourage research on herbal formulations. Integrating herbal preparations into the ICH regulatory framework facilitates the development of uniform, standardized guidelines for the products globally.Resolving inequalities in regulatory systems will improve not only trust in herbal preparations but also quality assurance systems, thereby improving accessibility of herbal preparations in the global market.

Finally, it is urgent to harmonize regulatory guidelines to ensure all herbal preparations are manufactured uniformly around the globe. In this way, these systems will enhance the trust, quality, and safety of herbal preparations in the global market [38, 39]. The following is the proposed framework for harmonized regulation of herbal cardiovascular drugs as showed in Figure 13.2.

## 13.7 CONCLUSION

Strong regulatory systems, evaluation approaches, and reliable authentication approaches are essential for the effective selection of herbal preparations in CVD management. Although WHO, USFA, EMA, and AYUSH achieved appreciable progress on regulations in preparation of herbal and traditional formulations, it is necessary to set unique specifications to get safety, quality, and authentication, and to achieve consistent drug effects of herbal preparations. Modern analytical equipment and molecular characterizing techniques are helpful in specific identification and detailed evaluation of phytochemical constituents and play a key role in enhancing authentication of herbal preparations. Science-based and globally coordinated regulatory systems strengthen the credibility, enhance product quality, and fosters reliability among physicians and patients. By coordinating modern science with traditional medical knowledge, herbal preparations can be effectively utilized for the management of CVDs. This not only expands the range of CVD management but also improves CV health patients. CVD management is progressively developed through adjuvant medical approaches that depend on traditional and modern combination medical systems. Continuous innovation, development, and international cooperation are urgently needed to achieve these transformational goals.

## REFERENCES

1. Shaito, A., Thuan, D.T.B., and Phu, H.T. (2020). Herbal medicine for cardiovascular diseases: efficacy, mechanisms, and safety. *Front. Pharmacol.* 11: 422.
2. Tiwari, P., Ahirwar, A., Singh, S. et al. (2022). Role of herbal medicines in the management cardiovascular diseases: a review. *J. Integr. Med.* 20 (2): 130–140.
3. World Health Organization (2003). *WHO guidelines on good agricultural and collection practices (GACP) for medicinal plants*. Geneva: World Health Organization.
4. World Health Organization (2019). *WHO Global Report on Traditional and Complementary Medicine 2019*. Geneva: World Health Organization.

5. World Health Organization (2004). *Guidelines for the Regulatory Assessment of Herbal Medicines*. Geneva: WHO.

6. Gostin, L.O., Meier, B.M., Thomas, R., and Magar, V. (2016). The normative authority of the World Health Organization. *Public Health* 132: 4–8.

7. U.S. Food and Drug Administration (2016). *Botanical Drug Development: Guidance for Industry*. Silver Spring, MD: FDA.

8. Dietary Supplement Health and Education Act of 1994, Pub. L. No. 103-417, 108 Stat. 4325 (Oct. 25, 1994).

9. Marcus, D.M. and Grollman, A.P. (2002). Botanical medicines – the need for regulations. *N. Engl. J. Med.* 347 (25): 2073–2076.

10. European Medicines Agency (2007). *Guideline on the Assessment of Clinical Safety and Efficacy in the Preparation of Community Herbal Monographs for Well-Established and Traditional Herbal Medicinal Products*. London: EMA.

11. European Medicines Agency (2023). *Herbal Medicinal Products*. London: EMA.

12. Tilburt, J.C. and Kaptchuk, T.J. (2008). Herbal medicine research and global health: an ethical analysis. *Bull. World Health Organ.* 86 (8): 594–599.

13. Ministry of AYUSH, Government of India (2008). *Good Manufacturing Practices (GMP) for Ayurveda, Siddha and Unani Medicines*. New Delhi: Ministry of AYUSH.

14. Pharmacopeial Commission for Indian Medicine and Homeopathy (PCIM&H) (2001–2023). *Ayurvedic Pharmacopeia of India*. New Delhi: Ministry of AYUSH.

15. Patwardhan, B. and Mashelkar, R.A. (2009). Traditional medicine-inspired approaches to drug discovery: can Ayurveda show the way forward. *Drug Discov. Today* 14 (15–16): 804–811.

16. Wallis, T.E. (2005). *Textbook of Pharmacognosy*, 5e. New Delhi: CBS Publishers &Distributors.

17. Khandelwal, K.R. (2014). *Practical Pharmacognosy Techniques and Experiments*, 25ee. Pune: Nirali Prakashan.

18. WHO (2004). *Quality Control Methods for Herbal Materials*. Geneva: World Health Organization.

19. Wagner, H. and Bladt, S. (2001). *Plant Drug Analysis: A Thin Layer Chromatography Atlas*, 2ee. Berlin: Springer-Verlag.

20. Reich, E. and Schibli, A. (2007). *High-Performance Thin layer Chromatography for the Analysis of Medicinal Plants*. New York: Thieme Medical Publishers.

21. Sethi, P.D. (2001). *High Performance Liquid Chromatography: Quantitative Analysis of Pharmaceutical Formulations*, 1e. New Delhi: CBS Publishers & Distributors.

22. Mandal, S.C., Mandal, V., and Konishi, T. (2018). *Natural Products and Drug Discovery: An Integrated Approach*. Amsterdam: Elsevier.

23. Bhutani, K.K. (2003). Fingerprint analysis of herbal products: a strategy for quality evaluation. *Phytomedicine* 10 (4): 249–258.

24. Devi, S., Dey, Y.N., De, S., and Ghosh, A.K. (2016). Spectroscopic techniques in quality control of herbal medicines. *J. Pharmacogn. Phytochem.* 5 (5): 325–330.

25. Kunle, O.F., Egharevba, H.O., and Ahmadu, P.O. (2012). Standardization of herbal medicines – a review. *Int. J. Biodivers. Conserv.* 4 (3): 101–112.

26. Kokate, C.K., Purohit, A.P., and Gokhale, S.B. (2015). *Pharmacognosy*, 50ee. Pune: Nirali Prakashan.

27. Trease, G.E. and Evans, W.C. (2009). *Pharmacognosy*, 16e. Edinburgh: Saunders Elsevier.

28. World Health Organization (2011). *Quality Control Methods for Herbal Materials*. Geneva: WHO.

29. Sucher, N.J. and Carles, M.C. (2008). Genome-based approaches to the authentication of medicinal plants. *Planta Med.* 74 (6): 603–623.

30. Serag, A., Zayed, A., Mediani, A. et al. (2023). Integrated comparative metabolite profiling via NMR and GC–MS analyses for Tongkat ali (*Eurycoma longifolia*) fingerprinting and quality control analysis. *Sci. Rep.* 13: 2533.

31. Gad, H.A., El-Ahmady, S.H., Abou-Shoer, M.I., and Al-Azizi, M.M. (2013). Application of chemometrics in authentication of herbal medicines: a review. *Phytochem. Anal.* 24 (1): 1–24.

32. Talwar, K.K., Dhar, K.L., Madan, A. et al. (1991). Beneficial effects of *Terminalia arjuna* in coronary artery disease. *J. Assoc. Physicians India* 39 (4): 395–399.

33. Bharani, A., Gupta, S., Kumar, R. et al. (2016). Clinical efficacy of water extract of stem bark of *Terminalia arjuna* (Roxb. ex DC.) Wight & Arn. in patients of chronic heart failure: a double-blind, randomized controlled trial. *Indian Heart J.* 68 (6): 773–778.

34. Ried, K., Frank, O.R., and Stocks, N.P. (2013). Aged garlic extract reduces blood pressure in hypertensives: a dose–response trial. *Eur. J. Clin. Nutr.* 67 (1): 64–70.

35. Borrelli, F., Capasso, R., and Izzo, A.A. (2003). No effect of garlic extract supplement on serum lipid levels in hypercholesterolemic subjects: a randomized, double-blind, placebo-controlled trial. *Thromb. Res.* 109 (2–3): 97–102.

36. Gardner, C.D., Zehnder, J.L., Rigby, A.J. et al. (2007). Effect of *G. biloba* (EGb 761) and aspirin on platelet aggregation and platelet function analysis among older adults at risk of cardiovascular disease: a randomized clinical trial. *Blood Coagul. Fibrinolysis* 18 (8): 787–793.

37. Snitz, B.E., O'Meara, E.S., Carlson, M.C. et al. (2009). *G. biloba* for preventing cognitive decline in older adults: a randomized trial. *JAMA* 302 (24): 2663–2670.

38. Li, Q., Schmitt, A., Zhao, L. et al. (2025). Advancing herbal medicine safety: the need for a global pharmacovigilance approach. *Naunyn-Schmiedeberg's Arch. Pharmacol.* 398 (5): 545–553.

39. World Health Organization (2004). *WHO Guidelines on Safety Monitoring of Herbal Medicines in Pharmacovigilance Systems*. Geneva: WHO.

CHAPTER 14

# Transforming Drug Delivery Systems Through Artificial Intelligence and Machine Learning

Mohan Gandhi Bonthu[1], Veera R. Bitra[2], Alluri Pavani Gayatri[3], and Balakrishna Talamanchi[4]

[1] *Department of Pharmaceutical Analysis, JSS College of Pharmacy, JSS Academy of Higher Education and Research, Ooty, The Nilgiris, Tamil Nadu, India*

[2] *Department of Pharmacology, School of Pharmacy, Faculty of Health Sciences, University of Botswana, Gaborone, Botswana, South Africa*

[3] *Department of Pharmacology, JSS College of Pharmacy, JSS Academy of Higher Education and Research, Ooty, The Nilgiris, Tamil Nadu, India*

[4] *Department of Pharmaceutics, VV Institute of Pharmaceutical Sciences, Gudlavalleru, Andhra Pradesh, India*

## 14.1 INTRODUCTION

### 14.1.1 OVERVIEW OF DRUG DELIVERY SYSTEMS

Drug delivery systems (DDS) are the backbone of modern pharmaceutics; they are engineered to deliver pharmaceutical products to the target site in a controlled, effective, and safe manner. The main role of any form of drug delivery is to increase the therapeutic index. This comprises improved drug concentration at the target site while simultaneously reducing concentration and exposure duration to nontarget organs to prevent side effects [1]. The concept of drug delivery has grown over the decades, developing from simple conventional delivery systems such as tablets, capsules, and injections to complex and engineered delivery systems such as nanoparticles, liposomes, microneedles, and transdermal patches [2]. This growth assures optimal drug stability, bioavailability, and patient adherence. For example, the understanding of pharmacokinetics and pharmacodynamics and improvements in material science have expanded drug release monitoring abilities by changing the rate, time, or position of drug release [3]. The 21st century has seen the merger of nanotechnology, biotechnology, and material science to develop a new class of pharmacy referred to as smart and targeted DDS, which can adapt to body or environmental factors like pH, temperature, enzymes, or magnetic parameters [4].

### 14.1.2 EVOLUTION FROM CONVENTIONAL TO INTELLIGENT DRUG DELIVERY

With traditional methods focusing majorly on passive diffusion and nonspecific distribution, clear limitations, including lack of efficacy and adverse issues, come at play. Furthermore, bioactive compounds—particularly those derived from phytomedicinal sources—often exhibit unpredictable pharmacological behavior due to poor solubility, instability, and complex composition. These limitations make it necessary to go for intelligent or responsive DDS that allow for site-specific delivery [5]. This concept has been further fostered by the technological advancements in computational tools, modeling techniques, and the invention of smart materials that can sense and adapt to external environments. When data science, artificial intelligence (AI), and machine learning (ML) systems are integrated with materials, a paradigm shift occurs from data-driven optimization and precise design to empirical formulations [6]. Such systems can predict drug behavior, optimize carrier selections and design, and adjust release dynamics based on patient-specific and time-dependent variable. Thus, there is a high predictable form known and personalized medicine signaled in the formulation science [7].

### 14.1.3 RELEVANCE OF DDS IN CARDIOVASCULAR AND PHYTOMEDICINE THERAPY

Cardiovascular diseases contribute to more deaths than any other cause globally, accounting for nearly one-third of the deaths. Traditional therapies available for the treatment of cardiovascular diseases experience obstacles, including low oral bioavailability and systemic toxicity, and the patients must adhere to them lifelong [8]. In the recent past, phytomedicines, which are plant-derived bioactive compounds with cardioprotective, antioxidant, as well as anti-inflammatory features, have received renewed interest because of the treatment potential to manage cardiovascular risk factors such as hypertension, dyslipidemia, and oxidative stress [9]. However, most of the phytoconstituents like curcumin, resveratrol, quercetin, and berberine have low solubility, poor stability, and high first-pass metabolism, which make their administration

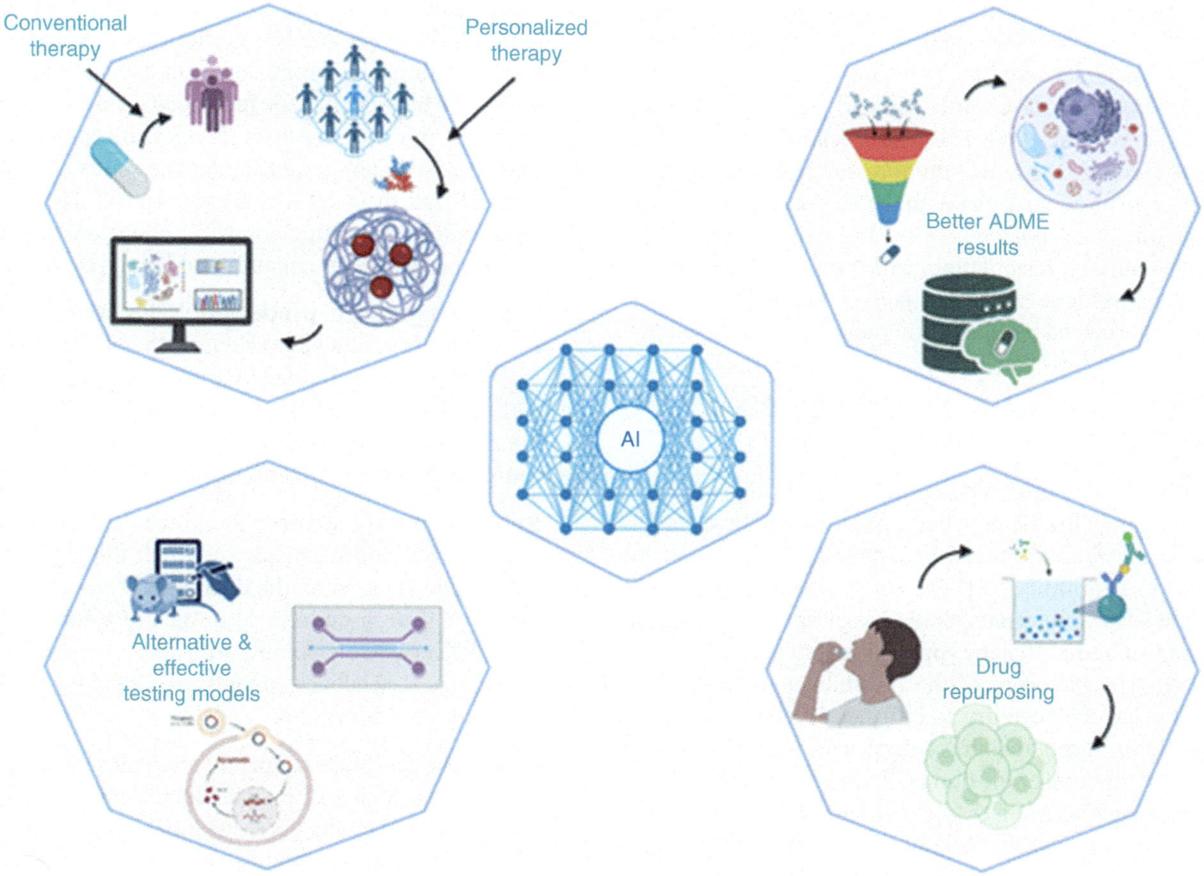


**FIGURE 14.1** Leveraging AI to transform drug development and personalized therapy.

difficult and challenging. Therefore, there is a general need to custom-design DDS that can help in improving the pharmacokinetic profile and facilitate site-specific delivery to the cardiovascular system [10]. In biomedical studies, AI integrated with ML can help in predictive modeling of formulation behavior, the simulation of pharmaceutical release kinetics, and design optimization, which move phytomedicine from traditional to evidence-based precision therapeutics [11].

### 14.1.4 THE NEED FOR COMPUTATIONAL TRANSFORMATION IN DDS

Nevertheless, to date, most of the DDS products are formulated using labor-intensive, trial-and-error methods. While these approaches are effective, there are highly inefficient, time-consuming, and costly. In contrast, AI and ML algorithms can analyze vast databases of experimental and biological knowledge to systematically detect previously unseen trends, predict outcomes, and formulate new optimized formulations within a matter of seconds, compared to the months or years needed for this with traditional methodologies [12]. Specialized deep learning algorithms can infer the solubility, permeability, and toxicity profiles of compounds. Furthermore, ML-based optimization can be used to fine-tune formulation parameters, such as excipient proportions, particle size, and film thickness, to achieve ideal release profiles [13]. Cardiovascular phytomedicine is the field where computational transformation can be most notable, as it can connect the ancient empirical herbal formulations with modern precision delivery. AI technologies can be used to examine the complex phytochemical composition-expression-activity narratives, simulate the ADME behavior, and decode bioactive cardio-target interaction networks. As such, computational intelligence may transform the contemporary artisan to a quantitative, replicable, and predictive science. This chapter summarizes how AI and ML are revolutionizing the field of DDS, with a special case of phytomedicine in CV health [14] (Figures 14.1 and 14.2).

## 14.2 FUNDAMENTALS OF ARTIFICIAL INTELLIGENCE AND MACHINE LEARNING IN PHARMACEUTICAL SCIENCES

AI refers to the capability of computer systems to perform human cognitive functions such as reasoning, learning, problem-solving, and decision-making. ML is a critical subset of AI that allows systems to learn from data and improve their performance with little or no explicit programming. ML models are designed to identify patterns, relationships, and predictive insights from large datasets, a capability that is pivotal in the pharmaceutical field because both experimental and biological data are voluminous and complex [15].

AI and ML are revolutionizing drug development and have implications at every step of the drug development pipeline, from target identification and molecular design to formulation optimization, drug dosage design, and post-marketing surveillance [16]. These two technologies are being adopted to facilitate the reduction of research timelines, minimize costs, and promote drug therapy precision. Application of AI in drug dosage necessitates the shift from empirical formulation to data-driven formulation, which enables rational prediction of the influence of dosage factors on the pharmacokinetics and pharmacodynamics of therapeutic outcomes [17].

### 14.2.1 EVOLUTION AND RELEVANCE OF AI IN MEDICINE AND PHARMACEUTICS

Historically, the era of computer-based digital algorithms in medicine began in the 1960s, when early mathematical models were used to create a logic model for addressing the development of diagnostic algorithms [18]. The early systems, which were mostly rule-based, interpreted clinical logic through the prism of determinism rather than by applying adaptive learning techniques [19]. The discovery of the possibilities of neural networks in the late 20th century and further development of this technology into the paradigm of deep learning, wherein the structure and function of the human brain's neural architecture were directly imitated with the help of DL, has radicalized this trend [20]. Modern deep learning systems, such as convolutional neural networks and recurrent neural networks, autonomously extract features from diverse data types—including imaging, signal, and molecular data—yielding highly accurate and rapid results compared to traditional models [21].

In a pharmaceutical connotation, AI development grew concurrent with the steady complexity of formulation and biological systems; thus, the development of AI in this field distinctly reflects these altering complexities. With the micropower of mathematical computation, both through power application and the rapid increase in computationally generated data, AI has passed from an advisory calculation to an autonomous thinking engine of innovation in molecular design and personalized therapy and, finally, dosage form optimization [22].

### 14.2.2 MAJOR SUBFIELDS OF AI AND THEIR PHARMACEUTICAL RELEVANCE

AI is a multi-faceted field that has multiple subfields, which each provide unique tools to aid research and innovation in pharmaceuticals and drug delivery. These subfields include:

- **Machine learning:** ML is the process of learning from data with the help of algorithms that can make predictions or classifications. In pharmaceutics, this helps predict drug–excipient compatibility, formulation stability, and release kinetics. For instance, it is possible to train random forest or support vector machines to predict the solubility or permeability of herbal compounds according to the availability of several physiology-based molecular descriptors [23].
- **Deep learning:** This involves neural networks with several hidden layers that can model very complex and nonlinear relationships. Applications of deep learning in pharmaceutics have been made in image-based particle analysis of drugs, microscopic drug dosages, morphology prediction, and biosignal processing for the control of release for personalized drug release. Moreover, DL can be used to model molecular interactions of phytoconstituents with CV targets using 3D structural modeling [24].
- **Natural language processing:** This aims to generate knowledge from the huge scientific literature. For instance, databases can be examined for traditional herbal knowledge without human intervention, then employing the acquired information autonomously to bring up potential therapeutic compounds for AI-based optimization [25].
- **Reinforcement learning:** Reinforcement learning occurs through trial and feedback, in which the algorithm optimizes actions based on the outcomes of reward. One of its uses in CV drug delivery is in adaptive control loops in drug delivery, like changing infusion rates in response to physiological feedback signals like blood pressure and heart rate variability [26].
- **Predictive and prescriptive analytics:** Essentially, AI incorporates predictive analytics forecasting likely outcomes into prescriptive analytics, which recommends optimal actions. The future demands such an AI-enabled systems, specifically for developing personalized dosing regimens for CV patients receiving phytopharmaceuticals [27].

### 14.2.3 CATEGORIES OF MACHINE LEARNING IN PHARMACEUTICAL APPLICATIONS

ML can be divided into three broad paradigms that broadly apply to different areas of drug delivery sciences.

**a) Supervised learning:** In supervised learning, models are trained on labeled data where both the inputs and the expected outputs are known. In the case of DDS, supervised learning is seen in:

- Prediction of drug-release profiles based on formulation variables
- Estimation of bioavailability or dissolution rates
- Classification of nanoparticles, excipients, etc., based on performance metrics

The primary algorithms involved are linear regression, decision trees, random forests, and neural networks [28].

**b) Unsupervised learning:** Unsupervised learning is useful for finding hidden patterns or clusters within unlabeled data. In the case of DDS, the applications include:

- Structural similarity discovery for phytoconstituents
- Clustering of excipients or natural actives based on chemical and physical properties

- Discovering a hidden relationship between formulation parameters and pharmacological responses

Additionally, the methods involved are k-means clustering, principal component analysis, autoencoders, etc. [29].

**c) Reinforcement learning:** Reinforcement learning is increasingly beneficial for adaptive drug delivery. For example, a feedback-driven release system is developed where an implantable or wearable device modulates the release rate of a phytomedicine from blood glucose, heart rate, oxygen saturation, etc., [30].

### 14.2.4 INTEGRATION OF BIG DATA, OMICS, AND AI IN PHARMACEUTICS

The promising confluence of omics sciences mentioned above and big data forms an excellent platform to employ AI-powered research. AI can analyze the high-dimensional datasets generated by laboratory studies, clinical trials, and pharmacovigilance systems to develop inferences and predictions targeted at drug performance and safety [31] (Figure 14.2).

## 14.3 AI AND ML IN DRUG DISCOVERY AND FORMULATION DESIGN

AI and ML have completely transformed the time-honored approach to pharmaceutical research and modified established models of drug preparation and discovery [36]. Traditional formulation development approaches and drug discovery models depended heavily on serendipity. Generally, these traditional approaches utilize an empirical technique in which the investigator conducts systematic studies to ascertain what happens when certain excipient ratios, methodological parameters, and distribution routes are combined [37]. These endeavors are labor-intensive and frequently less successful, primarily with complicated natural mixtures. AI and ML offer data-driven resolution, in which algorithms are instructed on experimental, molecular, and clinical datasets to project formation behavior, determine ideal formulations, and calculate therapy outcomes [38]. For phytomedicine, which usually entails finding natural concoctions with unstable and reasonably confused compositions and composite physical characteristics, AI-powered modeling might spell the difference between existing methods and completely reproducible formulations tailored to the patient [39].

### 14.3.1 AI IN DRUG DISCOVERY AND LEAD OPTIMIZATION

Before their use in the pharmaceutical sector, AI applications as drug discovery and lead optimization arose in developing new compounds or identifying bioactive compounds. Techniques such as quantitative structure–activity relationship (QSAR) modeling, deep learning-based molecular docking, and GANs are employed nowadays to design new molecules or optimize existing ones [40].

In cardiovascular phytomedicine, AI tools can first screen phytochemical databases, such as IMPPAT (Indian Medicinal Plants, Phytochemistry And Therapeutics) database or TCMID (Traditional Chinese Medicine Integrated Database), based on predicted binding affinity to prominent targets like angiotensin-converting enzyme (ACE), HMG-CoA reductase, or tumor necrosis factor-alpha (TNF-$\alpha$) to select new cardioprotective building blocks [41–44]. Second, they predict structure–function connections of endogenous compounds using ML-based models trained on chemistry descriptors and biological activity [45, 46]. Third, deep neural networks are utilized to simulate receptor–ligand on-target effects for molecules like curcumin, quercetin, or resveratrol, thereby enhancing their functionalization profile and optimizing their selective therapeutic index [47–49]. All such predictive methodologies significantly reduce the workloads and enable formulators to prioritize the testing of compounds based on their DDS [50].

### 14.3.2 ML-BASED PREDICTION OF DRUG–EXCIPIENT COMPATIBILITY AND STABILITY

One of the most important steps in designing a formulation is establishing drug–excipient compatibility and stability under varying circumstances. While traditional evidence-gathering techniques, such as differential scanning calorimetry and Fourier transform infrared spectroscopy (FTIR) spectroscopy, can provide valuable information, they are time-consuming and subject to bias based on the particular sample collection [51].

With AI-based predictive techniques, multivariate datasets consisting of information such as particle size, zeta potential, thermal profiles, pH, and solubility may predict formulation stability. The modeling of such datasets is now common, which might entail offering a prediction of the degradation kinetics using random forests and support vector machines to detect incompatible excipients and visualization of the formulated multivariate data in PCA [52–55].

### 14.3.3 AI IN FORMULATION OPTIMIZATION

In contrast, traditional formulation optimization is based on design of experiments (DoE) methodologies, such as Box–Behnken or central composite designs. Although DoE is extremely powerful, it is severely limited when the number of variables increases [56]. AI models avoid this limitation by utilizing nonlinear, multidimensional modeling instead, which enables simultaneous optimization of multiple formulation and process parameters like artificial neural networks (ANNs) for correlating input variables, like polymer concentration, mixing speed, surfactant type, with output responses, such as particle size, entrapment efficiency, and release rate. Genetic algorithms and particle swarm optimization are used for an iterative search of global optimum formulation conditions. Response surface methodology can be integrated with ML to predict optimal operating points based on large experimental datasets [56–58].

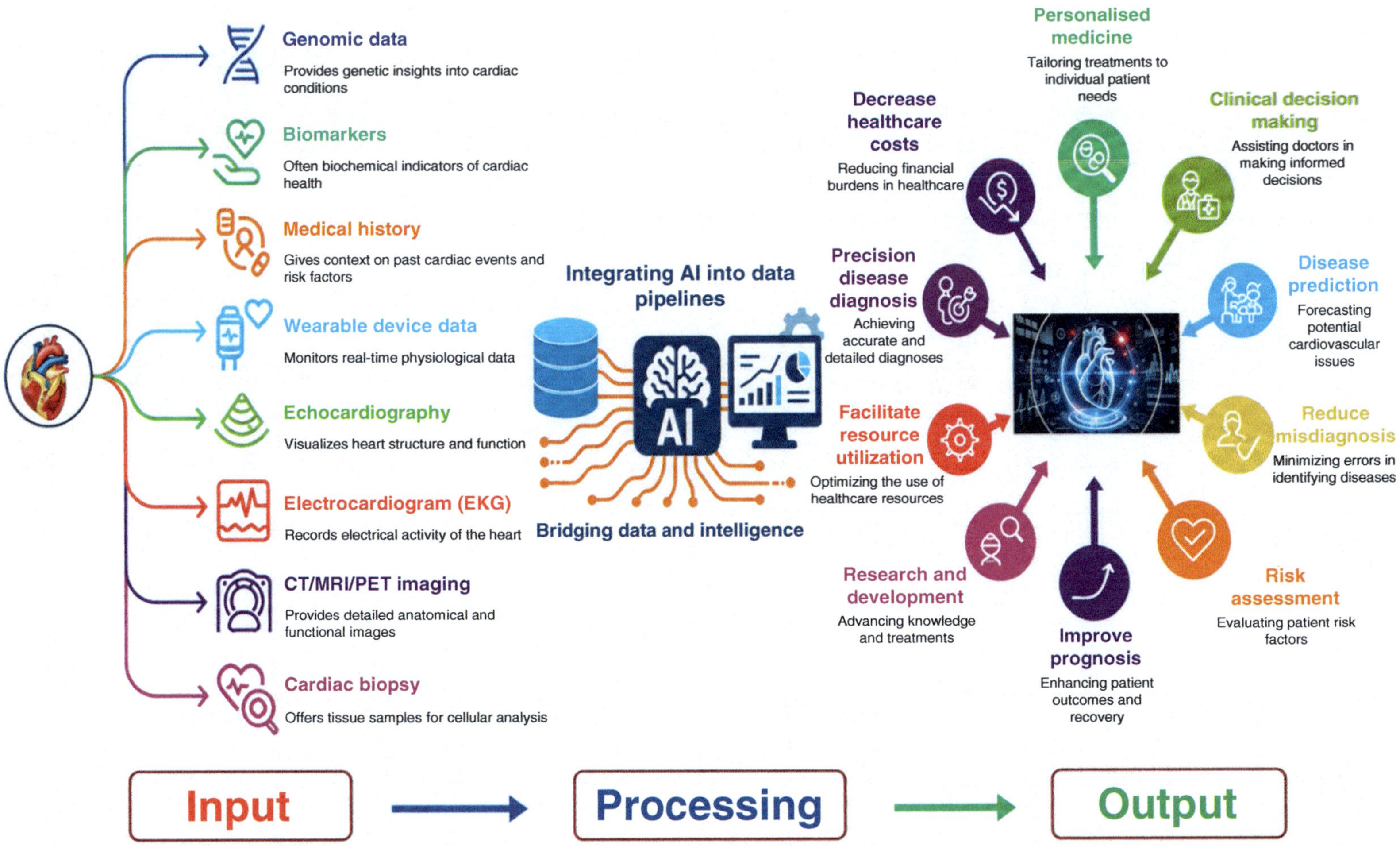


FIGURE 14.2 Integration of AI into cardiovascular data pipelines, illustrating how diverse diagnostic inputs such as genomic data, biomarkers, imaging, and wearable device information are processed through AI and ML frameworks to generate clinically valuable outputs, including personalized medicine, disease prediction, precision diagnosis, risk assessment, and improved healthcare outcomes. This model demonstrates the transformative role of AI in bridging data intelligence with cardiovascular decision-making and patient-centered therapy [32–35].

### 14.3.4 PREDICTIVE MODELING FOR SOLUBILITY, PERMEABILITY, AND BIOAVAILABILITY

Two fundamental challenges toward clinical use of phytochemicals are poor solubility and low permeability. Yet, AI algorithms can guide modification of molecular- or formulation-level parameters that affect both the above-mentioned issues [59]. Here large datasets such as AqSolDB allow for modeling aqueous solubility with deep learning methods [60]. In the meantime, ML-assisted permeability models can rely on *in silico* assessment of a molecule's absorbed intestine absorption or blood–brain barrier penetration, which, for example, should be estimated for compounds that would be applied in cardiovascular and neuroprotective medication [61]. Furthermore, reformulation steps permit evaluation of such computational models as pkCSM or DeepTox, which assess their absorption, distribution, metabolism, excretion, and toxicity [62].

### 14.3.5 CASE STUDIES: AI IN FORMULATION DEVELOPMENT

**a) AI-optimized nanoparticles for curcumin:** For instance, curcumin is a nontoxic natural antioxidant and anti-inflammatory drug candidate with poor water solubility and rapid metabolism. Optimization of the curcumin-loaded PLGA nanoparticle preparation using AI models like hybrid ANN–PSO systems was carried out. The following parameters, like polymer concentration, surfactant type, and homogenization speed, were optimized. The result was the development of an optimized system with increased EE% and 48-hour sustained release, as predicted with 95% accuracy by the ML model [63].

**b) ML-driven formulation of resveratrol liposomes:** Poor oral bioavailability and stability constrain the cardioprotective effect of resveratrol. The ML-based regression models for response surface methodology (RSM) and SVM on the lipid–cholesterol ratio predicted the optimal proportion for liposomal entrapment. Bioavailability was fivefold higher than that of the commercially available preparation [64].

**c) Predictive modeling for herbal polyherbal combinations:** ML algorithms of such complex phytomedicines working on models predict synergistic effects of the actives. Clustering analysis and regression were applied to predict the best combination of *Terminalia arjuna* extract and *Withania somnifera* for cardioprotective effect, namely to correlate their chemical composition with the results of *in vitro* antioxidative activity [65].

### 14.3.6 AI AND ML IN PROCESS CONTROL AND SCALE-UP

In adjunct to formulation development, AI is an escort in process monitoring and scale-up. In the context of smart manufacturing systems, AI synchronizes real-time PAT (Process Analytical Technology) with PAT testing for matching batches. Controllers based on the neural networks induce variations in temperature, stirring velocity, or the concentration of the solvents to reach the fixed particle size, or EE of the herbal nanoparticle during the scale-up process [66].

### 14.3.7 AI IN REGULATORY AND QUALITY BY DESIGN

Integration of AI complements quality by design (QbD) and amplifies its ability to provide predictions for critical quality attributes and process parameters. The risk tool associates how changes in the formulation predict the four critical quality attributes (CQAs), such as the dissolution rate and stability [67].

## 14.4 ROLE OF AI AND ML IN MODERN DRUG DELIVERY SYSTEMS

The DDS landscape has shifted from conventional dosage forms to smart, adaptive, and intelligent platforms that respond to biological stimuli, predict drug release patterns, and dynamically enhance therapeutic delivery. AI and ML have facilitated data-driven design, real-time control, and personalized delivery strategies, accelerating the development of AI-enabled DDS. In cardiovascular phytomedicine, this method allows for increased bioavailability and targeted action of active ingredients derived from plants by overcoming key limitations such as instability, poor solubility, and variable pharmacokinetics. It is no longer sufficient to deliver a medicament only. These have marked the shift from passive drug carriers to active, self-optimizing delivery systems.

### 14.4.1 ADVANCED DRUG DELIVERY SYSTEMS [68–70]

The modern DDS consists of various types of technology designed to enable controlled drug administration.

- Nanoparticles include polymeric, lipid-based, and metallic nanoparticles, which improve drug solubility and stability, allow easier targeting, and reduce exposure of nontarget tissues.
- Liposomes and phytosomes are systems of vesicles that serve to encapsulate phytochemicals and improve their absorption and bioavailability.
- Hydrogels and stimuli-responsive polymers are designed to be excreted and allow pH- and temperature-based release or enzymatic reaction-based release.
- Microneedles and transdermal patches are employed to provide noninvasive drug administration with controlled systemic absorption.
- Implantable and wearable drug delivery systems facilitate long-term therapeutic outcomes and enable feedback-controlled drug delivery.

### 14.4.2 AI-ASSISTED NANOCARRIER DESIGN FOR ENHANCED TARGETING

Although nanotechnology-based delivery systems represent one of the most revolutionary innovations in pharmaceutical technology, the optimal design of a nanocarrier with complex relationships between physicochemical and physiological variables is the biggest challenge. This range of variables or factors that include particle size, surface charge, polymer characteristics, and drug–carrier interactions affect the biodistribution and subsequent efficacy of nanosystems. AI and ML models can help developers optimize these multiparametric factors. In particular, supervised learning models can draw relationships between formulation parameters and outcomes such as encapsulation efficiency, stability of nanoparticles, and release kinetics. Deep learning models, in turn, can predict the fundamentals of molecular interaction between the phytoconstituents and the carrier materials to predict the most compatible matrices commanding encapsulation potential. Reinforcement learning models can be used to optimize the process parameters such as homogenization speed and solvent ratio. Through these feedback models, the process parameters will be iteratively improved through trial and error, improving the formulation performance [71].

### 14.4.3 AI IN CONTROLLED AND SUSTAINED DRUG RELEASE MODELING

The above shortcoming is largely overcome by AI and ML algorithms, given the ability of such systems to learn from sufficiently large amounts of data, incorporating physicochemical properties, *in vitro* release patterns, and *in vivo* pharmacokinetics. Thus, ANNs and SVMs demonstrate impressive accuracy in predicting the drug release profiles that are based not only on the specific formulation attributes but also on a wide range of physiological variations. Since the above variations may significantly change the relative effects of each parameter, deep learning offers an opportunity to integrate multiple inputs, such as diffusion coefficients, polymer degradability, and pH sensitivity, and predict sustained-release behavior. Finally, hybrid AI–mechanistic models, which combine the learn mode of ML methods with the theoretical approach of traditional release equations, are proposed for use [72–74].

### 14.4.4 AI IN STIMULI-RESPONSIVE AND SMART DELIVERY SYSTEMS

Alternatively, stimuli-responsive DDS releases the drug once it comes across specific physiological structures in a spatiotemporal manner. Physiological triggers may associate with acidity level around pH = 7.40, temperature, oxidative environment, or enzymatic activity. Thus, in CVD, these systems might operate on oscillations of localized oxidative equilibrium or inflammation. AI implementation allows one to predict and adjust responses by reinforcement learning algorithms, allowing for real-time adaptation of drug release patterns based on the integration of physiological data flow and feedback control; predictive analytics correlates drug release rate and cumulative dose with the patients' biomarkers, allowing for adaptive patient-oriented formulations. Additionally, Internet of Things (IoT)-based smart systems employing ML analyze biosensor data and trigger microactuators for controlled release [75].

### 14.4.5 MACHINE LEARNING FOR PHARMACOKINETIC AND PHARMACODYNAMIC PREDICTION

AI connects the gap between IVR (In Vitro Release) and IPP (Intellectual Property Protection) using pharmacokinetic/pharmacodynamic (PK/PD) modeling. ML algorithms developed on experimental datasets could accurately predict the ADME and D kinetics of a wide range of phytochemicals. Utilization of AI algorithms integrated with physiologically based pharmacokinetic (PBPK) models enables precise oral exposure and target-site concentration. Deep neural networks imitate intraindividual variability and are appropriately utilized to recommend adjustments in dose on an individual basis [76].

### 14.4.6 INTEGRATION OF AI WITH EMERGING TECHNOLOGIES [77–79]

AI and ML cannot work in sequestration and are fully employed only when interacting with corollary technologies in DDS:

- **The internet of things:** Real-time monitoring of physiological indicators using wearables and biosensors implements closed-loop control of drug release.
- **Blockchain:** Provides secure treatment for patient data and traceability in AI-sustained decision systems.
- **3D printing and additive manufacturing:** AI approaches can design and print an obligation dosage form with serialized release profiles.
- **CRISPR (Clustered Regularly Interspaced Short Palindromic Repeats) and gene editing:** In collaboration with AI-guided delivery vectors, these allow focused genetic moderation for cardiovascular disease (Tables 14.1 and 14.2).

## 14.5 TRANSFORMING PHYTOMEDICINE DELIVERY THROUGH ARTIFICIAL INTELLIGENCE AND MACHINE LEARNING

Phytomedicine, an ancient and resurged living therapy, has once again become an important part of the pharmacopoeia utilized to treat chronic diseases, including cardiovascular disorders. The distinctively bioactive constituents – curcumin, resveratrol, quercetin, berberine, catechins, and astragalosides – have displayed distinct cardioprotective success, which may entail antioxidant and anti-inflammatory patterns or a pattern modification on considerations like lipid dose and endothelial role [85].

### 14.5.1 CHALLENGES IN CONVENTIONAL PHYTOMEDICINE DELIVERY

Scientific and technological challenges make it hard for phytomedicine use to demonstrate consistent efficiency or to be translated to mainstream cardiotherapy. Most phytomedicine active constituents are multicomponent materials. Hence,

**Table 14.1** Applications of artificial intelligence and machine learning across stages of drug delivery system development [80–84].

| Stage of development | AI/ML techniques applied | Key applications/functions | Examples in phytomedicine or cardiovascular therapy |
|---|---|---|---|
| Drug discovery and screening | Deep learning, QSAR modeling, Generative adversarial networks (GANs) | Predicting bioactive molecules, virtual screening, target identification | Identification of cardioprotective phytoconstituents (e.g., resveratrol, curcumin) based on receptor-binding affinity |
| Formulation design | Artificial neural networks (ANN), support vector machines (SVM), random forest (RF) | Predicting solubility, permeability, stability, excipient compatibility | Optimization of polymer–drug ratios in curcumin or berberine nanoparticles |
| Optimization and process control | Genetic algorithms (GA), reinforcement learning (RL), response surface methodology (RSM) | Process parameter optimization, real-time control in nanoformulation scale-up | AI-optimized lipid-to-drug ratio in quercetin-loaded liposomes |
| Drug release and kinetics modeling | Deep neural networks (DNN), hybrid mechanistic-AI models | Predicting and simulating controlled or sustained release profiles | Predictive release modeling for *Terminalia arjuna* phytosomes in cardiovascular therapy |
| Toxicity and ADMET (Absorption, Distribution, Metabolism, Excretion, and Toxicity) prediction | Machine learning regression, pkCSM, DeepTox | Predicting absorption, metabolism, excretion, and toxicity of phytoconstituents | *In silico* safety profiling of berberine and ginsenosides |
| Clinical development and surveillance | Natural language processing (NLP), predictive analytics | Virtual trials, pharmacovigilance, safety signal detection | AI-assisted trial simulations for herbal antioxidants in heart disease |

their pharmacological activity as bioactive agents may involve synergistic enhancement or antagonistic interactions. Moreover, there are several potential variations in manufacturing origin, such as the harvest situation or extraction. Many biologically active phytomedicine components are lipophilic in nature and have important first-pass metabolism. Unless the method can be rapidly passed, common oral treatments are usually not powerful, and their systemic emphasis is not quick enough. The development of new medicine occurs largely by a hit-and-miss approach. Complicating matters is the fact most actively controlled phytomedicine substances have little or no stability in the gastrointestinal system. Since the formulation or its metabolite is more bioactive, precise administration time is critical [86].

### 14.5.2 AI IN HERBAL NANOCARRIERS AND ADVANCED DELIVERY SYSTEMS

AI integration with nanotechnology has transformed herbal formulation design. AI-surrounded nanocarrier systems offer advanced solubility, protect volatile phytoconstituents, and allow site-specific targeting in cardiovascular tissues. ML algorithms can predict: the ideal lipid-to-drug ratio to maximize encapsulation efficiency, and drug loading; surfactant and solvent composition and their effect on stability and release kinetics; and the biodistribution pattern of nanoparticles considering particle size and zeta potential at the same time. For instance, quercetin-loaded liposomes show improved oxidative stability and increased endothelial uptake following ML-based optimization. This instance provides evidence that such systems hold potential as preventive measures against atherosclerotic plaque formation. AI frameworks can predict polymer–drug interaction, degradation rates, and encapsulation efficiency. During nanoparticle synthesis, reinforcement learning models optimize manufacturing parameters in real time. In a recent case, deep learning predicted the interaction of berberine with five different polymer nanoparticles using volumetric cross-entropy to identify biodegradable carriers. Oral PK enhanced over 300% compared to the free drug in experimental pharmacokinetics. AI can simulate hydrogel matrix diffusion and swelling behavior to predict sustained release of phytochemicals like astragalosides and ginsenosides. ML-regulated emulsion stability ensures minimal coalescence and phase separation and is hence directly responsible for delivery performance [87–90].

### 14.5.3 PREDICTIVE TOXICITY, ADME, AND SAFETY PROFILING FOR HERBAL ACTIVES

Furthermore, limited systemic evaluation of ADMET prevents the ability to develop a biological response safety profile. The bioinformatics-driven approach, AI-based computational toxicology, employs earlier laboratory and clinical data for predictive toxicities. It makes use of algorithms to analyze both the structural and biological knowledge available in existing large databases. DeepTox and pkCSM models can predict the hepatotoxicity, cardiotoxicity, and bioaccumulation risk of phytoconstituents. Prospective structural analogues derived from herbal molecules are usually predicted using QSAR-based ML models in which the safer derivatives with better pharmacokinetic properties are identified. The available PBPK (Physiologically Based Pharmacokinetic) model was integrated with AI to simulate the concentration-dependent tissue distribution and predict the dose-induced interactions with conventional cardiovascular drugs [91].

### 14.5.4 PERSONALIZED PHYTOTHERAPY AND AI-ENABLED PRECISION DELIVERY

The convergence of AI-driven predictive modeling and personalized medicine creates novel opportunities for phytotherapy. AI, which combines patient-specific data like genomic, metabolomic, and lifestyle information, can be used to optimize dosing and formulation type. For example, ML can be used to estimate interpatient differences in the absorption or metabolism of phytoconstituents, such as resveratrol, or epigallocatechin gallate. Digital twin models can function as multipurpose simulators of individual cardiovascular profiles, allowing for forecasting of optimal dose–response curves for herbal formulations. Adaptive feedback systems can synchronize with external wearables and change delivery rates in real time, using indicators like heart rate variability or oxidative stress levels [92].

### 14.5.5 AI-GUIDED COMBINATION THERAPY AND SYNERGY PREDICTION

AI-based modeling of combination therapies involving multiple phytochemicals or the integration of phytomedicines (PhM) with synthetic cardiovascular (CV) drugs utilizes a combination of advanced computational approaches. Network pharmacology helps map and elucidate the multi-target interactions across cardiovascular pathways, providing a systems-level understanding of therapeutic mechanisms. ML algorithms identify synergistic combinations that modulate multiple targets simultaneously, enhancing therapeutic efficacy. Systems pharmacology integrates molecular and physiological data to capture the complex interactions within biological networks, while deep learning (DL) models predict additive, synergistic, or antagonistic effects of these combinations at both molecular and systemic levels, thereby optimizing combination therapy design in cardiovascular medicine [93].

## 14.6 AI AND ML IN CARDIOVASCULAR DRUG DELIVERY

Cardiovascular diseases are the leading causes of morbidity and mortality worldwide, claiming nearly 18 million lives annually. Frequently, conventional modalities, including antihypertensives, anticoagulants, and lipid-lowering agents, experience hitches in patients, including the poor patient adherence, systemic side effects, mainly targeting normal tissues, and inability to target pathological tissues such as atherosclerotic plaques, or ischemic myocardium [94].

### 14.6.1 AI IN PREDICTION OF CARDIOVASCULAR DISEASES AND DRUG TARGETING

The predictive power of AI and ML in cardiovascular diagnostics is well validated. For example, trained algorithms using ECG, echocardiography, and imaging database accurately predict arrhythmias, MI, and structural heart abnormality. This predictive ability is strategically combined with DDS for smart targeting. ECG, echocardiography, and imaging data are analyzed by deep learning models, such as convolutional neural networks (CNNs), to identify regions of ischemia and inflammation and generate target maps for drug deposition. Predictive analytics using machine learning (ML) estimates disease progression risk and enables adjustment of drug dosing frequency or release kinetics. Endogenous AI-driven models can further predict levels of endothelial dysfunction (ED) and guide the controlled release of antioxidant or anti-inflammatory agents [95].

### 14.6.2 AI-ENHANCED NANOCARRIER DELIVERY FOR CARDIOVASCULAR THERAPY [96]

Nanocarrier technology presents a versatile platform for site-specific and sustained release drug delivery. AI enhances the nanocarrier technology by optimizing the design for vascular selectivity and circulation control.

- **Supervised ML:** Physicochemical parameters influencing the nanocarrier vascular retention and parameters, e.g., particle size, zeta potential, ligand density.
- **Reinforcement learning:** Dynamically adjusting the formulation or infusion rates to maintain the optimized immediate drug levels.
- **Multi-scale simulations:** Prediction of nanoparticle interactions with vasculature from molecular, cellular, and hemodynamic data.

### 14.6.3 SMART AND RESPONSIVE CARDIOVASCULAR DDS PROGRESSIVE CARDIOVASCULAR DISORDERS [97]

Progressive cardiovascular disorders involve oscillating physiological parameters such as blood pressure, oxidative stress, or inflammatory cytokines. AI-based smart DDS can ascertain these biological cues and modulate drug release

- **Wearable-connected systems:** AI-integrated transdermal patches or micro-pumps detect and analyze data from heart rate and blood pressure sensors and adjust the dose in real time.
- **Stimuli-responsive nanoparticles:** ML algorithms correlate oxidative or enzymatic markers to drug-release triggers to allow on-demand antioxidant or nitric oxide donor.
- **Closed-loop implants:** Reinforcement learning algorithms within the microdevice learn from the feedbacks and patient-specific patterns and adjust therapeutic delivery over a period of time.

### 14.6.4 AI IN PHARMACOKINETIC/PHARMACODYNAMIC MODELING FOR CARDIOVASCULAR DRUGS [98, 99]

AI reformulates PK/PD modeling by incorporating real-world data and variability of patients.

- **Physiologically based pharmacokinetic:** The PBPK model is combined with ML for simulation of drug absorption and distribution in cardiovascular tissues.

- **Deep learning regression:** Used for prediction of plasma concentration–time profiles under different physiological conditions, such as age, comorbidities, and lifestyle.
- **Hybrid mechanistic-AI models:** To enhance the prediction accuracy of dosing by blending mathematical equations with learning from data.

### 14.6.5 AI AND DIGITAL BIOMARKERS FOR ADAPTIVE DRUG DELIVERY [100]

AI-enabled systems can process a continuous stream of digital biomarkers from ECGs, wearable sensors, and smartwatches to modulate drug delivery.

- **Predictive ML models:** AI systems can detect early signs of arrhythmia or hemodynamic instability and automatically adjust the drug-release rate in advance to prevent complications.
- **Reinforcement learning:** Learns optimal timing and dosing pattern based on a longitudinal method of how patients interact with the system.
- **Digital twin model:** Virtually duplicate patients' cardiovascular systems will virtually predict scenarios and suitable delivery formulations or regimens.

### 14.6.6 INTEGRATION WITH PHYTOMEDICINE FOR CARDIOVASCULAR HEALTH

Phytochemicals provide pluripotent cardioprotective effects, but their clinical translation demands precision delivery and modulation. AI integrates molecular, clinical, and sensor inputs to maximize these advantages.

AI and network pharmacology together help identify how herbal actives interact with multiple targets in cardiovascular pathways. AI-guided combination models can predict synergistic effects between molecules, such as resveratrol and astragaloside. ML further aids in optimizing formulations to ensure sustained and effective drug release, maintaining therapeutic plasma levels with fewer doses [101].

### 14.6.7 FEDERATED LEARNING AND MULTICENTER CARDIOVASCULAR DATA INTEGRATION

Nevertheless, the main limitation of AI-driven cardiovascular DDS development remains privacy and data heterogeneity. However, federated learning (FL) resolves it by retaining separate institutions while training models on one problem based on patient data. The FL model can evaluate patient-specific pharmacokinetics of herbal formulation across the center with the incorporation of regional variations in phytomedicine activity based on diet or genetics into the learning process. It ensures learning model improvement through global collaboration while still conforming to privacy regulations such as GDPR( General Data Protection Regulation) and HIPAA (Health Insurance Portability and Accountability Act) [102].

### 14.6.8 CASE STUDY AND FUTURE TRENDS [103–105]

**a) AI-guided nitric oxide transporter:** ML optimizes the release of nitric oxide (NO) nanoparticles used as vasodilators. These nanoparticles enhance E-selectin stability under pulsatile flow and reduce systemic vasodilator-related toxicity.

**b) Cardioprotective polyherbal scheme:** A deep learning (DL)-based hybrid AI model integrating phytochemical networks and preclinical pharmacology has shown strong synergistic cardioprotective effects of *Arjuna* bark extract combined with related bioactives, improving nonischemic cardiac function.

**c) IoT-enabled cardiovascular drug delivery:** AI-driven wearable pumps, connected to heart rate monitors, enable closed-loop delivery of herbal vasodilators such as resveratrol or EGCG, ensuring balanced and responsive therapeutic administration.

## 14.7 CLINICAL DEVELOPMENT AND REGULATORY APPLICATIONS OF AI IN DRUG DELIVERY AND PHYTOMEDICINE

First, although the incorporation of AI and ML in drug design and delivery has shown promise in laboratory and early clinical studies, the pharmaceutical development process, from clinical trials and regulatory approval to post-market surveillance, necessitates validation, transparency, and reproducibility.

### 14.7.1 AI IN CLINICAL TRIAL DESIGN AND OPTIMIZATION

Traditional clinical trials are expensive, long, and subject to unproductive recruitment and inflexible research designs. These innovations will be reoriented and enhanced through the power of AI and ML, enabling smarter, more precise, and adaptive cardiovascular therapies. Patient enrolment forecasts will predict the past data from patients' electronic health records (EHRs), genetic information, and lifestyle habits, identifying the most likely candidates to join a heart cardiovascular phenome trial. Reinforcement learning will help us adjust the dose or factors with each intermediary finding. Digital twin simulations help us generate *in silico* patient avatars, each with distinct physiological profiles, in order to test phytomedicines formulations before using them on human patients. Lastly, natural language processing is used to scour clinical trials literature and databases for the best endpoint and safety markers for cardiovascular phytotherapy [106].

### 14.7.2 VIRTUAL CLINICAL TRIALS AND *IN SILICO* MODELING

AI-supported clinical trials integrate *in vivo* dose–response studies with *in silico* efficacy and safety evaluations, transforming how pharmacological evidence is generated.

AI-powered virtual and hybrid trials mark a new era in drug development by enabling faster, more efficient, and cost-effective testing. Through AI-simulated studies, the dose–response, affinity, and safety profiles of plant-based formulations can be accurately predicted. The use of digital twins allows personalized, variable delivery simulations, optimizing therapeutic outcomes. These approaches make trials more affordable, accelerate development timelines, and reduce exposure risks during early-phase (phase I) studies [107].

### 14.7.3 AI-DRIVEN PHARMACOVIGILANCE AND POST-MARKETING SURVEILLANCE

AI equips pharmacovigilance with real-time detection and prediction of adverse events. Spontaneous adverse event reports, social media data, and wearable device feedback are closely scrutinized via ML for early-stage potential safety signals. NLP sorts similar adverse event patterns from unstructured reports, boosting herbal drug safety databases' precision. Predictive models identify heart attacks after equal changes in formulation, helping confirm that changes have been made in a safe manner [108].

### 14.7.4 AI IN REGULATORY SCIENCE AND QUALITY ASSURANCE

Agencies and committees now routinely integrate AI into their guidelines to enhance the quality, safety, and consistency of cannabis and psychotherapeutic product manufacturing. In regulatory science, AI is utilized to improve data analysis, predict product risks, ensure compliance, and support evidence-based decision-making. Regulatory agencies are increasingly encouraging the use of AI in the medical field to enable real-time quality monitoring, automated documentation, risk-based inspections, and faster approval processes, ultimately strengthening public health protection [109].

### 14.7.5 DATA GOVERNANCE, PRIVACY, AND ETHICAL CONSIDERATIONS

AI integration brings new legal and ethical sides to clinical and regulatory practices. In case of federated learning or AI integrated with a wearable, recording patient data is needed, and this should be done in accordance with the GDPR and other applicable laws at the state level (e.g., HIPAA, India's DPDP of 2023). In the event of geographic and genetic data imbalance, maldistribution in ML models survives unchecked for which global sourcing and representation in phytomedicine-encompassed ML are essential. "Black-box AI" models should be substituted, in combination or in total, with explanatory AI like XAI that supports their choices. Regulatory computer systems now support HITL AI, where automatic model-dictated strategies are approved and authenticated continuously by medical professionals to guarantee that the computational system is utilized responsibly [110].

### 14.7.6 CHALLENGES AND LIMITATIONS IN AI-BASED CLINICAL IMPLEMENTATION [111]

Despite significant progress, several barriers currently prevent full-scale adoption of AI-driven drug delivery methods.

- **Data fragmentation and standardization:** Clinical and herbal pharmacology data are frequently incongruous and insufficient.
- **Limited interpretability:** The majority of deep learning program mechanisms function as "black boxes," adopting a regulator is considered necessary.
- **Validation complexity:** A great deal of forthright and appropriate validation will be required to demonstrate that *in silico* predictions can be transformed into clinical outcomes in a rigorous and reproducible manner.
- **Infrastructure constraints:** The accommodation of AI technologies in phytopharmaceutical study will necessitate investment in digital infrastructure and appropriations personnel.
- **Cross-disciplinary disconnect:** Pharmacists, pharmacologists, data scientists, clinicians, and regulators will be afforded limited individual exposure to the possibility of small, collaborative silos.

It is necessary to identify a thoughtful structure that will mesh technical validation, regulator's compliance, and ethical oversight.

## 14.8 ETHICAL, SAFETY, AND IMPLEMENTATION CHALLENGES IN AI-BASED DRUG DELIVERY SYSTEMS

While AI and ML are dramatically reshaping the drug development and delivery industry, their integration comes with significant ethical, safety, and implementation obstacles. First, unlike the conventional course of pharmacological evolution, which can be relatively easily tracked, AI-based systems exist at the juncture of data science, biology, and clinical decision-making. Second, the utilization of AI and ML for drug reprofiling has raised many questions, such as data reliability and the transparency of algorithms and regulatory responsibility. Data quality and bias are crucial aspects of AI models, as they directly impact the accuracy, fairness, and generalizability of AI predictions. Ultimately, an AI model is only as good as the data it is trained on. In pharmaceuticals and herbal sciences, data come from several sources, specifically analytical studies, preclinical models, clinical trials, and ethnobotanical records, and are generally not standardized. In addition to the variety of these sources of input, herbal formulations differ between regions, as do chemical substances, which change due to cultivation conditions, extraction methods and storage. Such diversity can cause uncertainty in the model and exaggerate its predictive ability. Due to poorly defined clinical and experimental datasets, the outputs might be inappropriate for

**Table 14.2** Ethical, safety, and implementation challenges in AI-based drug delivery systems and suggested solutions [116–120].

| Challenge area | Specific concern | Impact on drug delivery/ phytomedicine | Proposed AI-governance or technical solution |
|---|---|---|---|
| Data quality and bias | Incomplete, heterogeneous, or unbalanced datasets | Model inaccuracy; nonrepresentative outcomes | Data harmonization, multicentric datasets, bias detection algorithms |
| Model transparency | "Black-box" decision-making in deep learning | Reduced clinical and regulatory trust | Explainable AI (XAI), SHAP/LIME (SHapley Additive exPlanations/ Local Interpretable Model-agnostic Explanations) interpretability tools, AI audit trails |
| Validation and reproducibility | Lack of standardized validation protocols | Unverified model reliability | Adoption of Good Machine Learning Practice (GMLP), external validation datasets |
| Data privacy and ownership | Risk of patient data misuse or IP loss of traditional knowledge | Ethical and legal noncompliance | Block chain-based data security, federated learning, data governance frameworks |
| Infrastructure and accessibility | Limited digital capacity in LMICs (Low- and Middle-Income Countries) | Unequal AI adoption, digital divide | Low-cost data centers, open-access AI tools, interdisciplinary training programs |
| Environmental sustainability | High computational energy demand | Increased carbon footprint | Green computing, energy-efficient AI models, circular pharmaceutics approaches |
| Ethical oversight | Algorithmic bias, consent, and autonomy issues | Potential loss of patient trust | Ethical AI frameworks, human-in-the-loop decision systems, continuous monitoring |

certain demographics. Training a biased model will result in a further propagated set, meaning that incorrect predictions, if left unattended, can be assumed as valid predictions. This can include certain geographical areas that are disproportional when using a model. Ethical problems can stem from the fact that an algorithm does not show how it arrives at a prediction and functions as a "black box." In a pharmaceutical scenario, this can be difficult to get regulatory approval or for a doctor to use an ML model's output. Relying on AI-based DDS, especially those that involve adaptive and feedback system models, requires rigorous validation to achieve a safe and repeatable outcome. For phytomedicines, two adverse responses might be not applicable due to both pathological variability in raw species and stochastic variation for computational models. The legal aspects of data control are important due to the large datasets that are used for feeds. In such instances as electronic-based therapeutics and IoT-based drug handovers, sensors continuously collect patient data. AI should assist humanity and not subdue its judgment. In essence, this means human control over the model decision and a patient's clear understanding, in addition to diversity in gender and ethnicity-centric data [112–115] (Table 14.2).

## 14.9 FUTURE PERSPECTIVES AND OPPORTUNITIES

The next half decade will not only see incremental gains but a near-total transformation that will swing the pendulum from effective, functional to intelligent, autonomous, and sustainable DDS. The convergence of AI and ML technology with pharmaceutical and phytomedicine sciences heralds a new dawn of health innovation, where data-driven intelligence, precision design, and adaptive delivery work together to achieve improved patient outcomes. The following fields are likely to experience massive changes as technology enhances their respective efforts in advancing the role and application of DDS [121].

## 14.10 CONCLUSION

The convergence of AI and ML with drug delivery science has transcended automation, influencing all aspects of modern phytomedicine, ranging from the science of discovery, formulation, and clinical translation, to surveillance of unexpected adverse drug reactions. This approach to integration combines the classic findings of phytomedicine with future therapeutic design, yielding distinct science-based systems capable of learning, anticipating, and adjusting to circumstances in real time. AI-based algorithms, such as neural networks and deep learning models, aid in the optimization of formulation design, predicting specific solubility, permeability, and stability ratios, optimizing excipient ratios, and speeding development. They are utilized in nanocarriers, liposomes, hydrogels, and microneedle systems to improve targeted, sustained, and feedback-regulated delivery, which is particularly effective in cardiovascular therapy. In phytomedicine, AI ensures that there are standardization, safety profiling, and readiness for regulatory inspection, which is done through advanced modeling and prediction of ADMET, resulting in better reproducible herbal formulations. AI simplifies clinical trial design, digital simulations, and pharmacovigilance in a clinical trial; however, obstacles such as data privacy, algorithmic prejudice, and ethical confidentiality remain persistent challenges. Federated learning, explainable AI, and international cooperation paradigms are new tools that greatly help solve AI encryption. Today's emerging tools are likely to establish further advanced opportunities. Smart digital twins, bioinformatics, interoperability, IoMT (Internet of Medical Things), and pharmacogenomics establish self-sustaining, globally linked drug delivery architectures that can prophesy and prevent disease. Broadly defined, AI in phytomedicine is not confined to technological development but also represents a shift in attitude to intelligent, fair, and caring medicine that meets the demands of humanity.

## REFERENCES


1. Khera R., Oikonomou E.K., Nadkarni G.N., Morley J.R., Wiens J., Butte A.J., Topol E.J. Transforming cardiovascular care with artificial intelligence: from discovery to practice. *J. Am. Coll. Cardiol.* 2024; 84(1): 97–114. https://doi.org/10.1016/j.jacc.2024.05.003
2. Mathur P., Srivastava S., Xu X., Mehta J.L. Artificial intelligence, machine learning, and cardiovascular disease. *Clin. Med. Insights Cardiol.* 2020; 14: 1–9. https://doi.org/10.1177/1179546820927404
3. Armoundas A.A., Narayan S.M., Arnett D.K., et al. Use of artificial intelligence in improving outcomes in heart disease: a scientific statement from the American Heart Association. *Circulation* 2024; 149: e1028–e1050. https://doi.org/10.1161/CIR.0000000000001201
4. Chowdhury M.A., Rizk R., Chiu C., Zhang J.J., Scholl J.L., Bosch T.J., Singh A., Baugh L.A., McGough J.S., Santosh K., Chen W.C. The heart of transformation: exploring artificial intelligence in cardiovascular disease. *Biomedicine* 2025; 13(2): 427. https://doi.org/10.3390/biomedicines13020427
5. Jena, G.K., Patra, C.N., Jammula, S. et al. (2024). Artificial intelligence and machine learning implemented drug delivery systems: a paradigm shift in the pharmaceutical industry. *J. Bio-X Res.* 7: 0016. https://doi.org/10.34133/jbioxresearch.0016.
6. Vora L.K., Gholap A.D., Jetha K., Thakur R.R.S., Solanki H.K., Chavda V.P. Artificial intelligence in pharmaceutical technology and drug delivery design. *Pharmaceutics* 2023; 15(7): 1916. https://doi.org/10.3390/pharmaceutics15071916
7. Topol, E.J. (2019). High-performance medicine: the convergence of human and artificial intelligence. *Nat. Med.* 25 (1): 44–56.
8. Moor, M., Banerjee, O., Abad, Z.S.H. et al. (2023). Foundation models for generalist medical artificial intelligence. *Nature* 616 (7956): 259–265.
9. Howell, M.D., Corrado, G.S., and KB., D.S. (2024). Three epochs of artificial intelligence in health care. *JAMA* 331 (3): 242–244.
10. Fogo, A.B., Kronbichler, A., and Bajema, I.M. (2024). AI's threat to the medical profession. *JAMA* 331 (6): 471–472.
11. Attia, Z.I., Kapa, S., Lopez-Jimenez, F. et al. (2019). Screening for cardiac contractile dysfunction using an artificial intelligence-enabled electrocardiogram. *Nat. Med.* 25 (1): 70–74.
12. Sangha, V., Nargesi, A.A., Dhingra, L.S. et al. (2023). Detection of left ventricular systolic dysfunction from electrocardiographic images. *Circulation* 148 (9): 765–777.
13. Goto, S., Solanki, D., John, J.E. et al. (2022). Multinational federated learning approach to train ECG and echocardiogram models for hypertrophic cardiomyopathy detection. *Circulation* 146 (10): 755–769.
14. Sangha, V., Dhingra, L.S., Oikonomou, E. et al. (2023). Identification of hypertrophic cardiomyopathy on electrocardiographic images with deep learning. *med Rxiv* https://www.medrxiv.org/content/10.1101/2023.12.23.23300490v1.
15. Bachtiger, P., Petri, C.F., Scott, F.E. et al. (2022). Point-of-care screening for heart failure with reduced ejection fraction using artificial intelligence during ECG-enabled stethoscope examination in London, UK: a prospective, observational, multicentre study. *Lancet Digit. Health* 4 (2): e117–e125.
16. Khunte, A., Sangha, V., Oikonomou, E.K. et al. (2023). Detection of left ventricular systolic dysfunction from single-lead electrocardiography adapted for portable and wearable devices. *NPJ Digit. Med.* 6 (1): 124.
17. Gibson, C.M., Mehta, S., Ceschim, M.R.S. et al. (2022). Evolution of single-lead ECG for STEMI detection using a deep learning approach. *Int. J. Cardiol.* 346: 47–52.
18. Narang, A., Bae, R., Hong, H. et al. (2021). Utility of a deep-learning algorithm to guide novices to acquire echocardiograms for limited diagnostic use. *JAMA Cardiol.* 6 (6): 624–632.
19. Ouyang, D., He, B., Ghorbani, A. et al. (2020). Video-based AI for beat-to-beat assessment of cardiac function. *Nature* 580 (7802): 252–256.
20. Kamel, P.I., Yi, P.H., Sair, H.I., and Lin, C.T. (2021). Prediction of coronary artery calcium and cardiovascular risk on chest radiographs using deep learning. *Radiol. Cardiothorac. Imaging* 3 (3): e200486.
21. Ueda, D., Yamamoto, A., Ehara, S. et al. (2022). Artificial intelligence-based detection of aortic stenosis from chest radiographs. *Eur. Heart J. Digit. Health* 3 (1): 20–28.
22. Ueda, D., Matsumoto, T., Ehara, S. et al. (2023). Artificial intelligence-based model to classify cardiac functions from chest radiographs: a multi-institutional, retrospective model development and validation study. *Lancet Digit. Health* 5 (8): e525–e533.
23. Avram, R., Barrios, J.P., Abreau, S. et al. (2023). Automated assessment of cardiac systolic function from coronary angiograms with video-based artificial intelligence algorithms. *JAMA Cardiol.* 8 (6): 586–594.
24. Chao, H., Shan, H., Homayounieh, F. et al. (2021). Deep learning predicts cardiovascular disease risks from lung cancer screening low-dose computed tomography. *Nat. Commun.* 12 (1): 2963.
25. Iribarren, C., Chandra, M., Lee, C. et al. (2022). Breast arterial calcification: a novel cardiovascular risk enhancer among postmenopausal women. *Circ. Cardiovasc. Imaging* 15 (3): e013526.
26. de Vos, B.D., Lessmann, N., de Jong, P.A., and Išgum, I. (2021). Deep learning-quantified calcium scores for automatic cardiovascular mortality prediction at lung screening low-dose CT. *Radiol. Cardiothorac. Imaging* 3 (2): e190219.
27. Kotanidis, C.P., Xie, C., Alexander, D. et al. (2022). Constructing custom-made radiotranscriptomic signatures of vascular inflammation from routine CT angiograms: a prospective outcomes validation study in COVID-19. *Lancet Digit. Health* 4 (10): e705–e716.
28. Duffy, G., Clarke, S.L., Christensen, M. et al. (2022). Confounders mediate AI prediction of demographics in medical imaging. *NPJ Digit. Med.* 5 (1): 188.
29. Wirth, F.N., Meurers, T., Johns, M., and Prasser, F. (2021). Privacy-preserving data sharing infrastructures for medical research: systematization and comparison. *BMC Med. Inform. Decis. Mak.* 21 (1): 242.
30. Ferrari F, van Dijck J, van den Bosch A. Observe, inspect, modify: three conditions for generative AI governance. *New Media Soc.* 29, 2023. https://doi.org/10.1177/14614448231214811
31. Department for Science, Innovation and Technology, Office for Artificial Intelligence (2023). A pro-innovation approach to AI regulation. https://www.gov.uk/government/publications/ai-regulation-a-pro-innovation-approach/white-paper (accessed 20 June 2023)

32. Jadon, A., and Kumar, S. (2023). Leveraging generative AI models for synthetic data generation in healthcare: Balancing research and privacy. ar Xiv [cs. LG]. https://doi.org/10.48550/arXiv.2305.05247
33. Ghosheh, G., Li, J., and Zhu, T. (2023). A review of generative adversarial networks for electronic health records: applications, evaluation measures and data sources. ar Xiv [cs. LG]. https://doi.org/10.48550/arXiv.2203.07018 (accessed 21 May 2023).
34. Chen, Y. and Esmaeilzadeh, P. (2024). Generative AI in medical practice: in-depth exploration of privacy and security challenges. *J. Med. Internet Res.* 26: e53008.
35. Cai, Y., Cai, Y.Q., Tang, L.Y. et al. (2024). Artificial intelligence in the risk prediction models of cardiovascular disease and development of an independent validation screening tool: a systematic review. *BMC Med.* 22 (1): 56.
36. Ramspek, C.L., Jager, K.J., Dekker, F.W. et al. (2021). External validation of prognostic models: What, why, how, when and where? *Clin. Kidney J.* 14 (1): 49–58.
37. Kamran, F., Tang, S., Otles, E. et al. (2022). Early identification of patients admitted to hospital for COVID-19 at risk of clinical deterioration: model development and multisite external validation study. *BMJ* 376: e068576.
38. Blumenthal, D. (2022). A step toward interoperability of health IT. *N. Engl. J. Med.* 387 (24): 2201–2203.
39. Hripcsak, G., Duke, J.D., Shah, N.H. et al. (2015). Observational health data sciences and informatics (OHDSI): opportunities for observational researchers. *Stud. Health Technol. Inform.* 216: 574–578.
40. Suchard, M.A., Schuemie, M.J., Krumholz, H.M. et al. (2019). Comprehensive comparative effectiveness and safety of first-line antihypertensive drug classes: a systematic, multinational, large-scale analysis. *Lancet* 394 (10211): 1816–1826.
41. Khera, R., Dhingra, L.S., Aminorroaya, A. et al. (2023). Multinational patterns of second-line antihyperglycaemic drug initiation across cardiovascular risk groups: federated pharmacoepidemiological evaluation in LEGEND-T2DM. *BMJ Med.* 2 (1): e000651.
42. Sangha, V., Mortazavi, B.J., Haimovich, A.D. et al. (2022). Automated multilabel diagnosis on electrocardiographic images and signals. *Nat. Commun.* 13 (1): 1583.
43. Aiello, M., Esposito, G., Pagliari, G. et al. (2021). How does DICOM support big data management? Investigating its use in the medical imaging community. *Insights Imaging* 12 (1): 164.
44. Cochrane, G., Akhtar, R., Bonfield, J. et al. (2009). Petabyte-scale innovations at the European nucleotide archive. *Nucleic Acids Res.* 37: D19–D25.
45. McDonough, C.W. (2021). Pharmacogenomics in cardiovascular diseases. *Curr. Protoc.* 1 (7): e189.
46. Claassens, D.M.F., Vos, G.J.A., Bergmeijer, T.O. et al. (2019). A genotype-guided strategy for oral P2Y12 inhibitors in primary PCI. *N. Engl. J. Med.* 381 (17): 1621–1631.
47. Alreshq, R. and Ruberg, F.L. (2021). Clinical approach to genetic testing in amyloid cardiomyopathy: from mechanism to effective therapies. *Curr. Opin. Cardiol.* 36 (3): 309–317.
48. Coorey, G., Figtree, G.A., Fletcher, D.F., and Redfern, J. (2021). The health digital twin: advancing precision cardiovascular medicine. *Nat. Rev. Cardiol.* 18 (12): 803–804.
49. Klarin, D. and Natarajan, P. (2022). Clinical utility of polygenic risk scores for coronary artery disease. *Nat. Rev. Cardiol.* 19 (5): 291–301.
50. Kent, D.M., van Klaveren, D., Paulus, J.K. et al. (2020). The predictive approaches to treatment effect heterogeneity (PATH) statement: explanation and elaboration. *Ann. Intern. Med.* 172 (1): W1–W25.
51. Oikonomou, E.K., Van Dijk, D., Parise, H. et al. (2021). A phenomapping-derived tool to personalize the selection of anatomical vs. functional testing in evaluating chest pain (ASSIST). *Eur. Heart J.* 42 (26): 2536–2548.
52. Oikonomou, E.K., Suchard, M.A., McGuire, D.K., and Khera, R. (2022). Phenomapping-derived tool to individualize the effect of canagliflozin on cardiovascular risk in type 2 diabetes. *Diabetes Care* 45 (4): 965–974.
53. Thangaraj PM, Shankar SV, Oikonomou EK, Khera R. RCT-Twin-GAN generates digital twins of randomized control trials adapted to real-world patients to enhance their inference and application. *med Rxiv*. 15, 2023. https://doi.org/10.1101/2023.12.06.23299464
54. Edward, J.A., Josey, K., Bahn, G. et al. (2022). Heterogeneous treatment effects of intensive glycemic control on major adverse cardiovascular events in the ACCORD and VADT trials: a machine-learning analysis. *Cardiovasc. Diabetol.* 21 (1): 58.
55. Athey, S. and Imbens, G. (2016). Recursive partitioning for heterogeneous causal effects. *Proc. Natl. Acad. Sci. USA* 113 (27): 7353–7360.
56. Hernán, M.A., Wang, W., and Leaf, D.E. (2022). Target trial emulation: a framework for causal inference from observational data. *JAMA* 328 (24): 2446–2447.
57. He, X., Liu, X., Zuo, F. et al. (2023). Artificial intelligence-based multi-omics analysis fuels cancer precision medicine. *Semin. Cancer Biol.* 88: 187–200.
58. Wang, R.S., Maron, B.A., and Loscalzo, J. (2023). Multiomics network medicine approaches to precision medicine and therapeutics in cardiovascular diseases. *Arterioscler. Thromb. Vasc. Biol.* 43 (4): 493–503.
59. Multiomic Health Limited. Leveraging deep omics data to tackle a global health challenge with precision. Springer Nature; 11 April 2022. Available at: https://www.nature.com/articles/d43747-022-00110-9 (accessed 27 April 2024).
60. Brown, D.G., Wobst, H.J., Kapoor, A. et al. (2022). Clinical development times for innovative drugs. *Nat. Rev. Drug Discov.* 21 (11): 793–794.
61. Liu, R., Rizzo, S., Whipple, S. et al. (2021). Evaluating eligibility criteria of oncology trials using real-world data and AI. *Nature* 592 (7855): 629–633.
62. Woodcock, J. and LaVange, L.M. (2017). Master protocols to study multiple therapies, multiple diseases, or both. *N. Engl. J. Med.* 377 (1): 62–70.
63. Cunningham, J.W., Singh, P., Reeder, C. et al. (2024). Natural language processing for adjudication of heart failure in a multicenter clinical trial: a secondary analysis of a randomized clinical trial. *JAMA Cardiol.* 9 (2): 174–181.
64. Nargesi AA, Adejumo P, Dhingra L, et al. Automated identification of heart failure with reduced ejection fraction using deep learning–based natural language processing. *med Rxiv*, 11, 2023. https://doi.org/10.1101/2023.09.10.23295315
65. LeCun Y, Bengio Y, Hinton G. Deep learning. *Nature* 2015; 521: 436–444. https://doi.org/10.1038/nature14539
66. Silver, D., Schrittwieser, J., Simonyan, K. et al. (2017). Mastering the game of Go without human knowledge. *Nature* 550: 354–359.
67. Aikins, J.S., Kunz, J.C., Shortliffe, E.H., and Fallat, R.J. (1983). PUFF: an expert system for interpretation of pulmonary function data. *Comput. Biomed. Res.* 16: 199–208.
68. Deo, R.C. (2015). Machine learning in medicine. *Circulation* 132: 1920–1930.
69. Johnson, K.W., Torres Soto, J., Glicksberg, B.S. et al. (2018). Artificial intelligence in cardiology. *J. Am. Coll. Cardiol.* 71: 2668–2679.
70. McCulloch, W.S. and Pitts, W. (1943). A logical calculus of the ideas immanent in nervous activity. *Bull. Math. Biophys.* 5: 115–133.
71. Massachusetts Institute of Technology. (2017) Explained: neural networks and deep learning. http://news.mit.edu/2017/explained-neural-networks-deep-learning-0414 (accessed 12 April 2020).
72. Nautilus. (2015) The man who tried to redeem the world with logic. http://nautil.us/issue/21/information/the-man-who-tried-to-redeem-the-world-with-logic (accessed 12 April 2020).

73. Illinois State University. McP neuron model tutorial. n.d. http://www.mind.ilstu.edu/curriculum/mcp_neurons/mcp_neuron_5.php? mod GUI=212& comp GUI=1749& item GUI=3022 (accessed 12 April 2020).
74. Dilsizian ME, Siegel EL. Machine meets biology: a primer on artificial intelligence in cardiology and cardiac imaging. *Curr. Cardiol. Rep.* 2018; 20: 139. https://doi.org/10.1007/s11886-018-1074-8
75. Kalinin, A.A., Higgins, G.A., Reamaroon, N. et al. (2018). Deep learning in pharmacogenomics: from gene regulation to patient stratification. *Pharmacogenomics* 19: 629–650.
76. Cavallari, L.H. and Weitzel, K. (2015). Pharmacogenomics in cardiology—genetics and drug response: 10 years of progress. *Futur. Cardiol.* 11: 281–286.
77. Sibbing, D., Aradi, D., Alexopoulos, D. et al. (2019). Updated expert consensus statement on platelet function and genetic testing for guiding P2Y12 receptor inhibitor treatment in percutaneous coronary intervention. *JACC Cardiovasc. Interv.* 12: 1521–1537.
78. Kitzmiller, J.P., Mikulik, E.B., Dauki, A.M. et al. (2016). Pharmacogenomics of statins: understanding susceptibility to adverse effects. *Pharmgenomics Pers. Med.* 9: 97–106.
79. Pirmohamed, M., Burnside, G., Eriksson, N. et al. (2013). A randomized trial of genotype-guided dosing of warfarin. *N. Engl. J. Med.* 369: 2294–2303.
80. Shah, S.J. (2017). Precision medicine for heart failure with preserved ejection fraction: an overview. *J. Cardiovasc. Transl. Res.* 10: 233–244.
81. Shameer, K., Johnson, K.W., Glicksberg, B.S. et al. (2018). Machine learning in cardiovascular medicine: Are we there yet? *Heart* 104: 1156–1164.
82. Lee, K.T., Hour, A.L., Shia, B.C., and Chu, P.H. (2017). The application and future of big database studies in cardiology: a single-center experience. *Acta Cardiol. Sin.* 33: 581–587.
83. Krittanawong, C., Bomback, A.S., Baber, U. et al. (2018). Future direction for using artificial intelligence to predict and manage hypertension. *Curr. Hypertens. Rep.* 20: 75.
84. Constantinides P, Fitzmaurice DA. Artificial intelligence in cardiology: applications, benefits and challenges. *Br. J. Cardiol.* 2018; 25: 86–87. https://doi.org/10.5837/bjc.2018.024
85. Laser, K.T., Horst, J.P., Barth, P. et al. (2014). Knowledge-based reconstruction of right ventricular volumes using real-time three-dimensional echocardiographic as well as cardiac magnetic resonance images: comparison with a cardiac magnetic resonance standard. *J. Am. Soc. Echocardiogr.* 27: 1087–1097.
86. Kirschbaum, S., Aben, J.P., Baks, T. et al. (2008). Accurate automatic papillary muscle identification for quantitative left ventricle mass measurements in cardiac magnetic resonance imaging. *Acad. Radiol.* 15: 1227–1233.
87. Gao, S., R, v.'t.K., Brandts, A. et al. (2017). Quantification of common carotid artery and descending aorta vessel wall thickness from MR vessel wall imaging using a fully automated processing pipeline. *J. Magn. Reson. Imaging* 45: 215–228.
88. Thompson WR, Reinisch AJ, Unterberger MJ, Schriefl AJ. Artificial intelligence-assisted auscultation of heart murmurs: validation by virtual clinical trial. *Pediatr. Cardiol.* 2019; 40: 623–629. https://doi.org/10.1007/s00246-018-2036-z
89. Nirschl, J.J., Janowczyk, A., Peyster, E.G. et al. (2018). A deep-learning classifier identifies patients with clinical heart failure using whole-slide images of H & E tissue. *PLoS One* 13: e0192726.
90. Jung, S., Song, S.W., Lee, S. et al. (2018). Metabolic phenotyping of human atherosclerotic plaques: metabolic alterations and their biological relevance in plaque-containing aorta. *Atherosclerosis* 269: 21–28.
91. GDPR.eu. (2018) General data protection regulation (GDPR). https://gdpr.eu/ (accessed 12 April 2020).
92. The White House. (2016) Preparing for the future of artificial intelligence. https://obamawhitehouse.archives.gov/blog/2016/10/12/administrations-report-future-artificial-intelligence (accessed 12 April 2020).
93. The White House. (2016) Big risks, big opportunities at the intersection of big data and civil rights. https://obamawhitehouse.archives.gov/blog/2016/05/04/big-risks-big-opportunities-intersection-big-data-and-civil-rights (accessed 12 April 2020).
94. Petersen, S.E., Abdulkareem, M., and Leiner, T. (2019). Artificial intelligence will transform cardiac imaging—opportunities and challenges. *Front. Cardiovasc. Med.* 6: 133.
95. Khadela A., Popat S., Ajabiya J., Valu D., Savale S., Chavda V.P. AI, ML and other bioinformatics tools for preclinical and clinical development of drug products. In: *Bioinformatics Tools for Pharmaceutical Drug Product Development.* Wiley, Hoboken, NJ; 2023: 255–284. Editors: Chirag Patel, Vivek P. Chavda.
96. Times of India. (2025) Pharmaceutical supply chain management: crises and innovations. https://timesofindia.indiatimes.com/blogs/voices/pharmaceutical-supply-chain-management-crises-and-innovations/ (accessed 15 October 2025).
97. Sharma, R.; Shishodia, A.; Gunasekaran, A.; Min, H.; Munim, Z.H. The role of artificial intelligence in supply chain management: mapping the territory. *Int. J. Prod. Res.* 2022, 60, 7527–7550. https://doi.org/10.1080/00207543.2022.2034142.
98. Grilo, A.L.; Mantalaris, A. The increasingly human and profitable monoclonal antibody market. *Trends Biotechnol.* 2019, 37, 9–16. https://doi.org/10.1016/j.tibtech.2018.05.014.
99. Sarpatwari, A.; Barenie, R.; Curfman, G.; Darrow, J.J.; Kesselheim, A.S. The US biosimilar market: stunted growth and possible reforms. *Clin. Pharmacol. Ther.* 2019, 105, 92–100. https://doi.org/10.1002/cpt.1289.
100. Daka, A.; Peer, D. RNAi-based nanomedicines for targeted personalized therapy. *Adv. Drug Deliv. Rev.* 2012, 64, 1508–1521. https://doi.org/10.1016/j.addr.2012.03.003.
101. Colombo, S.; Zeng, X.; Ragelle, H.; Foged, C. Complexity in the therapeutic delivery of RNAi medicines: an analytical challenge. *Expert Opin. Drug Deliv.* 2014, 11, 1481–1495. https://doi.org/10.1517/17425247.2014.930451.
102. Müller, R.H.; Junghanns, A.H. Nanocrystal technology, drug delivery and clinical applications. *Int. J. Nanomed.* 2008, 3, 295–310. https://doi.org/10.2147/ijn.s595.
103. Jain, K.K. Nanomolecular diagnostics. In : Kewal K. Jain *The Handbook of Nanomedicine*; Springer: Berlin/Heidelberg, 2017; 133–200. https://doi.org/10.1007/978-3-662-53707-3_9.
104. Kalepu, S.; Nekkanti, V. Insoluble drug delivery strategies: review of recent advances and business prospects. *Acta Pharm. Sin. B* 2015, 5, 442–453. https://doi.org/10.1016/j.apsb.2015.07.003.
105. Deloitte. (2022) Using AI to accelerate clinical trials. https://www2.deloitte.com/us/en/blog/health-care-blog/2022/using-ai-to-accelerate-clinical-trials.html (accessed 1 May 2023).
106. Dickherber, A.; Morris, S.A.; Grodzinski, P. NCI investment in nanotechnology: achievements and challenges for the future. *Wiley Interdiscip. Rev. Nanomed. Nanobiotechnol.* 2015, 7, 251–265. https://doi.org/10.1002/wnan.1304.
107. National Nanotechnology Initiative (NNI). Budget supplements and strategic plans. n.d. https://www.nano.gov/NNIBudgetSupplementsandStrategicPlans (accessed 1 May 2023).
108. Colombo, S.; Beck-Broichsitter, M.; Bøtker, J.P.; Malmsten, M.; Rantanen, J.; Bohr, A. Transforming nanomedicine manufacturing toward quality by design and microfluidics. *Adv. Drug Deliv. Rev.* 2018, 128, 115–131. https://doi.org/10.1016/j.addr.2017.09.016.

109. Troiano, G.; Nolan, J.; Parsons, D.; Van Geen Hoven, C.; Zale, S. A quality by design approach to developing and manufacturing polymeric nanoparticle drug products. *AAPS J.* 2016, 18, 1354–1365. https://doi.org/10.1208/s12248-016-9953-0.
110. Puri, M., Pathak, Y., Sutariya, V.K. et al. (2015). *Artificial Neural Network for Drug Design, Delivery and Disposition*. Cambridge, MA: Academic Press.
111. Vyas, M., Thakur, S., Riyaz, B. et al. (2018). Artificial intelligence: the beginning of a new era in pharmacy profession. *Asian J. Pharm.* 12: 72–76.
112. Kumar, Y.; Koul, A.; Singla, R.; Ijaz, M.F. Artificial intelligence in disease diagnosis: a systematic literature review, synthesizing framework and future research Agenda. *J. Ambient. Intell. Humaniz. Comput.* 2023, 14, 8459–8486. https://doi.org/10.1007/s12652-022-04203-9.
113. Chapman, A.B.; Peterson, K.S.; Alba, P.R.; DuVall, S.L.; Patterson, O.V. Detecting adverse drug events with rapidly trained classification models. *Drug Saf.* 2019, 42, 147–156. https://doi.org/10.1007/s40264-018-0761-9.
114. Elkin, M.E.; Zhu, X. Predictive modeling of clinical trial terminations using feature engineering and embedding learning. *Sci. Rep.* 2021, 11, 3446. https://doi.org/10.1038/s41598-021-83291-0.
115. Chavda, V.P.; Sorathiya, A.; Valu, D.; Marwadi, S. Role of data mining in bioinformatics. In : Vivek P. Chavda, Hitesh A. Solanki *Computation in Bioinformatics: Multidisciplinary Applications*; John Wiley & Sons: Hoboken, NJ, 2021; 69–84. https://doi.org/10.1002/9781119785519.ch5.
116. Parikh, S., Patel, R., Khunt, D. et al. (2023). Data analytics and data visualization for the pharmaceutical industry. In: *Bioinformatics Tools for Pharmaceutical Drug Product Development* (ed. C. Patel and V.P. Chavda), 55–76. Hoboken, NJ: John Wiley & Sons, Ltd.
117. Karim, M.R.; Beyan, O.; Zappa, A.; Costa, I.G.; Rebholz-Schuhmann, D.; Cochez, M.; Decker, S. Deep learning-based clustering approaches for bioinformatics. *Brief. Bioinform.* 2021, 22, 393–415. https://doi.org/10.1093/bib/bbz170.
118. Vamathevan, J.; Clark, D.; Czodrowski, P.; Dunham, I.; Ferran, E.; Lee, G.; Li, B.; Madabhushi, A.; Shah, P.; Spitzer, M.; et al. Applications of machine learning in drug discovery and development. *Nat. Rev. Drug Discov.* 2019, 18, 463–477. https://doi.org/10.1038/s41573-019-0024-5.
119. Goldstein, M.; Uchida, S. A comparative evaluation of unsupervised anomaly detection algorithms for multivariate data. *PLoS One* 2016, 11, e0152173. https://doi.org/10.1371/journal.pone.0152173.
120. Noguchi, Y.; Ueno, A.; Otsubo, M.; Katsuno, H.; Sugita, I.; Kanematsu, Y.; Yoshida, A.; Esaki, H.; Tachi, T.; Teramachi, H. A new search method using association rule mining for drug–drug interaction based on spontaneous report system. *Front. Pharmacol.* 2018, 9, 197. https://doi.org/10.3389/fphar.2018.00197.
121. Liu, L.; Tang, L.; Dong, W.; Yao, S.; Zhou, W. An overview of topic modeling and its current applications in bioinformatics. *Springer Plus* 2016, 5, 1608. https://doi.org/10.1186/s40064-016-3252-8

CHAPTER 15

# Future Challenges and Opportunities in Herbal-Based Cardiovascular Therapy

Gummadi Veda Priya[1], Saurabh Gupta[2], Karri Swathi Priya[3], and Arya Lakshmi Marisetti[4]

[1] *Aditya College of Pharmacy, Jawaharlal Nehru Technological University, Kakinada, Surampalem, Andhra Pradesh, India*

[2] *Chameli Devi Institute of Pharmacy, Rajiv Gandhi Proudyogiki Vishwavidyalaya University, Indore, Madhya Pradesh, India*

[3] *Srinivasarao College of Pharmacy, Andhra University, Visakhapatnam, Andhra Pradesh, India*

[4] *School of Pharmaceutical Sciences, Delhi Pharmaceutical Sciences and Research University, New Delhi, India*

## 15.1 INTRODUCTION

Cardiovascular diseases, or CVDs, include conditions like heart or blood vessel problems. Examples of these diseases are peripheral vascular diseases, heart disease, heart failure, strokes, heart attacks, cardiomyopathies, high cholesterol, and high blood pressure. These conditions are all considered as CVDs [1, 2]. Every year, more than 17 million people die from CVDs worldwide. Because of this, CVDs are the main cause of death around the world and cause a big burden on health and the economy [3]. According to World Health Organization, 31% of all deaths each year are because of CVDs. For instance, problems with blood vessels can lead to a stroke in the brain or a heart attack in the heart. Some main causes of vascular diseases are atherosclerosis, blood clots, and high blood pressure. Other common risk factors for CVDs include smoking, eating poorly, having diabetes, abundant levels of bad cholesterol (low-density lipoprotein [LDL]), insufficient levels of good cholesterol (high-density lipoprotein [HDL]), and high blood pressure [4]. Although many natural product-based medicines have been successfully used to produce drugs over the centuries or decades, the advent of the field of combinatorial chemistry in the late 1980s shifted the focus of drug discovery from natural products to synthetic chemistry in laboratory settings. However, natural products as drugs or sources for drug discovery are still a valuable and active area of research in the 21st century [5]. Indeed, with advances in science both on the research front and also in conventional medical practice, traditional herbal medications and plant-derived products have regained popularity for their contributions to the prevention and treatment of diseases [6]. There is substantial scientific evidence, advances in technological processes, and trends resulting from evidence-based research demonstrating that naturally derived products will be a major source of new medicines [7, 8]. This has reenergized herbal medicine in research, and many journals have published studies demonstrating the use and effectiveness of herbal medicines. Despite the significant advancements in combinatorial chemical synthesis and the development of modern synthetic medicines, herbal medicine has gained widespread social and medical recognition due to a better understanding of its health and quality-of-life benefits [9]. The leading cause of mortality and disability worldwide in diagnosis, treatment, as well as prevention in CVD remains even with progress in molecular medicine [10]. Across all cultures and civilizations, herbal remedies have been used for centuries for the prevention and/or treatment of CVDs. In clinical practice guidelines, some of the active compounds derived from herbal medicines (HMs) are now included. The global market for herbal medicines was estimated approximately one hundred fifty-one billion in 2021 and expected to reach three hundred forty-seven billion by 2029, representing an annual growth rate of 11%. The usage of HMs in Western countries is 33%, as per WHO, while 30–50% of population in China rely on traditional remedies for medicinal consumption. HMs are considered as the primary or sole source of healthcare for 80% of the population in developing countries, as shown in Figure 15.1.

According to the World Health Organization (WHO), 33% in Western countries use herbal medicines, whereas a total of 11% is recorded in China. Herbal medicines rely as their primary or sole source of healthcare in developing countries [11]. Acceptance of herbal medicine has expanded within the medical field over the last decade due to increased understanding of how herbs can contribute to health and improve quality of life [9]. Worldwide CVDs are considered as a source of death rate and fatality as one of the leading and fast-developing public health challenges in recent years [12]. CVDs have remained the most common cause of mortality for the past several decades [13].

## 15.2 SELF-CARE THROUGH BEHAVIORAL AND LIFESTYLE CHANGE

A critical aspect of an individualized, integrative practice is helping patients change lifestyle, behavioral, and self-care. Several studies indicate that 70% of chronic diseases can be prevented by quitting smoking, drinking moderately, healthy diet, exercise, and managing social and emotional stress [14, 15].

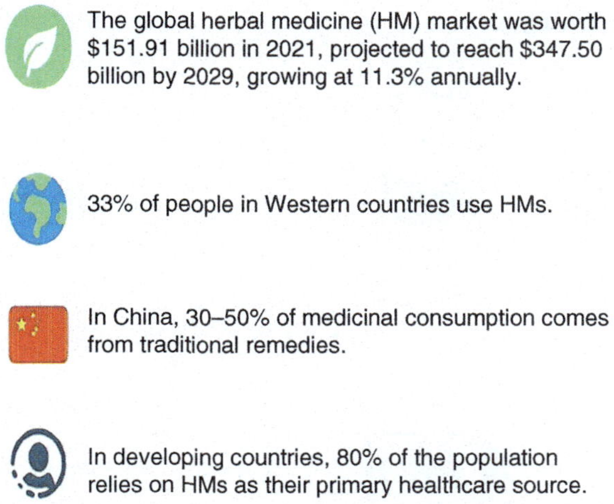


**FIGURE 15.1** WHO estimation of herbal medicines.

Integrative health recasts the association between practitioner and patient to include the entire individual and the whole community. It is guided by scientific research and utilizes all relevant preventative, therapeutic, and palliative practices, healthcare providers, and disciplines to support maximum health and well-being. This envelops the integration of ordinary, complementary/alternative, and lifestyle/self-care.

### 15.2.1 INTEGRATIVE MEDICINE MODELS

Health and well-being are optimum when all determinants of health are considered, such as medical care, individual behaviors, mental and spiritual aspects, as well as societal, economic and environmental factors.

### 15.2.2 INTEGRATIVE HEALTH

Integrative health focuses on personal health and well-being as the top priority while also addressing disease when necessary. Using this approach, a health team supports all proven methods of preventing and treating diseases, including conventional, complementary, and self-care practices.

### 15.2.3 CONVENTIONAL MEDICINE

Conventional medicine delivers proof-based methods. These methods are taught, provided and paid by the mainstream healthcare system.

### 15.2.4 INTEGRATIVE MEDICINE

Integrative medicine uses proven complementary and alternative medicine (CAM) to help improve health and overall well - being.

### 15.2.5 LIFE STYLE MEDICINE

Life style medicine uses healthy, proven self-care and behavior changes, with regular medical practice, to enhance health and healing of the body.

## 15.3 DIET IMPACT ON CARDIOVASCULAR HEALTH

A healthy diet is necessary to control elevated levels of blood pressure, which is a chronic risk for heart and blood vessel problems. For lowering blood pressure, the Dietary Approaches to Stop Hypertension (DASH) diet is good, which focuses on fruits, vegetables, whole grains, and low-fat dairy products. [16]. Blood pressure can be kept in check by including foods with less intake of salt and potassium, magnesium, and calcium in more quantities. For reducing the risk of heart problems, keeping a healthy weight is important. Common risk factors are shown in Figure 15.2. A heart-healthy diet chooses foods that are rich in nutrients but have fewer calories, unhealthy fats, and added sugars. Controlling portion sizes, including proteins and fiber-rich foods, should be focused. These eating habits help manage weight and prevent obesity when combined with regular exercise, which is a major risk for heart and blood vessels [17].

The two eating styles, such as Mediterranean diet and the DASH diet, have been closely studied and are known to offer important benefits for a healthy heart.

**Mediterranean diet:** It is based on traditional eating habits in places like Greece, Italy, and Spain. The main type of fat used in this diet is olive oil. Research shows that a Mediterranean diet that includes extra-virgin olive oil with a mix of nuts has a lower chance of having heart or blood vessel problems compared to those who follow a low-fat diet [18].

**DASH diet:** It is based on consuming more fruits, veggies, whole grains, and dairy products with low fat content and lean proteins, while eating less salt. It has been widely researched for how it affects blood pressure [19]. Cholesterol levels are improved in recent studies, and those who follow this diet have a lower risk of heart and blood vessel problems and a decreased chance of getting non-insulin-dependent diabetes mellitus.

**Plant-based diets:** People who completely base their diets on non-animal products (vegetarians), and vegan diets, are connected to a lower chance of developing heart and blood vessel problems. A detailed study that reviewed a lot of research found that these diets helps in lowering blood pressure, improving levels of cholesterol, leading to weight loss, and contributing to CVD prevention by improving blood flow compared to diets that include meat [20].

**Dietary approaches:** The American Heart Association suggests eating in a way that helps your heart. They recommend diets like the Mediterranean or DASH diet, eating less salt, avoiding extra sugars, and not using hydrogenated oils. The "Life's Simple 7" includes things like eating well, staying active, quitting smoking, keeping a healthy weight, managing blood pressure, taking care of cholesterol, and keeping blood sugar levels under control [21].

Following these guidelines is connected with a much lower chance of developing CVDs, as shown in Table 15.1. Although these eating patterns have been found to help heart health, each person is different, and factors like culture health and personal health issues should be taken into account when choosing what to eat.

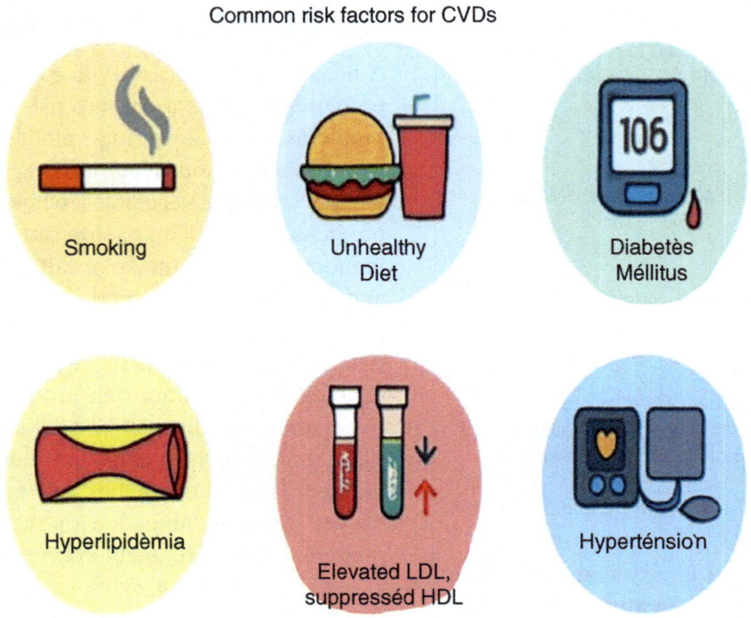


**FIGURE 15.2** Common risk factors for cardiovascular diseases.

**Table 15.1** Current recommendations and guidelines for lifestyle changes in cardiovascular health.

| S.no | Association | Guidelines |
|---|---|---|
| 1 | WHO | **Diet:** A balanced diet that involves vegetables, cereals, and unsaturated fats. Lowering of consumption of compounds containing free sugars is suggested.<br>**Physical activity:** WHO recommends 150 minutes of moderate-intensity aerobic activity or 75 minutes of vigorous-intensity aerobic activity per week, along with muscle-strengthening activities.<br>**Control of tobacco:** Smoke-free areas, tobacco taxes, and assistance in quitting tobacco are the comprehensive measures promoted by WHO. |
| 2 | The American Heart Association (AHA) | **Diet:** Everyone of us follow a diet, but a healthy diet prioritizes low fat foods. It promotes reducing added sugars, sodium and limiting saturated and trans fats.<br>**Physical activity:** Muscle-strengthening activities twice a week, in addition to 150 minutes of moderate-intensity aerobic activity. The AHA also suggests 75 minutes of vigorous-intensity aerobic activity per week .<br>**Smoking cessation:** The AHA strongly adheres to and gives advises against smoking and supports comprehensive smoking-cessation programs [22]. |
| 3 | The European Society of Cardiology (ESC) | **Lifestyle modifications**: Lifestyle changes play a major role and are the cornerstone for CVD prevention, as suggested by the ESC guidelines, which inculcate quitting smoking, maintaining a healthy diet, weight management and regular physical exercise.<br>**Dietary patterns:** It mainly emphasizes on fruits, vegetables, fish, legumes, whole grains, and olive oil. The optimal dietary pattern recommended by ESC is the Mediterranean diet.<br>**Physical activity:** It also suggests engaging in muscle-strengthening activities as a daily lifestyle in addition to 150 minutes or more of vigorous-intensity aerobic exercise [23]. |

## 15.4 GROWING GLOBAL INTEREST IN NATURAL THERAPIES

As populations age and urbanization increases, lifestyles become more sedentary. A rise in hypertension, dyslipidemia, coronary artery disease, heart failure, and obesity rates contributes to unhealthy diet. It is particularly evident in Asia, Latin America, and Africa. For preventive and complementary approaches, a growing need for not just treatments is required. Many individuals worry about the side effects of conventional drugs, their costs, accessibility, and long-term safety [24, 25]. Natural therapies are often viewed as safer and more holistic. They are considered more suitable for long-term prevention instead of just treatment. There is significant growth in the market for cardiovascular health supplements. Natural supplements, such as omega-3s, herbs, botanicals, and coenzyme Q10, are a major focus. Natural therapies often have lower costs or are more accessible in below- and mid-poverty countries. For those with limited access to traditional healthcare or pharmaceuticals, herbal or natural therapies can provide primary or complementary care.

### 15.4.1 RICH SOURCE OF BIOACTIVE COMPOUNDS

As we know, because of the tremendous increase in awareness regarding medicinal plants in the recent years, medicinal plants have been used to treat CVD. For example, various parts of *Achillea Arabica* [26] and *Ageratum conyzoides* [27], along with the aerial parts (leaves, stalks, and stems) of *Artemisia absinthium* [28], flowers of *Chrysanthemum morifolium* [29] and leaves of *Clerodendrum volubile* have been utilized for this purpose. Certain species belonging to Lamiaceae family, such as *Ballota glandulosissima* [30] (Turkey), *Clerodendrum volubile* [31] (Nigeria), *Ajuga integrifolia* [32] (Ethiopia), *Leonurus cardiaca* [33] (Europe), and *Pogostemon elsholtzioides* [34] (Eastern Himalaya) are also used for treating cardiovascular conditions [35].

### 15.4.2 ADVANCEMENTS IN PHYTOCHEMISTRY

Phytochemicals, which are bioactive compounds derived from plants, play a pivotal role in various pathways and mechanisms in maintaining cardiovascular health.

**Polyphenols:** These are diversified compounds abundant in plants, mostly famous for their pharmacological effects. Some flavonoids include quercetin, catechins, and anthocyanins [36]. A well-known flavonoid quercetin, commonly found in plants, has shown tremendous results in lowering blood pressure, improving endothelial function, and reducing oxidation of LDL cholesterol. Its benefits arise from its antioxidant effects and its role in regulating inflammation [37]. Polyphenols are abundant in foods like artichoke, spinach, broccoli, chicory, flax, onion, apple, plum, pear, grape, and cherry [38].

**Carotenoids:** The color of many fruits and vegetables is due to the presence of these bioactive substances. Their antioxidant qualities, which promote heart health, are well known. Lycopene, β-carotene, and lutein are important carotenoids [39]. Clinical studies have demonstrated the ability of lycopene, which is present in tomatoes and other red fruits, to decrease LDL cholesterol oxidation, lower blood pressure, and enhance endothelial function. It preserves cardiovascular health and prevents atherosclerosis [40]. The following are examples of common carotenoids: lutein, zeaxanthin, lycopene, fucoxanthin, [41] α-carotene, β-carotene and β-cryptoxanthin.

**Phytosterols:** These plant sterols aid in the regulation of plant physiological processes. They can be found in almonds, peanuts, macadamia nuts, sunflower, corn, sesame, olive oil, and beans [42]. Campesterol, sitostanol, and stigmasterol are examples of plant sterols.

**Saponins:** These glycosides are found in various plants and are commonly found in legumes and herbs. Because of their efficient antioxidant and cholesterol-lowering properties, they benefit cardiovascular health [43]. For instance, soy saponins in soybeans help improve heart health by maintaining and regulating lipid levels, reducing cholesterol levels, and exhibiting antioxidant activities [44].

**Tannins:** Polyphenol compounds that are found in some exotic fruits. Tannins in red wine, along with other polyphenols, are mostly essential in improving cardiovascular health by reducing oxidative stress and inflammation in the body. Antioxidant and anti-inflammatory effects by few polyphenols, like resveratrol, kaempferol, and quercetin, can enhance cardiovascular health [45].

**Dietary fibers and polysaccharides:** Polysaccharides are compounds that contain sugar units linked together. Starch and glycogen are in abundant storage of energy or cellulose and pectin as non-digestible components collectively known as dietary fiber. Good sources of fiber are found in plant-based foods such as chicory, tamarind, beans, corn, and green beans [46].

## 15.5 KEY CHALLENGES FACING HERBAL-BASED THERAPIES FOR CARDIOVASCULAR DISEASES

### 15.5.1 INADEQUATE STANDARDIZATION AND QUALITY CONTROL

Herbal products have been used for centuries in many cultures as a primary form of healthcare. Materials derived from plants offer a wealth of bioactive substances that may have positive health effects. Herbal products have been popular for a long time because of their historical uses and perceived natural origin. However, the high demand also raises questions regarding their efficacy, safety, and quality [47–49]. For herbal products to be safe and effective, it is essential to maintain a consistent level of quality and standardization [50]. To safeguard the health of consumers, strict quality control procedures are required [51]. Safety can be ensured by implementing strict testing and quality assurance procedures to reduce risks such as contamination and the presence of dangerous materials. Customers could face significant danger due to insufficient quality control [52]. Herbal products that are tainted or improperly prepared can lead to adverse reactions and various health issues.

### 15.5.2 QUALITY CONTROL

Herbal products can display a range of active compounds due to inadequate quality control [53]. Providers feel that there is an issue with prescribing and treating patients safely due to this inconsistency, which may lead to varying therapeutic outcomes [54]. Quality control for these herbal products helps to deliver consistency in strength and composition. Knowledge and information about the concentration of active ingredients through standardized production and testing help achieve product outcomes in a consistent manner [55]. It conveys a level of commitment to the customers, providers, and government organizations.

### 15.5.3 NEED FOR THE STANDARDIZATION OF HERBAL MEDICINES

International standards for pharmacopeia, good manufacturing practices, and WHO guidance are being established [56]. Regulatory bodies are a requirement in providing safety, strength, quality, and efficacy of herbal products [57]. Establishing uniform standards of quality for herbal products will always be difficult due to their inherent complexity. Conventional formulations can provide challenges for established models of standardization, as sometimes active compounds are not palpable or well defined [58, 59]. This means that all the ingredients must be produced under any type of standardization with the following elements: selection of identified raw material, storage and handling, uniformity of sources of raw materials, and empirical evaluation of raw ingredients.

Current technologies such as high-performance liquid chromatography (HPLC), liquid chromatography–mass spectrometry (LC–MS), nuclear magnetic resonance (NMR), Fourier transform infrared spectroscopy (FTIR), and DNA barcoding have gained substantial importance in quality standards establishment. The WHO has made available detailed documents on the quality assurance of herbal medicines in the context of efficacy for therapeutic, professional, and research information.

### 15.5.4 ANALYTICAL TECHNIQUES FOR QUALITY CONTROL AND STANDARDIZATION

For ensuring the quality of finished herbal products, it is essential for including advanced techniques such as chromatography and spectroscopy. These methods are integrated into official guidelines for the quality control of herbal drugs. For assessing both raw materials and final products, significant measures have been adopted to enhance the quality control of herbal products and to develop robust analytical methods mentioned in Table 15.2.

**Table 15.2** Examples of herbal plants using analytical techniques.

| S.no | Technique | Application | Examples |
|---|---|---|---|
| 1. | TLC/HPTLC | Separation, fingerprinting | *Salvia officinalis* |
| 2. | TLC–MS | TLC + compound ID | *Punica granatum* |
| 3. | HPLC/UPLC | Quantitative analysis | *Piper longum* |
| 4. | LC–NMR | Structural elucidation | *Saraca asoca* |
| 5. | LC–MS/MS | Adulteration, multi-marker profiling | Ashwagandha |
| 6. | NMR and NMR-based metabolomics | Structural elucidation and metabolic profiling | *Withania somnifera*, *Ephedra* spp. |
| 7. | FTIR | Fingerprinting of plant species, identification of functional groups | *W. somnifera*, *Sida cordifolia* |

Analytical techniques applied in the quality control and standardization of herbal drugs include the following:

1. Spectroscopy
2. IR, UV, FTIR, two-dimensional infrared spectroscopy (2DIR)
3. Hyperspectral imaging, short-wavelength infrared
4. NMR-based metabolomics in quality control
5. Chromatographic techniques
6. TLC
7. High-performance thin layer chromatography (HPTLC)
8. HPLC
9. Ultra-performance liquid chromatography (UPLC)
10. TLC–MS
11. Liquid chromatography–mass spectrometry (LC–MS), liquid chromatography–selected reaction monitoring–mass spectrometry (LC–SRM–MS), LC–MS–MS
12. LC–NMR
13. GC–MS
14. DNA fingerprinting

### 15.5.5 WHO STANDARDIZATION PARAMETERS AND PHARMACOGNOSTICAL QUALITY CONTROL PARAMETERS FOR HERBAL DRUGS

All the ancient and herbal medicines considered by the WHO and promoted in national programs because they are available at a cheaper cost, are safely usable, and are widely recommended by people. They stress the importance of the qualitative and quantitative methods for identifying samples and quantifying the markers and fingerprint profiles [60]. The WHO assembly has underscored the necessity for contemporary methodologies and appropriate standards to guarantee the quality of medical and herbal goods [61]. The important standard parameters are illustrated in Figure 15.3.

To guarantee the stability of herbal formulations, thorough studies are essential to determine their shelf life and to maintain standards of efficacy and safety. These can be categorized into two types:

**Stability studies** assess how a product's components degrade under normal storage conditions to determine its expiration date and storage instructions.

**Accelerated stability studies:** By subjecting products to stress from higher temperature, humidity, and light, accelerated stability tests rapidly predict shelf life, uncover degradation problems, establish quality control measures, and guide packaging development.

- Herbal remedies are frequently self-prescribed, lacking professional guidance and quality assurance.

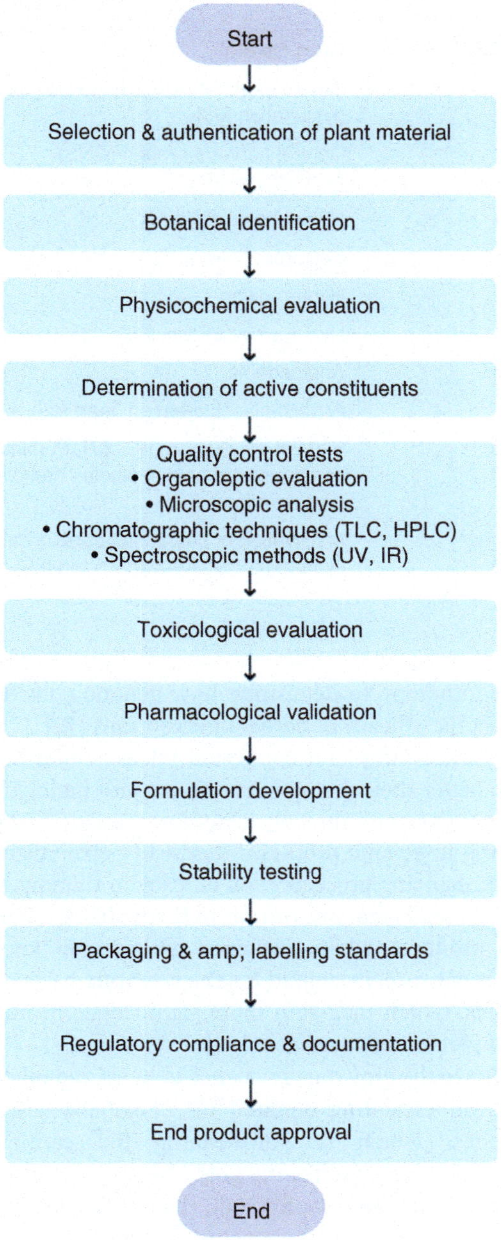


**FIGURE 15.3** Standardization of herbal drugs.

- Cultural or traditional beliefs may contribute to the misuse of herbal products. These are just a few of the drawbacks and contraindications associated with herbal medicines.
- Pharmacologically active substances that can cause drug–drug interactions are frequently found in herbal remedies.
- Because of inadequate pharmacodynamic and pharmacokinetic data, excessive use can cause serious hepatic and renal toxicity.
- It can be difficult to determine which ingredients are causing beneficial or negative effects in complex formulations with several ingredients. The lack of standardized formulas is one of the few drugs that is mentioned in Table 15.3.

### 15.5.6 SCIENTIFIC VALIDATION AND CLINICAL TRIALS

Clinical trials, preclinical research, and phytochemical analysis are some of the steps involved in the scientific validation of herbal medicine. Preclinical trials assess toxicity, biological effectiveness, and pharmacokinetic analysis [70]. Phytochemical research helps identify active compounds that yield therapeutic effects. Clinical trials offer further evidence of the safety and efficacy of herbal formulations in humans, conducted under closely monitored conditions to ensure their reliability as medical treatments. Herbal medicine faces numerous challenges in obtaining regulatory approval and scientific validation, even with its promising potential. Notable issues arise from changes in plant composition caused by environmental factors, inconsistent processing techniques, and contamination or adulteration [71]. Moreover, to ensure patient safety, herb–drug interactions and potential toxicity must be carefully examined.

## 15.6 CHALLENGES FACED BY HERBAL MEDICAL PRACTITIONERS

Herbal remedies remain integral to many healthcare systems and form the foundation of some modern medications, or allopathic medications. Although they are commonly used, there is still a significant gap between medical professions that rely on evidence-based practice and roots of herbal medicine. The most critical barrier is the lack of scientific scope and evidence, rendering the profession skeptical toward herbal medicine. As many herbal formulations do not have uniform dosage, standardized quality assurance systems, or classified and rigorous clinical studies, practitioners also raise concerns about safety, potential efficacy, and interactions, between herbal medicine and pharmaceuticals. Meanwhile, regulatory bodies that oversee medical practice, like the WHO and United States regulatory agencies, have developed established guidelines for herbal medicine under the European Medicine Agency (EMA) and the Food and Drug Administration (FDA). However, the establishment of herbal medicine in practice is complicated by changes in environmental conditions affecting plant composition and expulsion of herbal remedy from practice. In addition to environmental influences on plant preparation, due to inconsistency in quality assurance and method of preparation, healthcare providers are further constrained by a lack of substantial clinical trials that pave the way for commercialization. With the increased global interest in natural and holistic medicine, the gap between practiced herbals and government-trusted pharmacological studies must be addressed quickly.

**1) Bridging the gap between tradition and science**
Many of the plant-based treatments, due to limited strong clinical evidence, have been offering invaluable therapeutic benefits. By the way of phytochemical characterization and their integration into contemporary medicine, herbal constituents require confirmation of pharmacological activity, scientific validation, preclinical testing, and clinical trials.

**Table 15.3** List of some herbs with adverse effects.

| S. no. | Name of the herb | Adverse effects | Cases reported |
|---|---|---|---|
| 1. | *Allium sativum* | Increased bleeding tendency. | Case reports of hemorrhage [62], platelet dysfunction [63] |
| 2. | *Ginkgo biloba* | Bleeding, platelet dysfunction | Central nervous system (CNS) hemorrhage [64] |
| 3. | *Camellia sinensis* | Arrhythmias, increased heart rate | Hypercholesterolemia |
| 4. | *Ephedra sinica* | Hypertension, irregular heart rate | Seizures, heart attacks |
| 5. | *Citrus aurantium* | Obesity | Hypertension |
| 6. | *Ginseng* | Hypertension | Hypotensive effects [65] |
| 7. | *Punica granatum* | Hypertension | Angioedema |
| 8. | *Ilex paraguariensis* | Obesity | Arrhythmias, increased heart rate |
| 9. | *Zingiber officinale* | Platelet dysfunction, hypertension | Platelet antagonism [66, 67], Purified ginger compounds in animal studies demonstrate pressor effects [68] |
| 10. | Liquorice | Cardiomyopathy, pulmonary edema, hypertension | Inactivation of decreased cortisol causing symptoms of mineralocorticoid [69] |

**2) Ensuring safety and efficacy**

The lack of consistency in the composition of plants because of environmental influences, differences in processing techniques, and possible contamination are the main concerns of herbal medicine. Patients can be subjected to ineffective or even harmful therapy without proper validation. The safety and reliability of herbal remedies play an important role for which strengthening the standardization and regulation is highly recommended.

**3) Meeting regulatory challenges**

U.S. FDA and the EMA for herbal products proposed certain guidelines. In commercialization and quality control, the absence of global uniform standards still poses problems. Regulatory systems need to be investigated to suggest methods to enhance approval procedures for herbal medicines.

**4) Promoting integrative medicine**

Chronic diseases, including diabetes, cancer, and neurodegenerative disorders, have been demonstrated to be controlled by herbal medicine. Providing greater options for treatment to patients by scientifically proving the efficacy of herbal remedies using modern research techniques, medical professionals can incorporate them into mainstream therapies with confidence.

**5) Leverage technological advances**

Transforming the discovery of herbal drugs, recent developments in biotechnology, nanotechnology, and artificial intelligence (AI) have been made. For novel and effective plant-based therapies, through these technologies we can improve the scientific assessment, preparation, and delivery of herbal medicines.

## 15.7 FUTURE TRENDS AND OPPORTUNITIES

Contemporary healthcare is the future of herbal medicine with its integration. Phytopharmacogenomics is the future trend, which integrates the research of pharmacogenomics and phytotherapy to determine how genetic considerations can affect the efficacy of herbal interventions [72].

Bioavailability and controlled release could be improvised to better their therapeutic effects, with nanotechnology breakthroughs on the horizon for herbal compounds. According to genetic profiles, interest in personalized medicine in enhancing precision and efficacy in therapy opportunity for herbal medicines to be individualized. Further, for natural products, when combined with deeper knowledge, increases consumer demand for the scientific basis of herbal medicines, which may gain more significance in integrative and complementary medicine [73].

Due to the growing prevalence of heart and other CVDs, there is an escalating demand for personalized treatment approaches, which is transforming the cardiovascular MedTech domain significantly [74]. The rise of novel innovations such as wearable technology, remote monitoring equipment, and telemedicine is a reaction to a growing recognition of the need for a more individualized approach to caring for health, thereby indicating a trend toward for more engaged and responsive healthcare. These devices allow for real-time tracking of key health metrics [75].

The integration of machine learning and AI is transforming cardiovascular interventions by refining risk assessments, detecting early disease pathways, and creating personalized treatment plans [76]. AI, and specifically AI-based algorithms that review large datasets, are a valuable resource as decision aids for clinicians during procedures to predict patient outcomes. To customize patient therapies, these tools are applied to enhance clinical understanding of a patient's health status [77]. For example, these AI-based algorithms can support medicine dermatology [78]. The advancement of AI has the potential to impact significantly on the medical field by identifying areas or pathologies of interest so that life-saving interventions can be enhanced. AI algorithms can quickly process complex medical data and can be employed to promote an improved accuracy of medical diagnostics and treatment [79].

This targeted approach ultimately enhances outcomes for patients and consequently allows targeting and more efficient interventions. In the cardiovascular system, technologies such as Cydar Medical employ AI algorithms that can provide surgeons real-time insights and guidance, especially important to improve intraoperative decision-making and optimal navigation. In contrast, the practical and ethical implications of using AI technology in cardiovascular procedures must be evaluated. Although AI has the potential for benefitting personalized and efficacious therapies considerably, its application requires much consideration.

### 15.7.1 WEARABLE DEVICES

Functional information in concurrent time can be achieved and has the capacity to consistently monitor using high-tech sensors through wearable technology [79]. Assessing patients' cardiovascular state allows doctors to take instantly quick decisions during a medical operation [80]. Physiological parameters, such as pulse rate, hypertension, and oxygen saturation, are to be comprehended by medical professionals employing these technologies. For continuous monitoring of health, more personalized and holistic cardiovascular treatment can be possible by wearable devices such as T-line, chronic noncommunicable diseases (CNAP), and Nexfin. Other important vital parameters can be achieved through advanced sensors that are used precisely to monitor blood pressure, oxygen saturation, and heart rate. Extensive information through continuous pulse pressure can be achieved by "Nexfin HD" through noninvasive technology [81].

### 15.7.2 3D PRINTING TECHNOLOGY

Therapeutic applications and personalized medicine are emerging as significant applications of 3D printing technology. 3D printing provides the opportunity to precisely manufacture anatomical models in a manner that is tailored to each patient and offers invaluable opportunities for clinicians in surgical planning, medical education, and improved communication with patients [82]. However, the limitations and challenges facing the use of 3D printing technology in cardiovascular medicine must be addressed. One area that has not yet been widely adopted is bioprinting. The aim of existing tissue engineering technology is to produce biologically compatible structures, such as manufactured tissue constructs that have complex, multilayered designs. Products like stents, prosthetic valves, and vascular grafts could be more closely tailored to the specific anatomical shape [83].

### 15.7.3 BIOENGINEERING AND REGENERATIVE MEDICINE

The rapid development of bioengineering and regenerative medicine is paving the way for innovative strategies to treat heart disease [84]. These fields involve ideas from biology, engineering, and materials science to formulate new therapies for cardiovascular issues. Regenerative medicine emphasizes the body's inherent capacity to regenerate or promotes external modalities to restore damaged heart tissue. First in line to demonstrate innovative methods for heart repair include stem cell therapy, tissue engineering, and engineered scaffolds that mimic the structure of native tissue [85]. Both therapy options are designed to restore the structure and function of heart while stimulating the body's innate healing properties. The combination of bioengineering strategies with regenerative medicine could lead to advanced therapies that target the underlying causes of CVD. This approach surpasses addressing symptomatic treatment, which could lead to subsequent heart problems [86].

### 15.7.4 IMAGING TECHNOLOGIES AND DIGITAL SIMULATION

The landscape of interventional cardiology and vascular planning is evolving due to innovations in digital imaging and simulation. MRI today can acquire real-time, comprehensive views of the heart and vascular structures using 4D MRI [87]. Other imaging advancements that will improve evaluation of the heart structures include electron-beam computed tomography (CT), photon-counting CT, multidetector CT, iterative reconstruction CT, and myocardial CT perfusion. These technologies can providing diagnostic capabilities that enhance the ability of diagnosing the anatomical changes over time [88].

### 15.7.5 ROLE OF GENETIC PROFILING AND BIOMARKERS

It is the process of analyzing genetic variations that may influence an individual's DNA to identify how they respond to various treatments and how likely they are to develop CVDs. For instance, differences in genes such as PCSK9 and LDLR are linked to cardiovascular risk and cholesterol levels, which influence the use of statins and other drugs that lower cholesterol. Troponins and cardiac CRP are the two biomarkers that provide important information about inflammation and damage in the cardiovascular system [89]. In order to diagnose diseases like myocardial infarction (MI) and predict subsequent cardiovascular events, these markers are essential, enabling prompt and appropriate therapeutic interventions [90].

## 15.8 FUTURE RESEARCH DIRECTIONS

### 15.8.1 GENOMIC AND METABOLOMIC PROFILING OF MEDICINAL PLANTS

The contribution of secondary metabolites remains undiscovered, although hundreds of life-saving drugs have been discovered from and inspired by nature. Traditionally, for isolation and identifying individual compounds from mixture of natural products, researchers have relied on chemical-guided fractionation or bioassays. However, there has been a shift in recent years, with scientists increasingly favoring genomics, metabolomics, and other Big Data methodologies as the preferred approach in the quest for new natural products. These advanced techniques give a chance to explore deep into the previously untapped chemical spaces, assuring new directions in drug discovery concerned to natural products.

Natural product chemists are experiencing a new frontier, one characterized by abundance of data instead of shortage. Thousands of genome sequences and metabolite profiles of phylogenetically diverse sources can now be accessed, as opposed to past research [91, 92]. This is in big part a result of the reduced cost of sequencing DNA, which has revealed the biosynthetic potential of organisms once thought to be well characterized. These organisms have many biosynthetic genes that remain to be linked their corresponding metabolites products [93]. Furthermore, instrumentation for analytical purposes has greatly enhanced and is now able to easily detect and compare thousands of secondary metabolites with ease, thus enabling greater research ability. By employing the application for predictive algorithms automatically, scientists are making progress in unraveling the organized patterns of biosynthetic routes concerned with secondary metabolism [94] and in allowing the targeted breakthroughs of novel chemical compounds via combinatorial biosynthesis [95]. The study of metabolomics is being used more and more to depict the relationships between metabolites and predict their chemical characteristics.

### 15.8.2 PERSONALIZED HERBAL MEDICINE USING PHARMACOGENOMICS

Personalized herbal medicine is an innovative healthcare strategy that enables the prediction, prevention, treatment, and curing of disease on an individual basis, leading to individual and population well-being. It leverages targeted diagnostics, prognostics, and therapies to create lifelong wellness. A part of this strategy, pharmacogenomics, addresses the manner in which genetic differences affects drug absorption, distribution, metabolism, and response within the individual. Critical genes usually studied are those encoding drug-metabolizing enzymes such as cytochrome P450, carrier proteins such as SLCO1B1, and drug targets such as receptors, including VKORC1, which is pertinent to warfarin. Such genetic variations, termed polymorphisms, are capable of modifying protein activities, either reducing or increasing them. For instance, a particular genetic variant may hinder an enzyme's function, preventing a medication from transforming into its effective form, and thus making it useless; alternatively, this variant can cause toxicity with an active drug because the impaired clearance results in drug accumulation in the body. Although there have been significant advancements in cardiovascular pharmacogenomics, its widespread application faces numerous obstacles. A crucial challenge is the need for randomized controlled trials to demonstrate the clinical advantages of genetic testing, as detractors argue that observational studies and retrospective data are inadequate.

### 15.8.3 EXPLORING GUT MICROBIOTA MODULATION VIA HERBAL INTERVENTIONS

The gut microbiota and its metabolites, which are greatly impacted by dietary choices, and the novel CVD pathogenesis pathway have been the subject of numerous studies that have brought attention to this relationship [96]. A variety of CVD treatment approaches, including the use of antibiotics, enzyme inhibitors, and fecal microbiota transplantation, are emerging in response to this, with the goal of lowering the toxic metabolites. However, evidence regarding their effect on health and diseases is still lacking, and these treatments are still in the early stages of development [97]. Although it is anticipated that the gut microbiota and metabolites contribute as risk factors for CVDs, continuous research is anticipated to be a drawn-out process. Historically, diet and herbal remedies have been used in the management of CVD.

### 15.8.4 GREEN CHEMISTRY FOR ECO-FRIENDLY EXTRACTION OF BIOACTIVES

For the analysis of bioactive pharmaceuticals, green and sustainable analytical techniques in a variety of industries such as food, plants, medicines, and cosmetics have significantly increased in recent years. In order to lessen the adverse effects of the environment, this shift is essential. Thus, one of the main areas of research in this wide field at the moment is the creation of sustainable and environmentally friendly extraction techniques. Three key approaches are identified to successfully apply these techniques both on small scale and large scales, with an emphasis on energy, solvent, and raw material optimization.

- Phytochemical extraction and green solvents in food analysis
- Sustainable green analytical chemistry
- Micronutrients, cosmeceuticals and pharmaceuticals

### 15.8.5 SUSTAINABILITY AND ECO-CONSCIOUSNESS

The environmental consequences of synthetic drugs have sparked concerns related to their production and disposal methods. Synthetic drug manufacturing typically involves processes that generate significant pollution and leave enduring residues in the environment. On the other hand, herbal drugs, which are derived from plant sources, present a more sustainable alternative due to their natural origin and biodegradability. These medicines are usually cultivated using natural farming methods that are eco-friendly, and their processing involves lower levels of chemicals, reducing ecological damage [98]. The degradation of herbal medicines is hastened by microbial consortia, thus minimizing their effect in the environment over time due to their complicated chemical structures. Herbal medicines have served an important role in sustainable practice with meaningful influence to ecosystems and communities through traditional knowledge with contemporary scientific approaches for centuries [99]. Herbal medicines offer us opportunities for reducing the environmental footprint of pharmaceuticals due to their sustainable cultivation, biodegradability, and community empowerment; however, regulatory and market matters will be principle to unlocking their full eco-friendly potential.

## 15.9 POTENTIAL BENEFITS AND CHALLENGES

The increased focus on individualized healthcare is propelling innovation in research and the wider healthcare systems and industries. Stakeholders such as policymakers, healthcare providers, the population at large, and commercial business must take an active role in putting particular strategies in place to ensure they derive the maximum benefits of this revolutionary approach. To successfully achieve its potential, while many advantages promise tailored healthcare, there are challenges and exertions needed from policymakers and practitioners alike. There is a need to enhance genetic literacy of both healthcare professionals and the general public for encouraging active engagement of patients in healthcare deliberations to meet these requirements. Moreover, it is important to create enhanced governance framework, consent procedures, and trust-establishment practices within the healthcare system. Better health outcomes can be fostered by using the data–knowledge cycle effectively. The assessment of emerging technologies is also crucial for the uptake and adjustment of the health technology assessment framework. Lastly, humanistic values and promoting community participation in the provision of healthcare services are essential considerations, as noted in Figure 15.4.

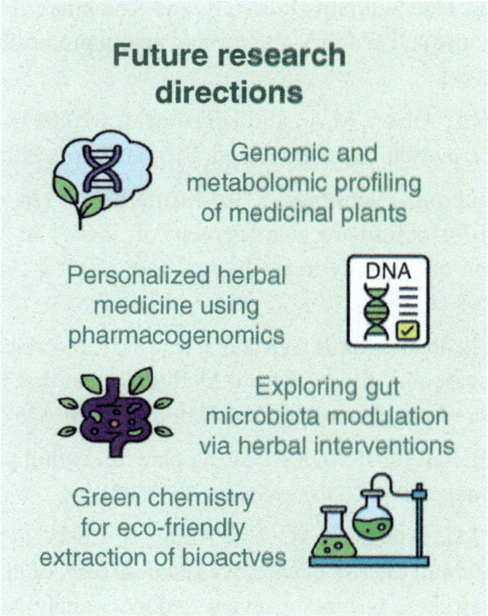


**FIGURE 15.4** Future research directions.

## 15.10 CONCLUSION

Herbal-based cardiovascular therapy offers a desirable option in the prevention and treatment of CVDs because it can simultaneously address many different mechanisms with less toxicity while providing more diversified health advantages. However, its progress is hindered by issues related to herb–drug interactions, insufficient standardization, lack of regulatory oversight, and lack of clinical validation. A co-participatory approach that integrates traditional knowledge with advanced analytical methodology, contemporary pharmacological techniques, and formally applied evidence-based clinical trials would benefit treatment progress. Globally recognized therapy can happen by building international partnerships to advance the herbal treatment of cardiovascular conditions into scientific validation with standardized herbal products and innovative technologies like nanodelivery systems and metabolomics. Ongoing scientific investigation and innovation are critical to create safe and effective herbal cardiovascular products in the future.

## REFERENCES


1. Toth, P.P. (2007). Making a case for quantitative assessment of cardiovascular risk. *J. Clin. Lipidol.* 1 (4): 234–241.
2. Reiner, Z., Laufs, U., Cosentino, F., and Landmesser, U. (2019). The year in cardiology 2018: prevention. *Eur. Heart J.* 40 (4): 336–344.
3. https://www.who.int/news-room/fact-sheets/detail/cardiovascular-diseases-(cvds)
4. Cragg, G.M. and Newman, D.J. (2013). Natural products: a continuing source of novel drug leads. *Biochim. Biophys. Acta* 1830 (6): 3670–3695.
5. Newman, D.J. and Cragg, G.M. (2016). Natural products as sources of new drugs from 1981 to 2014. *J. Nat. Prod.* 79 (3): 629–661.
6. Frishman, W.H., Beravol, P., and Carosella, C. (2009). Alternative and complementary medicine for preventing and treating cardiovascular disease. *Dis. Mon.* 55 (3): 121–192.
7. Davison, E.K. and Brimble, M.A. (2019). Natural product derived privileged scaffolds in drug discovery. *Curr. Opin. Chem. Biol.* 52: 1–8.
8. Otvos, R.A., Still, K.B.M., Somsen, G.W. et al. (2019). Drug discovery on natural products: from ion channels to nAChRs, from nature to libraries, from analytics to assays. *SLAS Discov.* 24 (3): 362–385.
9. Panda, V.S. and Naik, S.R. (2009). Evaluation of cardioprotective activity of *Ginkgo biloba* and *Ocimum sanctum* in rodents. *Altern. Med. Rev.* 14 (2): 161–171.
10. Liperoti, R., Davide, L., Vetrano, D.L. et al. (2017). Herbal medications in cardiovascular medicine. *J. Am. Coll. Cardiol.* 69 (9): 1188–1199.
11. Villaescusa, L., Zaragozá, C., Zaragozá, F., and Tamargo, J. (2023). Herbal medicines for the treatment of cardiovascular diseases: benefits and risks – a narrative review. *Int. J. Cardiol.* 385 (15): 44–52.
12. Shaito, A., Thuan, D.T.B., Phu, H.T. et al. (2020). Herbal medicine for cardiovascular diseases: efficacy, mechanisms, and safety. *Front. Pharmacol.* 11: 422.
13. Hesari, M., Mohammadi, P., Khademi, F. et al. (2021). Current advances in the use of nanophytomedicine therapies for human cardiovascular diseases. *Int. J. Nanomed.* 11 (16): 3293–3315.
14. McGinnis, J.M. and Foege, W.H. (1993). Actual causes of death in the United States. *JAMA* 270 (18): 2207–2212.

15. McGinnis, J.M., Williams-Russo, P., and Knickman, J.R. (2002). The case for more active policy attention to health promotion. *Health Aff.* 21 (2): 78–93.

16. Challa, H.J., Ameer, M.A., and Uppaluri, K.R. (2023). *DASH Diet to Stop Hypertension*. Treasure Island, FL: Stat Pearls Publishing.

17. De Bacquer, D., Jennings, C.S., Mirrakhimov, E. et al. (2022). Potential for optimizing management of obesity in the secondary prevention of coronary heart disease. *Eur. Heart J. Qual. Care Clin. Outcomes* 8: 568–576.

18. Estruch, R., Ros, E., Salas-Salvado, J. et al. (2018). Primary prevention of cardiovascular disease with a Mediterranean diet supplemented with extra-virgin olive oil or nuts. *N. Engl. J. Med.* 378 (25): e34.

19. Campbell, A.P. (2017). DASH eating plan: an eating pattern for diabetes management. *Diabetes Spectr.* 30: 76–81.

20. Dybvik, J.S., Svendsen, M., and Aune, D. (2023). Vegetarian and vegan diets and the risk of cardiovascular disease, ischemic heart disease and stroke: a systematic review and meta-analysis of prospective cohort studies. *Eur. J. Nutr.* 62: 51–69.

21. Lichtenstein, A.H., Appel, L.J., Vadiveloo, M. et al. (2021). 2021 dietary guidance to improve cardiovascular health: a scientific statement from the American Heart Association. *Circulation* 144: 0–87.

22. Piercy, K.L., Troiano, R.P., Ballard, R.M. et al. (2018). The physical activity guidelines for Americans. *JAMA* 320: 2020–2028.

23. Visseren, F.L., Mach, F., Smulders, Y.M. et al. (2021). ESC guidelines on cardiovascular disease prevention in clinical practice. *Eur. Heart J.* 42: 3227–3337.

24. Shoaib, S. (2010). Cardioprotective effect of gemmotherapeutically treated *Withania somnifera* against chemically induced myocardial. *Pak. J. Bot.* 2 (2): 1487–1499.

25. Jahan, N. and Ali, S. (2012). Cardioprotective and antilipidemic potential of *Cyperus rotundus* in chemically induced cardiotoxicity. *Int. J. Agric. Biol.* 14 (6): 989–992.

26. Mais, B., Yaser, A.M., and Ream, N. (2016). Hypolipidemic effect of *Achillea biebersteinii* ethanolic extract in hamsters with diet-induced hypercholesterolemia. *Int. J. Pharmacogn. Phytochem. Res.* 8 (9): 1555–1559.

27. Atawodi, S.E., Adepoju, O.A., and Nzelibe, H.C. (2017). Anti-hyperglycaemic and hypolipidemic effect of methanol extracts of *Ageratum conyzoides* L (Asteraceae) in normal and diabetic rats. *Trop. J. Pharm. Res.* 16 (5): 989–996.

28. Bora, K.S. and Sharma, A. (2011). Evaluation of antioxidant and free-radical scavenging potential of *Artemisia absinthium. Pharm. Biol.* 49 (12): 1216–1223.

29. Gao, T., Zhu, Z.Y., Zhou, X., and Xie, M.-L. (2016). *Chrysanthemum morifolium* extract improves hypertension-induced cardiac hypertrophy in rats by reduction of blood pressure and inhibition of myocardial hypoxia-inducible factor-1alphaexpression. *Pharm. Biol.* 54 (12): 2895–2900.

30. Akinpelu, B., Apata, J., Iwalewa, E., and Oyedapo, O. (2016). Evaluation of anti-hyperlipidemic potential of ethanolic leaf extract of *Clerodendrum volubile* P. Beauv. *IFE J. Sci.* 18 (3): 789–800.

31. Citoglu, G.S., Coban, T., Sever, B., and Iscan, M. (2004). Antioxidant properties of Ballota species growing in Turkey. *J. Ethnopharmacol.* 92 (2–3): 275–280.

32. Hailu, W. and Engidawork, E. (2014). Evaluation of the diuretic activity of the aqueous and 80% methanol extracts of *Ajuga remota Benth* (Lamiaceae) leaves in mice. *BMC Complement. Altern. Med.* 14 (1): 1–8.

33. Ritter, M., Melichar, K., Strahler, S. et al. (2010). Cardiac and electrophysiological effects of primary and refined extracts from *Leonurus cardiaca* L. (Ph. Eur.). *Planta Med.* 76 (6): 572–582.

34. Kumar, G.S., Kattimani, S., Sarkar, S., and Sekhar, S. (2017). Prevalence of depression and its relation to stress level among medical students in Puducherry. *Indian Ind. Psychiatry J.* 26 (1): 86–90.

35. Michel, J., Abd Rani, N.Z., and Husain, K. (2020). A review on the potential use of medicinal plants from Asteraceae and Lamiaceae plant family in cardiovascular diseases. *Front. Pharmacol.* 11: 852.

36. Asogwa, F.C., Okoye, C.O.B., Okechukwu, P.C.U. et al. (2015). Phytochemistry and antimicrobial assay of *Jatropha curcas* extracts on some clinically isolated bacteria—a comparative analysis. *Eur. J. Appl. Sci.* 7 (1): 12–16.

37. Anand David, A.V., Arulmoli, R., and Parasuraman, S. (2016). Overviews of biological importance of quercetin: a bioactive flavonoid. *Pharmacogn. Rev.* 10 (20): 84–89.

38. M, D.'.A., Filesi, C., Di Benedetto, R. et al. (2007). Polyphenols, dietary sources, and bioavailability. *Ann. Ist. Super. Sanita* 43 (4): 348–361.

39. Crupi, P., Faienza, M.F., Naeem, M.Y. et al. (2023). Overview of the potential beneficial effects of carotenoids on consumer health and well-being. *Antioxidants* 12 (5): 1069.

40. Przybylska, S. and Tokarczyk, G. (2022). Lycopene in the prevention of cardiovascular diseases. *Int. J. Mol. Sci.* 23 (4): 1957.

41. Quitério, E., Grosso, C., Ferraz, R. et al. (2022). A critical comparison of the advanced extraction techniques applied to obtain health-promoting compounds from seaweeds. *Marine Drug* 20 (11): 677.

42. Melton, L., Varelis, P., Sahahidi, F., and Bot, A. (2019). Phytosterols. In: *Encyclopedia of Food Chemistry* (ed. L. Melton, F. Shahidi, and P. Varelis), 225–228. Amsterdam: Elsevier.

43. Timilsena, Y.P., Phosanam, A., and Stockmann, R. (2023). Perspectives on saponins: food functionality and applications. *Int. J. Mol. Sci.* 24 (17): 135–138.

44. Sharma, K., Kaur, R., Kumar, S. et al. (2023). Saponins: a concise review on food related aspects, applications and health implications. *Food Chem. Adv.* 2: 100191.

45. Iqbal, I., Wilairatana, P., Saqib, F. et al. (2023). Plant polyphenols and their potential benefits on cardiovascular health: a review. *Molecules* 28 (17): 6403.

46. Dhingra, D., Michael, M., Rajput, H., and Patil, R.T. (2011). Dietary fibre in foods: a review. *J. Food Sci. Technol.* 49: 255–266.

47. Osman, A.G., Haider, S., Chittiboyina, A.G., and Khan, I.A. (2019). Utility of alkaloids as chemical and biomarkers for quality, efficacy, and safety assessment of botanical ingredients. *Phytomedicine* 54: 347–356.

48. Zhou, S.S., Hu, J.W., Kong, M. et al. (2019). Less SO (2) residue may not indicate higher quality, better efficacy and weaker toxicity of sulfur-fumigated herbs: Ginseng, a pilot study. *J. Hazard. Mater.* 364 (10): 376–387.

49. Tao, Y., Bao, J., Zhu, F. et al. (2023). Ethnopharmacology of *Rubus idaeus* Linnaeus: a critical review on ethnobotany, processing methods, phytochemicals, pharmacology and quality control. *J. Ethnopharmacol.* 302 (Pt A): 115870.

50. Kubra, I.R., Kumar, D., and Jagan Mohan Rao, L. (2016). Emerging trends in microwave processing of spices and herbs. *Crit. Rev. Food Sci. Nutr.* 56 (13): 2160–2173.

51. Deutch, M.R., Grimm, D., Wehland, M. et al. (2019). Bioactive candy: effects of licorice on the cardiovascular system. *Foods* 8 (10): 495.

52. Giacometti, J., Bursac Kovacevic, D., Putnik, P. et al. (2018). Extraction of bioactive compounds and essential oils from Mediterranean herbs by conventional and green innovative techniques: a review. *Food Res. Int.* 113: 245–262.

53. Liu, H., Lu, X., Hu, Y., and Fan, X. (2020). Chemical constituents of *Panax ginseng* and *Panax notoginseng* explain why they differ in therapeutic efficacy. *Pharmacol. Res.* 161: 105263.

54. Ma, P.Y., Li, X.Y., Wang, Y.L. et al. (2022). Natural bioactive constituents from herbs and nutraceuticals promote browning of white adipose tissue. *Pharmacol. Res.* 178: 106175.

55. Braga, F., Pasqualetti, S., Aloisio, E., and Panteghini, M. (2020). The internal quality control in the traceability era. *Clin. Chem. Lab. Med.* 59 (2): 291–300.

56. World Health Organization (2025). *Cardiovascular diseases (CVDs) [Internet]*. Geneva: World Health Organization Jul 31 [cited 2026 Apr 27]. Available from: Cardiovascular diseases (CVDs) fact sheet.

57. Folashade, K.O., Omoregie, E.H., and Ochogu, A.P. (2012). Standardization of herbal medicines – a review. *Int. J. Biodivers. Conserv.* 4 (3): 101–112.

58. Steinhoff, B. (2019). Quality of herbal medicinal products: state of the art of purity assessment. *Phytomedicine* 60: 153003.

59. Chaachouay, N. and Zidane, L. (2024). Plant-derived natural products: a source for drug discovery and development Drugs. *Drug Candid.* 3 (1): 184–207.

60. Dixit, V.K. and Yadav, N.P. (2008). Recent approaches in herbal drug standardization. *Integr. Biol.* 2 (3): 195–203.

61. Chaudhury, R.R. (1999). *Herbal Medicine for Human Health*. New Delhi, Geneva: CBS Publishers and Distributors LTD, World Health Organization.

62. Rose, K., Croissant, P., Parliament, C. et al. (1990). Spontaneous spinal epidural hematoma with associated platelet dysfunction from excessive garlic ingestion: a case report. *Neurosurgery* 26: 880–882.

63. Ali, M., Thomson, M., and Afzal, M. (2000). Garlic and onions: their effect on eicosanoid metabolism and its clinical relevance. *Prostaglandins Leukot. Essent. Fat. Acids* 62 (2): 55–73.

64. Rowin, J. and Lewis, S.L. (1996). Spontaneous bilateral subdural hematomas associated with chronic *Ginkgo biloba* ingestion. *Neurology* 46 (6): 1775–1776.

65. Han, K.H., Choe, S.C., Kim, H.S. et al. (1998). Effect of red ginseng on blood pressure in patients with essential hypertension and white coat hypertension. *Am. J. Chin. Med.* 26 (2): 199–209.

66. Lumb, A.B. (1994). Effect of dried ginger on human platelet function. *Thromb. Haemost.* 7: 110–111.

67. Janssen, P.L.T.M.K., Meyboom, S., van Staveren, W.A. et al. (1996). Consumption of ginger (*Zingiber officinale* roscoe) does not affect *ex vivo* platelet thromboxane production in humans. *Eur. J. Clin. Nutr.* 50 (11): 772–774.

68. Suekawa, M., Aburada, M., and Hosoya, E. (1986). Pharmacological studies on ginger. II. Pressor action of (6)-shogaol in anesthetized rats, or hindquarters, tail and mesenteric vascular beds of rats. *J. Pharmacobiodyn.* 9 (10): 842–852.

69. Walker, B.R. and Edwards, C.R.W. (1994). Liquorice-induced hypertension and syndromes of apparent mineralocorticoid excess. *Endocrinol. Metab. Clin. N. Am.* 23 (2): 359–377.

70. Heinrich, M., Barnes, J., Gibbons, S. et al. (2020). Herbal medicine in the treatment of neurodegenerative diseases. *Phytother. Res.* 34 (4): 728–748.

71. Süntar, I. (2020). Nanotechnology and herbal medicine: the way forward. *Curr. Top. Med. Chem.* 20 (10): 905–918.

72. Rottmann, M., Jacoby, D., and Müller, M. (2020). Phyto pharmacogenomics: a promising approach to precision herbal medicine. *Phytomedicine* 70: 153227.

73. Atanasov, A.G., Zotchev, S.B., Dirsch et al. (2021). Natural products in drug discovery: advances and challenges. *Nat. Rev. Drug Discov.* 20 (10): 756–773.

74. Vaduganathan, M., Mensah, G.A., Turco, J.V. et al. (2022). The global burden of cardiovascular diseases and risk: a compass for future health. *J. Am. Coll. Cardiol.* 80 (25): 2361–2371.

75. Steinhubl, S.R., Muse, E.D., and Topol, E.J. (2015). The emerging field of mobile health. *Sci. Transl. Med.* 7 (283): 283rv3.

76. Samant, S., Bakhos, J.J., Wu, W. et al. (2023). Artificial intelligence, computational simulations, and extended reality in cardiovascular interventions. *JACC Cardiovasc. Interv.* 16 (20): 2479–2497.

77. Gala, D., Behl, H., Shah, M., and Makaryus, A.N. (2024). The role of artificial intelligence in improving patient outcomes and future of healthcare delivery in cardiology: a narrative review of the literature. *Healthcare* 12 (4): 481.

78. Kuntz, S., Gangloff, H., Naamoune et al. (2021). Automated histological segmentation on micro computed tomography images of atherosclerotic arteries. *Eur. J. Vasc. Endovasc. Surg.* 61 (4): 714–715.

79. Guk, K., Han, G., Lim, J. et al. (2019). Evolution of wearable devices with real-time disease monitoring for personalized healthcare. *Nanomaterials* 9 (6): 813.

80. Haleem, A., Javaid, M., Singh, R.P., and Suman, R. (2021). Telemedicine for healthcare: capabilities, features, barriers, and applications. *Sens. Int.* 2: 100117.

81. Ariturk, C., Açil, M., Ulugol, H. et al. (2016). Is the Nexfin finger cuff method for cardiac output measurement reliable during coronary artery bypass grafting? A prospective comparison with the echocardiography and Flo Trac/vigileo methods. *Turk. J. Med. Sci.* 46 (2): 291–295.

82. Giannopoulos, A.A., Mitsouras, D., Yoo, S.J. et al. (2016). Applications of 3D printing in cardiovascular diseases. *Nat. Rev. Cardiol.* 13 (12): 701–718.

83. Bartel, T., Rivard, A., Jimenez, A. et al. (2018). Medical three-dimensional printing opens up new opportunities in cardiology and cardiac surgery. *Eur. Heart J.* 39 (15): 1246–1254.

84. Chingale, M., Zhu, D., Cheng, K., and Huang, K. (2021). Bioengineering technologies for cardiac regenerative medicine. *Front. Bioeng. Biotechnol.* 9: 681705.

85. Augustine, R., Dan, P., Hasan, A. et al. (2021). Stem cell-based approaches in cardiac tissue engineering: controlling the microenvironment for autologous cells. *Biomed. Pharmacother.* 138: 111425.

86. Haneke, T. and Sahara, M. (2022). Progress in bioengineering strategies for heart regenerative medicine. *Int. J. Mol. Sci.* 23 (7): 3482.

87. Bissell, M.M., Raimondi, F., Ait Ali, L. et al. (2023). 4D Flow cardiovascular magnetic resonance consensus statement: 2023 update. *J. Cardiovasc. Magn. Reson.* 25 (1): 40.

88. Counseller, Q. and Aboelkassem, Y. (2023). Recent technologies in cardiac imaging. *Front. Med. Technol.* 4: 984492.

89. Wang, J., Tan, G.J., Han, L.N. et al. (2017). Novel biomarkers for cardiovascular risk prediction. *J. Geriatr. Cardiol.* 14 (2): 135–150.

90. Haaf, P., Drexler, B., Reichlin, T. et al. (2012). High-sensitivity cardiac troponin in the distinction of acute myocardial infarction from acute cardiac noncoronary artery disease. *Circulation* 126 (1): 31–40.

91. Kang, K.B., Ernst, M., van der Hooft, J.J. et al. (2019). Comprehensive mass spectrometry-guided phenotyping of plant specialized metabolites reveals metabolic diversity in the cosmopolitan plant family Rhamnaceae. *Plant J.* 98: 1134–1144.

92. Nguyen, D.D., Melnik, A.V., Koyama, N. et al. (2017). Indexing the Pseudomonas specialized metabolome enabled the discovery of poaeamide B and the bananamides. *Nat. Microbiol.* 2: 16197.

93. Didelot, X., Bowden, R., Wilson, D.J. et al. (2012). Transforming clinical microbiology with bacterial genome sequencing. *Nat. Rev. Genet.* 13 (9): 601–612.

94. Blin, K., Shaw, S., Steinke, K. et al. (2019). anti SMASH 5.0: updates to the secondary metabolite genome mining pipeline. *Nucleic Acids Res.* 47 (W1): W81–W87.

95. Medema, M.H. and Fischbach, M.A. (2015). Computational approaches to natural product discovery. *Nat. Chem. Biol.* 11 (9): 639–648.

96. Beale, A.L., O'Donnell, J.A., Nakai, M.E. et al. (2021). The gut microbiome of heart failure with preserved ejection fraction. *J. Am. Heart Assoc.* 10 (13): e020654.

97. Witkowski, M., Weeks, T.L., and Hazen, S.L. (2020). Gut microbiota and cardiovascular disease. *Circ. Res.* 127 (4): 553–570.

98. Huang, Y., Xiao, L., Li, F. et al. (2018). Microbial degradation of pesticide residues and an emphasis on the degradation of cypermethrin and 3-phenoxy benzoic acid: a review. *Molecules* 23: 2313.

99. Fokunang, C.N., Ndikum, V., Tabi, O.Y. et al. (2011). Traditional medicine: past, present and future research and development prospects and integration in the National Health System of Cameroon. *Afr. J. Tradit. Complement. Altern. Med.* 8 (3): 284–295.

# Index

Wiley The manufacturer's authorized representative according to the EU General Product Safety Regulation is Wiley-VCH GmbH, Boschstr. 12, 69469 Weinheim, Germany, e-mail: Product_Safety@wiley.com.

Printed and bound by CPI Group (UK) Ltd, Croydon, CR0 4YY
15/09/2026
02217187-0001